Medical Radiology
Radiation Oncology

Series Editors

L.W. Brady, Philadelphia

H.-P. Heilmann, Hamburg

M. Molls, Munich

C. Nieder, Bodø

For further volumes:
http://www.springer.com/series/4353

Jiade J. Lu · Luther W. Brady (Eds.)

Decision Making in Radiation Oncology

Volume 1

Foreword by

L.W. Brady, H.-P. Heilmann, M. Molls, and C. Nieder

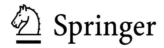 Springer

Jiade J. Lu, MD, MBA
Department of Radiation Oncology
National University Cancer Institute
National University Health System
National University of Singapore
1E Kent Ridge Road
NUHS Tower Block, Level 7
Singapore 119228
Republic of Singapore
Email: mdcljj@nus.edu.sg

Luther W. Brady, MD
Department of Radiation Oncology
Drexel University, College of Medicine
Broad and Vine Streets
Mail Stop 200
Philadelphia, PA 19102-1192, USA
Email: lbrady@drexelmed.edu

ISSN: 0942-5373
ISBN: 978-3-642-12462-4   e-ISBN: 978-3-642-13832-4

DOI: 10.1007/978-3-642-13832-4

Springer-Verlag Heidelberg Dordrecht London New York

Library of Congress Control Number: 2010937231

Cover design: eStudio Calamar, Figueres, Berlin

Printed on acid-free paper

Springer is part of Springer Science+Business Media (www.springer.com)

Foreword

With the development of the patterns of care study chaired by Dr. Simon Kramer, the decision tree concept was initiated for a number of tumor sites including the carcinomas of the larynx, base of the tongue, the anterior two-thirds of the tongue, prostate, bladder, etc. This led to the gathering of significant information in terms of clinical presentations, clinical work-up, and decision-making with regard to management during pretreatment, treatment, and post-treatment phases. This concept has been widely accepted in the community of oncologists and it has been the purpose of this book to strengthen that concept and to add the supporting data that make it a very useful clinical tool.

The authors have done a superb job in presenting the information that allows for innovative approaches to management and outcome analysis not only in clinical practice but in properly designed clinical trials, and for careful assessment of current practice based on solid and credible clinical research using the concept of the patterns of care but also the concepts of evidence-based outcome studies in oncology.

It is very important to have these kinds of information available in the clinical assessment of the patient in order to make the appropriate, proper decision relative to management.

It is important for oncologists to have a clear understanding of how the clinical and work-up information can be used to make the appropriate, proper decision relative to management.

The present volume is specifically aimed at identifying these resources and how they can be used along with evidence-based medicine not only in terms of outcome from radiation therapy treatment but also in terms of the appropriate, proper work-up that allows for appropriate decisions to be made. The book represents a significant and important standard by which all oncologists can design their treatment management.

Philadelphia - Luther W. Brady, M.D.
Hamburg – Hans Peter Heilman, M.D.
Munich – Michael Molls, M.D.
Bodø – Carsten Neider, M.D.

Volume 1

Volume 2

Contents of Volume 1

Contents of Volume 2

Contributors

Luther W. Brady, MD
Department of Radiation Oncology
Drexel University, College of Medicine
Broad and Vine Streets
Mail Stop 200
Philadelphia, PA 19102-1192, USA
Email: lbrady@drexelmed.edu

Manjeet Chadha, MD
Associate Chair, Department of Radiation Oncology
Beth Israel Medical Center, New York
Director of Breast and Gynecologic Cancer Programs -
Radiation Oncology
Continuum Cancer Centers of New York
Associate Professor, Radiation Oncology,
Albert Einstein College of Medicine, New York
10 Union Square East, Suite 4G
New York, NY 10003, USA
Email: mchadha@chpnet.org

Eric L. Chang, MD
Professor of Radiation Oncology
Department of Radiation Oncology
UT MD Anderson Cancer Center, Unit 97
1515 Holcombe Blvd.
Houston, TX 77030, USA
Email: echang@mdanderson.org

Joe Y. Chang, MD
Professor of Radiation Oncology
Clinical Service Chief, Thoracic Radiation Oncology
Department of Radiation Oncology
UT MD Anderson Cancer Center, Unit 97
1515 Holcombe Boulevard
Houston, TX 77030, USA
Email: jychang@mdanderson.org

Jay S. Cooper, MD
Director, Maimonides Cancer Center
Chair, Department of Radiation Oncology
6300 Eighth Avenue
Brooklyn, NY 11220, USA
Email: jcooper@maimonidesmed.org

Almond J. Drake III, MD
Professor of Medicine
Chief, Division of Endocrinology
Brody School Of Medicine at East Carolina University 3E-129
Greenville, NC 27834 USA
Email: drakea@ecu.edu

Alysa Fairchild, BSc, PGDip(Epi), MD, FRCPC
Assistant Professor
Department of Radiation Oncology
University of Alberta,
Faculty of Medicine, Cross Cancer Institute
11560 University Ave NW
Edmonton, AB T6G1Z2, Canada
Email: alysa.fairchild@albertahealthservices.ca

Steven Finkelstein, MD
Radiation Oncology
H. Lee Moffitt Cancer Center & Research Institute
12902 Magnolia Drive
Tampa, FL 33612, USA
Email: steven.finkelstein@moffitt.org

Shen Fu, MD
Professor and Chairman
Department of Radiation Oncology
The 6th Hospital of Jiao Tong University
600 Yishan Road
Shanghai 200233
People's Republic of China
Email: shen_fu@hotmail.com

Hiram Gay, MD
Assistant Professor of Radiation Oncology
Washington University in St. Louis
4554 Parkview Pl
Campus Box 8224
Saint Louis, MO 63110-6311, USA
Email: hgay@radonc.wustl.edu

Louis B. Harrison, MD
Professor and Chairman
Department of Radiation Oncology
Beth Israel Medical Center
10 Union Square East, Suite 4G
New York, NY 10003, USA
Email: lharrison@chpnet.org

Sarah E. Hoffe, MD
Assistant Member
GI Radiation Oncology
H. Lee Moffitt Cancer Center & Research Institute
12902 Magnolia Drive
Tampa, FL 33612, USA
Email: sarah.hoffe@moffitt.org

Kenneth S. Hu, MD
Associate Professor of Radiation Oncology
Beth Israel Medical Center
10 Union Square East, Suite 4G
New York, NY 10003, USA
Email: khu@chpnet.org

Edward Kim, MD
Assistant Professor of Radiation Oncology
University of Washington
1959 NE Pacific St
Box 356043
Seattle, WA 98195, USA
Email: edykim@u.washington.edu

Feng-Ming (Spring) Kong, MD, PhD, MPH
Chief, Radiation Oncology
Veteran Administration Health Center and University
Hospital Department of Radiation Oncology
University of Michigan
1500 E. Medical Center Drive
Ann Arbor, MI 48109, USA
Email: fengkong@med.umich.edu

Lin Kong, MD
Associate Professor of Radiation Oncology
Department of Radiation Oncology
Fudan University, Shanghai Cancer Center
270 Dong An Road
Shanghai 200032
People's Republic of China
Email: konglinj@gmail.com

Nancy Lee, MD
Associate Attending
Department of Radiation Oncology
Memorial Sloan Kettering Cancer Center
New York, NY 10021, USA
Email: leen2@mskcc.org

Zhongxing Liao, MD
Professor of Radiation Oncology
Department of Radiation Oncology
UT MD Anderson Cancer Center, Unit 97
1515 Holcombe Boulevard
Houston, TX 77030, USA
Email: zliao@mdanderson.org

Steven H. Lin, MD, PhD
Assistant Professor of Radiation Oncology
Department of Radiation Oncology
UT MD Anderson Cancer Center, Unit 97
1515 Holcombe Boulevard
Houston, TX 77030, USA
Email: shlin@mdanderson.org

Simon S. Lo, MD
Associate Professor of Radiation Oncology and Neurosurgery
Department of Radiation Oncology
Arthur G. James Cancer Hospital
Ohio State University Medical Center
300 West 10th Avenue
Columbus, OH 43210, USA
Email: simon.lo@osumc.edu

Jiade J. Lu, MD, MBA
Chief and Senior Consultant
Department of Radiation Oncology
National University Cancer Institute
National University Health System
National University of Singapore
1E Kent Ridge Road
NUHS Tower Block, Level 7
Singapore 119228
Republic of Singapore
Email: mdcljj@nus.edu.sg

Stephen Lutz, MD
Department of Radiation Oncology
Blanchard Valley Regional Cancer Center
15990 Medical Drive South
Findlay, OH 45840, USA
Email: slutz@bvha.org

Vivek K. Mehta, MD
Radiation Oncologist and Director
Center for Advanced Targeted Radiotherapies
Department of Radiation Oncology
Swedish Cancer Institute
1221 Madison Street, First Floor,
Seattle, WA 98104, USA
Email: vivek.mehta@swedish.org

Roger Ove, MD, PhD
Philip Rubin Professor and Vice Chair
Department of Radiation Oncology
Univerisity of South Alabama Mitchell Cancer Institute
1660 Springhill Avenue
Mobile, AL 36604, USA
Email: rove@usouthal.edu

Surjeet Pohar, MD
Radiation Oncology Services of Central New York
1088 Commons Ave
Cortland, NY 13045, USA
Email: spohar@netzero.net

Ugur Selek, MD
Department Chief of Radiation Oncology
American Hospital
Güzelbahçe Sokak, No. 20
Tesvikiye, 34365
Istanbul, Turkey
and
Adjunct Associate Professor of Radiation Oncology
University of Texas M.D. Anderson Cancer Center
1515 Holcombe Boulevard
Houston, TX 77030,USA
Email: uselek@mdanderson.org

Ravi Shridhar, MD, PhD
Assistant Member
GI Radiation Oncology
H. Lee Moffitt Cancer Center & Research Institute
12902 Magnolia Drive
Tampa, FL 33612, USA
Email: ravi.shridhar@moffitt.org

Jeremy Tey, MD
Consultant
Department of Radiation Oncology
National University Cancer Institute
National University Health System
National University of Singapore
1E Kent Ridge Road
NUHS Tower Block, Level 7
Singapore 119228
Republic of Singapore
Email: jeremy_tey@nuhs.edu.sg

Ivan W.K. Tham, MD
Consultant
Department of Radiation Oncology
National University Cancer Institute
National University Health System
National University of Singapore
1E Kent Ridge Road
NUHS Tower Block, Level 7
Singapore 119228
Republic of Singapore
Email: ivan_wk_tham@nuhs.edu.sg

Qing Zhang , MD
Associate Professor
Department of Radiation Oncology
The 6th Hospital of Jiao Tong University
600 Yishan Road
Shanghai 200233
People's Republic of China
Email: zhangqingcyw@hotmail.com

Zhen Zhang , MD
Professor and Chairman
Department of Radiation Oncology
Fudan University, Shanghai Cancer Hospital
270 Dong An Road
Shanghai 200032
People's Republic of China
Email: zhenzhang6@gmail.com

Section I
Palliative Treatment

1A

Radiation Therapy for Brain Metastasis

Ugur Selek[1], Simon S. Lo[2] and Eric L. Chang[3]

Key Points

- Metastasis to the brain is the most common intracranial tumor in adults.
- The most common sites of primary are lung, breast, melanoma, kidney, and colon.
- Common symptoms include headache, neurological deficit, and seizures.
- Parameters to predict prognosis include recursive partitioning analysis (RPA), score index for radiosurgery (SIR), and graded prognostic assessment (GPA).
- Standard treatment for patients with multiple metastases is whole-brain radiotherapy.
- For patients with single brain metastases, surgical resection followed by whole-brain radiotherapy can improve intracranial tumor control as compared with surgical resection alone, although no survival benefit has been demonstrated.
- For patients with one to four brain metastases, stereotactic radiosurgery (SRS) with or without whole-brain radiotherapy may be offered, although the latter approach will result in an increased risk of intracranial failure, without impacting survival.
- Compared with 30 Gy in ten fractions, none of the other whole-brain radiotherapy regimens yields additional benefits.
- Neurocognitive deficits can be caused by the presence of brain metastases, intracranial tumor progression, whole-brain radiotherapy, and chemotherapy ("chemobrain").

[1] Ugur Selek, MD
Email:
uselek@mdanderson.org

[2] Simon S. Lo, MD
Email:
simon.lo@osumc.edu

[3] Eric L. Chang, MD
Email:
echang@mdanderson.org

J. J. Lu, L. W. Brady (Eds.), *Decision Making in Radiation Oncology*
DOI: 10.1007/978-3-642-13832-4_1, © Springer-Verlag Berlin Heidelberg 2011

Epidemiology and Etiology

Metastasis to the brain is the most common intracranial tumor in adults, with an estimated incidence of as high as 200,000 cases per year in the USA alone. The most common primary tumors metastasizing to the brain includes lung, breast, melanoma, renal, and colon (Table 1A.1).

Table 1A.1 Relative probabilities of brain metastases according to diagnosis and anatomical parts of brain

Primary disease	Probability (%)	Brain metastasis	Probability (%)
Lung cancer	40–50 %	Cerebral hemispheres	80%
Breast cancer	15–25%	Cerebellum	15%
Melanoma	5–20 %	Brainstem	5%

Symptomatic brain metastases occur in eight to ten of all cancer patients

Brain metastases demonstrate the same gender predilection as the primary tumors do, as the most common source of metastases is lung cancer in males and breast cancer in females.

Routes of Spread and Pathophysiology

Although tumor cells are generally larger than capillary vessels are (diameters: capillaries 3–8 μm, tumor cells: 20 μm) and usually arrest in the first capillary bed such as in lung, liver or vertebral bodies related with their venous drainage (vena cava, portal vein, or Batson's plexus), some tumor cells reach the arterial circulation via their ability to distort and squeeze through capillaries, to be arrested in the capillary bed of other organs such as the brain. This is related to the recognition by tumor cells of surface molecules (called addressins) on the endothelium and organotropic factors.

Metastases are generally round and well-demarcated lesions at the junction of gray and white matter, with a zone of surrounding edema. Peritumoral edema is believed to start primarily with the leakage of plasma constituents across an injured blood–brain barrier, leading to an increase of extravascular space and with altered or newly formed capillaries. This process is mediated by release of vasoactive cytokines and mediators of tumor associated with angiogenesis. Brain edema is mainly within the white matter, which is roughly hypodense on computed tomography (CT) and hypointense on T_1-weighted magnetic resonance imaging (MRI) or hyperintense on T_2.

Diagnosis, Staging, and Prognosis

Clinical Presentation

Common symptoms include headache, neurological deficit, and seizures. Neurologic deficits are related to peritumoral edema, increased intracranial pressure, destruction of brain tissue, or vascular compromise.

Cognitive impairment was demonstrated in 65% of patients with brain metastases. Hemorrhage can be observed in 3–14% of metastases (melanoma, choriocarcinoma, renal, thyroid, lung, breast, germ-cell, etc) (*Chang EL, Wefel JS, Maor MH et al (2007) A pilot study of neurocognitive function in patients with one to three new brain metastases initially treated with stereotactic radiosurgery alone. Neurosurgery 60:277–283, discussion 283–284; Mehta MP, Rodrigus P, Terhaard CH et al (2003) Survival and neurologic outcomes in a randomized trial of motexafin gadolinium and WBRT in brain metastases. J Clin Oncol 21:2529–2536*).

Diagnosis and Staging

The development of above-mentioned symptoms and signs in patients with a diagnosis of cancer prompts investigation with diagnostic imaging. CT or MRI of the brain is used to confirm the diagnosis of brain metastasis.

Compared with CT, MRI has a higher resolution and is able to detect smaller metastatic lesions. Brain metastases typically appear as contrast-enhanced lesions on CT or MRI axial T_1 or spoiled gradient-recalled acquisition in the steady state (GRASS) volume sequence with gadolinium. The spoiled GRASS volume sequence has a better ability to detect very small metastases. Double-dose gadolinium is used in stereotactic MRI when Gamma Knife–based stereotactic radiosurgery (SRS) is performed. On axial fluid-attenuated inversion recovery (FLAIR) sequence, brain metastases may show high signal intensity. Blood can be seen in hemorrhagic brain metastases on non-contrast CT or MRI axial T_1 sequence without gadolinium.

No formal staging system exists for brain metastasis, but a few systems are in use to categorize prognostic groups.

Prognosis

Appropriate assessment of independent prognostic factors, demographic, and clinical variables is required to predict survival and neurologic function.

Performance status (major determinant of survival: the Karnofsky performance status [KPS] score), age, number of brain metastases (single versus multiple), primary tumor type (lymphoma, germ cell, and breast versus other), systemic tumor activity (controlled versus uncontrolled), and time to develop brain metastases (longer is favorable, especially for breast and melanoma) are essential (*Lagerwaard FJ, Levendag PC, Nowak PJ et al (1999) Identification of prognostic factors in patients with brain metastases: a review of 1,292 patients. Int J Radiat Oncol Biol Phys 43:795–803; Yates JW, Chalmer B, McKegney FP (1980) Evaluation of patients with advanced cancer using the Karnofsky Performance Status. Cancer 45:2220–2224*).

The Recursive Partitioning Analysis (RPA) is the first effective predictive tool studied in patients pooled from three Radiation Therapy and Oncology Group (RTOG) trials between 1979 and 1993, receiving WBRT in various fractionation schedules to suggest three classes for overall survival duration (Table 1A.2). Additional prognostic value within classes 1 and 2 for single versus multiple brain metastases was revealed afterward.

Table 1A.2 Overall survival duration

Class	Recursive partitioning analysis (RPA)	Median survival (months)
I	KPS ≥ 70, <65 years of age with controlled primary, no extracranial metastases	7.1
II	Remaining populace	4.2
III	KPS < 70	2.3

Sources: Gaspar L, Scott C, Rotman M et al (1997) Recursive partitioning analysis (RPA) of prognostic factors in three RTOG brain metastases trials. Int J Radiat Oncol Biol Phys 37:745–751; Gaspar LE, Scott C, Murray K et al (2000) Validation of the RTOG recursive partitioning analysis (RPA) classification for brain metastases. Int J Radiat Oncol Biol Phys 47:1001–1006; Agboola O, Benoit B, Cross P et al (1998) Prognostic factors derived from recursive partition analysis (RPA) of RTOG brain metastases trials applied to surgically resected and irradiated brain metastatic cases. Int J Radiat Oncol Biol Phys 42:155–159

The Score Index for Radiosurgery (SIR) is an alternative prognostic scoring system derived from patients undergoing SRS, including lesion number and largest lesion volume in addition to age, KPS score, and systemic disease status (Table 1A.3). SIR is the sum of the values of each factor, ranging from 0 to 10. Median survival was shown to change from 2.9 months, with scores of 1–3 to 31.4 months with scores of 8–10.

Table 1A.3 Score Index for Radiosurgery (*SIR*)

Parameter	Score		
	0	1	2
Age (years)	≥60	51–59	≤50
KPS	≥50	60–70	80–100
Systemic disease	Progressive	Stable	Complete response or no evidence of disease
No. of lesions	≥3	2	1
Volume of largest lesion (ml)	>13	5–13	<5

Sources: Weltman E, Salvajoli JV, Brandt RA et al (2000) Radiosurgery for brain metastases: a score index for predicting prognosis. Int J Radiat Oncol Biol Phys 46:1155–1161; Lorenzoni J, Devriendt D, Massager N et al (2004) Radiosurgery for treatment of brain metastases: estimation of patient eligibility using three stratification systems. Int J Radiat Oncol Biol Phys 60:218–224

The Graded Prognostic Assessment (GPA) is the newest quantitative index based on RTOG databases (Tables 1A.4 and 1A.5).

Table 1A.4 Graded Prognostic Assessment (*GPA*)

Parameter	Score		
	0	0.5	1
Age (years)	>60	50–59	<50
KPS	<70	70–80	>80
No. of brain metastases	>3	2–3	1
Extracranial metastases	Present	Not applicable	None

Source: Sperduto CM, Watanabe Y, Mullan J et al (2008) A validation study of a new prognostic index for patients with brain metastases: the Graded Prognostic Assessment. J Neurosurg 109:S87–S99

Table 1A.5 GPA scores in terms of survival

GPA	Median survival (months)
3.5–4	11
3	6.9
1.5–2.5	3.8
0–1	2.8

Source: Sperduto PW, Berkey B, Gaspar LE et al (2008) A new prognostic index and comparison to three other indices for patients with brain metastases: an analysis of 1,960 patients in the RTOG database. Int J Radiat Oncol Biol Phys 70:510–514

Treatment

Principles and Practice

Various factors determine the most appropriate therapy for brain metastasis (Table 1A.6). Treatment strategy is usually guided by the number of lesions present. Single brain metastasis is one brain metastasis without regard to status of the extracranial disease, while solitary metastasis is single brain metastasis in the absence of extracranial disease.

Table 1A.6 Factors determining therapy

Factor	Description
Patient	■ Neurological deficits ■ Age ■ KPS ■ Patient input
Disease	■ Number of metastases ■ Size of lesion(s) ■ Location ■ Primary tumor status ■ Extracranial disease status

Treatment options include whole-brain radiotherapy (WBRT) alone, WBRT with or without surgery, WBRT with or without SRS, surgery with or without radiation (localized or WBRT), and SRS alone (Table 1A.7).

Table 1A.7 Treatment modalities used in brain metastasis

Type	Description
Surgery[a]	
Indications	■ Surgery is indicated for symptomatic lesions with mass effect ■ Particularly considered in case of requiring a tissue diagnosis, resecting a single, easily accessible lesion without extensive systemic disease, or reducing symptomatic mass effect for tumors generally >3 cm ■ Used to address brain metastases failing SRS or radiation necrosis
Facts/issues	■ Resection in solitary metastasis (with radiation therapy) improves overall survival ■ Controversial for multiple lesions ▶

Table 1A.7 (*continued*)

Type	Description
Radiation therapy[b]	
Indication	■ Stands as the initial approach for deep-seated tumors and tumors at eloquent brain locations (brainstem, basal ganglia, speech areas, receptive language areas, motor cortex, and visual cortex)
Techniques	■ Whole-brain radiation therapy (WBRT) is currently the standard treatment of brain metastases ■ WBRT improves survival over supportive care and neurologic function ■ SRS may be precluded or dose-limited for lesions located <5 mm from optic chiasm ■ If the suspected brain metastasis is ambiguous, observation is not suitable if the tumor exceed a diameter of 1 cm for radiosurgical control of small brain metastases[c]
Other treatments[d,e]	
Indication	■ Medical treatment for symptomatic management is usually needed in addition to radiation therapy and/or surgery
Medications	■ Corticosteroids for brain edema ■ Anticonvulsants for seizure ■ Medications improving cognition and mood such as methylphenidate and donepezil

[a]*Source: Martin JJ, Kondziolka D (2005) Indications for resection and radiosurgery for brain metastases. Curr Opin Oncol 17:584–587*
[b]*Source: Borgelt B, Gelber R, Kramer S et al (1980) The palliation of brain metastases: final results of the first 2 studies by RTOG. Int J Radiat Oncol Biol Phys 6:1–9*
[c]*Source: Chang EL, Hassenbusch SJ 3rd, Shiu AS et al (2003) The role of tumor size in the radiosurgical management of patients with ambiguous brain metastases. Neurosurgery 53:272–280, discussion 280–281*
[d]*Source: Meyers CA, Weitzner MA, Valentine AD et al (1998) Methylphenidate therapy improves cognition, mood, and function of brain tumor patients. J Clin Oncol 16:2522–2257*
[e]*Source: Shaw EG, Rosdhal R, D'Agostino RB Jr et al (2006) Phase II study of donepezil in irradiated brain tumor patients: effect on cognitive function, mood, and quality of life. J Clin Oncol 24:1415–1420*

Figure 1A.1 outlines the best therapeutic approaches based on various factors.

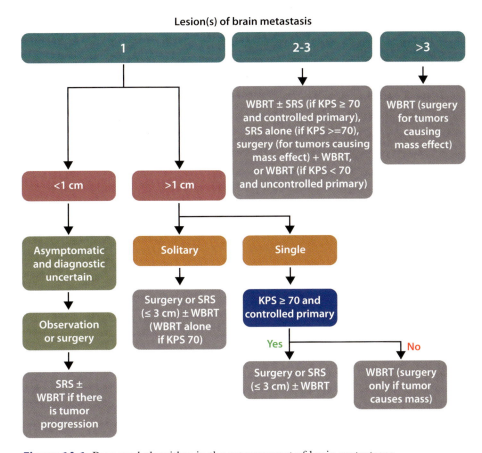

Figure 1A.1 Proposed algorithm in the management of brain metastases.

Source: Chang EL, Lo S (2003) Diagnosis and management of central nervous system metastases from breast cancer. Oncologist 8:398–410

Treatment of Solitary or Single Brain Metastasis

WBRT after surgical resection or SRS is considered the standard of care option for solitary brain metastasis. The survival benefit of additional local treatment such as surgery or SRS to WBRT in solitary and single metastasis has been identified (Table 1A.8).

Table 1A.8 Clinical evidence comparing single-modality treatment (surgery or WBRT) versus combined modality (surgery and WBRT) for single brain metastasis

Study	Results
Patchell et al[a]	■ 95 Patients with single brain metastasis were randomized to receive surgery alone or surgery and WBRT ■ No difference in survival was found, while patients treated by surgery and WBRT had fewer deaths due to neurologic causes and fewer local relapses at the original site (10 versus 46%), as well as elsewhere in the brain (14 versus 37%) ■ Complete resection without WBRT leads to 70% actuarial relapse, which is a relative risk of 3
Patchell et al[b]	■ 48 Patients with single brain metastasis were randomized and received WBRT alone or WBRT plus surgical resection ■ Surgical resection provides longer survival (median, 40 versus 15 weeks) ■ Fewer recurrences of cancer in the brain in comparison to radiotherapy alone in patients with single brain metastasis
Vecht et al[c]	■ Randomized trial compared patients with solitary or single brain metastasis (i.e., progressive extracranial disease, stratified) treated with surgery plus WBRT or WBRT alone ■ The combined treatment compared with radiotherapy alone led to a longer survival ($p = 0.04$) and a longer functionally independent survival (FIS) ($p = 0.06$) ■ Improvement was most pronounced in patients with single brain metastasis and stable extracranial disease: MS were 12 versus 7 months, and median FIS were 9 versus 4 months ■ Patients with progressive extracranial cancer had a median overall survival of 5 months and a FIS of 2.5 months irrespective of given treatment ■ Improvement in functional status occurred more rapidly and for longer periods after neurosurgical excision and radiotherapy than after radiotherapy alone

[a]*Source: Patchell RA, Tibbs PA, Regine WF et al (1998) Postoperative radiotherapy in the treatment of single metastases to the brain: a randomized trial. JAMA 280:1485–1489*
[b]*Source: Patchell RA, Tibbs PA, Walsh JW et al (1990) A randomized trial of surgery in the treatment of single metastases to the brain. N Engl J Med 322:494–500*
[c]*Source: Vecht CJ, Haaxma-Reiche H, Noordijk EM et al (1993) Treatment of single brain metastasis: radiotherapy alone or combined with neurosurgery? Ann Neurol 33:583–590*

Furthermore, results of retrospective series showed SRS is comparable to and can replace surgery (with WBRT) for treatment of solitary or single brain metastasis (Table 1A.9).

Table 1A.9 Retrospective series compared surgical resection versus SRS in the treatment of solitary or single brain metastasis

Study	Results
Muacevic et al[a]	▪ A retrospective study compared surgery plus WBRT (52 patients) versus SRS alone (56 patients) in patients with solitary brain metastases <3.5 cm in diameter ▪ The 1-year survival rate and median survival was 53% and 68 weeks in the surgical plus WBRT group, versus 43% and 35 weeks, respectively, in the SRS group ($p = 0.19$) ▪ The 1-year local tumor control rates after surgery and radiosurgery were 75 and 83%, respectively ($p = 0.49$); the 1-year neurological death rates in these groups were 37 and 39% ($p = 0.8$) ▪ Results from this retrospective study suggest surgery and SRS are comparable in the treatment of solitary and small brain metastasis.
O'Neill BP et al[b]	▪ A retrospective study compared surgical resection (74 patients) versus SRS (23 patients) in patients with solitary brain metastases ▪ There was no significant difference in the percentage of patients received WBRT in the 2 groups ▪ 1-Year survival rate was 56% for the patients received SRS, and 62% for those received surgery ($p = 0.15$) ▪ However, local tumor control was 100% in patients treated with SRS, as compared to 19 (58%) after surgical resection ($p = 0.020$)
Schoggl et al[c]	▪ A retrospective study on 133 patients with single brain metastasis treated with microsurgery or SRS ▪ All patientsreceived additional WBRT ▪ The median survival for patients after RS was 12 months, and 9 months for patients after microsurgery ($p = 0.19$) ▪ SRS and microsurgery combined with WBRT are comparable modalities in treating single brain metastasis

[a]*Source: Muacevic A, Kreth FW, Horstmann GA et al (1999) Surgery and radiotherapy compared with gamma knife radiosurgery in the treatment of solitary cerebral metastases of small diameter. J Neurosurg 91:35–43*
[b]*Source: O'Neill BP, Iturria NJ, Link MJ et al (2003) A comparison of surgical resection and stereotactic radiosurgery in the treatment of solitary brain metastases. Int J Radiat Oncol Biol Phys 55:1169–1176*
[c]*Source: Schoggl A, Kitz K, Reddy M et al (2000) Defining the role of stereotactic radiosurgery versus microsurgery in the treatment of single brain metastases. Acta Neurochir (Wien) 142:621–626*

Treatment of Oligometastasis (One to Three)

Combined Treatment for Oligometastasis of the Brain

WBRT with SRS is considered as the standard of care for patients with one to three brain metastases. The efficacy of combined treatment has been demonstrated in a randomized clinical trial (Table 1A.10).

Table 1A.10 Clinical evidence supported the use of combined SRS plus WBRT over WBRT alone in patients with one to three brain metastases

Study	Results
RTOG 9508	■ 333 Patients with 1–3 brain metastases were randomized to WBRT versus WBRT plus SRS ■ Patients were stratified by number of metastases and status of extracranial disease ■ Univariate analysis showed that there was a survival advantage in the WBRT and stereotactic radiosurgery group for patients with a single brain metastasis (median survival time 6.5 versus 4.9 months, $p = 0.0393$) ■ Patients in the stereotactic surgery group were more likely to have a stable or improved KPS score at 6 months' follow-up than were patients allocated WBRT alone (43 versus 27%, respectively; $p = 0.03$) ■ By multivariate analysis, survival improved in patients with an RPA class 1 ($p < 0.0001$) or a favorable histological status ($p = 0.0121$) ■ WBRT and stereotactic radiosurgery should, therefore, be standard treatment for patients with a single unresectable brain metastasis and considered for patients with two or three brain metastases

Source: Andrews DW, Scott CB, Sperduto PW et al (2004) WBRT with or without SRS boost for patients with 1–3 brain metastases: phase III results of the RTOG 9508 randomised trial. Lancet 363:1665–1672

Based on published clinical evidence (levels I–III), the American Society of Therapeutic Radiology and Oncology (ASTRO) summarized the findings as detailed in Table 1A.11. The findings were further supported by the results of a meta-analysis (Table 1A.12).

Table 1A.11 Summary of the ASTRO evidence-based review of the role of SRS for brain metastases

Scenario	Clinical outcome
Patients with small (<4 cm) oligometastases of brain	The addition of SRS boost to WBRT improves brain control as compared with WBRT alone
Patients with single or solitary brain metastasis	The addition of SRS boost to WBRT improves survival, despite a small risk of toxicity associated with SRS as compared with WBRT alone
If treated with SRS alone for newly diagnosed brain metastases	Overall survival is not altered. However, local and distant brain control is significantly poorer with omission of upfront WBRT (levels I–III evidence)

Source: Mehta MP, Tsao MN, Whelan TJ et al (2005) The ASTRO evidence-based review of the role of radiosurgery for brain metastases. Int J Radiat Oncol Biol Phys 63:37–46

Table 1A.12 Results of meta-analysis–compared single- or multiple-treatment modalities of various combinations

Meta-analysis	Results
Stafinski et al	▪ The review identified 3 RCTs and one cohort study on: SRS versus SRS with WBRT, SRS versus WBRT with or without surgical resection, SRS versus surgical resection only, or SRS and WBRT versus WBRT ▪ Among patients with multiple metastases, no difference in survival between those treated with WBRT and SRS and those treated with WBRT alone was found ▪ In patients with single metastasis, a statistically significant difference, favoring those treated with WBRT plus SRS, was observed ▪ Intracranial tumor control at 2 years was improved regardless of the number of brain lesions if SRS is added to WBRT

Source: Stafinski T, Jhangri GS, Yan E et al (2006) Effectiveness of SRS alone or in combination with WBRT compared to conventional surgery and/or WBRT for the treatment of one or more brain metastases: a systematic review and meta-analysis. Cancer Treat Rev 32:203–213

SRS as a Single-Treatment Modality

Although WBRT with or without SRS has been the standard for palliative treatment in patients with multiple brain metastases, in cases of four or fewer brain metastases, results from both randomized and retrospective studies showed that SRS alone is also a reasonable option in well-selected patients (Tables 1A.13 to 1A.15).

SRS alone with close follow-up should be considered for high-functioning patients who wish to preserve neurocognitive function in terms of learning and memory. These individuals should be motivated, willing, and able to undergo close follow-up with serial neuroimaging, preferably with MRI and subsequent salvage therapies. Conversely, patients who are unreliable follow-up candidates should probably be treated with SRS plus WBRT.

Table 1A.13 Results of randomized trials on SRS alone for oligo-metastases of brain (one to four lesions) versus SRS plus WBRT

Trial	Results
Hokkaido University (Japan)[a]	▪ Randomized controlled trial of 132 patients with 1 to 4 brain metastases (all <3 cm in diameter) treated with WBRT plus SRS (65 patients) or SRS alone (67 patients) ▪ Median survival time and the 1-year actuarial survival rate were 7.5 months and 38.5% for combined treatment versus 8.0 months and 28.4% for SRS alone ($p = 0.42$) ▪ The 12-month brain tumor recurrence rate was 46.8% in the WBRT plus SRS group and 76.4% for SRS alone group ($p < 0.001$)
Chang EL et al[b]	▪ Randomized trial of 58 patients treated with SRS alone (30 cases) or SRS plus WBRT (28 cases) ▪ SRS plus WBRT were significantly more likely to show a decline in learning and memory function (mean posterior probability of decline 52%) at 4 months than patients assigned to receive SRS alone (mean posterior probability of decline 24%) ▪ At 4 months there were 4 deaths (13%) in the group that received SRS alone, and 8 deaths (29%) in the group that received SRS plus WBRT

[a]*Source: Aoyama H, Shirato H, Tago M et al (2006) SRS plus WBRT vs SRS alone for treatment of brain metastases: a randomized controlled trial. JAMA 295:2483–2491*
[b]*Source: Chang EL, Wefel JS, Hess KR et al (2009) Neurocognition in patients with brain metastases treated with SRS or SRS plus WBRT: a randomized controlled trial. Lancet Oncol 10:1037–1044*

Table 1A.14 Results of retrospective studies on SRS alone for oligometastases of brain versus WBRT or SRS plus WBRT

Trial	Results
University of Heidelberg (Germany)[a]	■ 158 Patients received SRS, 78 patients received SRS and WBRT ■ Overall median survival was 5.5 months, with control of CNS disease achieved in 92% of the treated brain metastases ■ The results were not significantly different between patients treated by RS with or without WBRT ■ Patients without evidence of extracranial disease, median survival was increased for patients who received WBRT (15.4 versus 8.3 months, $p=0.08$)
Multi-institutional review[b]	■ 569 Evaluable patients, 268 had SRS alone initially (24% of whom ultimately had salvage WBRT), and 301 had RS plus up-front WBRT ■ The median survival times for patients treated with RS alone initially versus RS plus WBRT were 14.0 versus 15.2 months for RPA class 1 patients, 8.2 versus 7.0 months for class 2, and 5.3 versus 5.5 months for class 3, respectively ■ With adjustment by RPA class, there was no survival difference comparing RS alone initially with RS plus up-front WBRT ($p = 0.33$, hazard ratio = 1.09)
Rades et al[c]	■ Retrospective study of 186 patients in RPA classes 1 and 2 who had 1–3 brain metastases treated with SRS or WBRT ■ Total dose of WBRT was 30–40 Gy, and that of SRS was 18–25 Gy ■ SRS alone was associated with improved local control as compared to WBRT, although overall survival were not significantly different

[a]Source: Pirzkall A, Debus J, Lohr F et al (1998) Radiosurgery alone or in combination with whole-brain radiotherapy for brain metastases. J Clin Oncol 16:3563–3569
[b]Source: Sneed PK, Suh JH, Goetsch SJ et al (2002) A multi-institutional review of radiosurgery alone versus radiosurgery with WBRT as the initial management of brain metastases. Int J Radiat Oncol Biol Phys 53:519–526
[c]Source: Rades D, Pluemer A, Veninga T et al (2007) WBRT versus SRS for patients RPA classes 1 and 2 with 1 to 3 brain metastases. Cancer 110:2285–2292

Table 1A.15 SRS alone versus resection plus WBRT for 1 or 2 brain metastases

Study	Results
Rades et al	■ Retrospective study included 206 patients in RPA classes 1 and 2 who had 1–2 brain metastases and treated with SRS alone or surgery plus WBRT ■ The comparison did not reveal significantly significant difference in overall survival ($p = 0.19$), brain control ($p = 0.52$), or local control ($p = 0.25$) ■ SRS alone appeared to be as effective as resection plus WBRT in the treatment of 1 or 2 brain metastases for patients in RPA classes 1 and 2

Source: Rades D, Bohlen G, Pluemer A et al (2007) SRS alone versus resection plus WBRT for 1 or 2 brain metastases in RPA class 1 and 2 patients. Cancer 109:2515–2521

SRS as an Adjuvant-Treatment Modality

SRS to the surgical cavity after resection of brain metastases also improves local control in comparison to surgery alone. Local control rate at the surgical cavity at 1 year is found to be 79% in a Stanford University series and 94% in a University of Virginia series, which is satisfactory in comparison to historic results with observation alone (54%) and postoperative WBRT (80–90%) (Table 1A.16).

Table 1A.16 Retrospective studies support the use of SRS as an adjuvant treatment modality

Study	Results
University of Virginia series[a]	■ 47 Patients with pathologically confirmed metastatic disease underwent SRS to the postoperative resection cavity following gross–total resection of the tumor ■ The mean volume of the treated cavity was 10.5 cm³ (range of 1.75–35.45 cm³), and the mean dose to the cavity margin was 19 Gy ■ With a median radiographic follow-up duration was 10 months (range of 4–37 months), local tumor control at the site of the surgical cavity was achieved in 44 patients (94%) ■ SRS appears to be effective in terms of providing local tumor control at the resection cavity after resection of a brain metastasis
Stanford University series[b]	■ 72 Patients with 76 cavities treated ■ Average tumor volume of 9.8 cm³ (range of 0.1–66.8 cm³), and median marginal dose of 18.6 Gy (range of 15–30 Gy) ■ With a median follow-up of 8.1 months, actuarial local control rates at 6 and 12 months were 88 and 79%, respectively

[a]*Source: Jagannathan J, Yen CP, Ray DK et al (2009) GammaKnife radiosurgery to the surgical cavity following resection of brain metastases. J Neurosurg 111:431–438*
[b]*Source: Soltys SG, Adler JR, Lipani JD et al (2008) SRS of the postoperative resection cavity for brain metastases. Int J Radiat Oncol Biol Phys 70:187–193*

Radiation Therapy Techniques

Whole Brain Radiation Therapy

Simulation and Field Arrangements

WBRT radiation fields should have adequate coverage of all intracranial contents by ensuring inclusion of the anterior cranial fossa, middle cranial fossa, and skull base.

Typical beam arrangement is right and left lateral opposing fields. Cerrobend blocks or multileaf collimator can be used to shape the fields. To eliminate hotspots, a field-in-field plan can be used when three-dimensional (3D) computer planning is performed (Figure 1A.2).

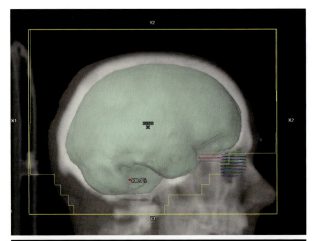

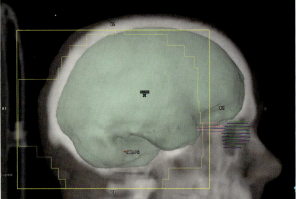

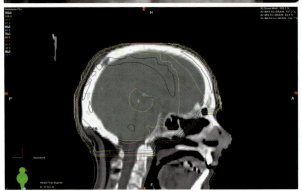

Figure 1A.2 A right and left lateral opposing field arrangement is used for WBRT; a field–in–field technique is used to minimize the hotspots

Dose and Treatment Delivery

Standard dose of WBRT is considered 30 Gy in ten daily fractions or 20 Gy in five daily fractions. Dose escalation of whole brain beyond 30 Gy in ten daily fractions was not associated with improved outcome in patients with brain metastasis. The Cochrane review demonstrated that none of the randomized clinical trials with altered dose-fractionation schemes as compared with standard delivery of 30 Gy found a survival, neurologic function, or symptom control benefit. Table 1A.17 shows the standard dose regimens used for WBRT.

Table 1A.17 Commonly used WBRT regimens

Dose (Gy)	No. of fractions
40	20
37.5	15
30	10
20	5

Sources: Tsao MN, Lloyd N, Wong R et al (2006) Whole-brain radiotherapy for the treatment of multiple brain metastases. Cochrane Database Syst Rev 3:CD003869; Tsao MN, Lloyd NS, Wong RK (2005) Clinical practice guideline on the optimal radiotherapeutic management of brain metastases. BMC Cancer 5:34; Tsao MN, Lloyd NS, Wong RK et al (2005) Radiotherapeutic management of brain metastases: a systematic review and meta-analysis. Cancer Treat Rev 31:256–273

Stereotactic Radiosurgery

Stereotactic radiosurgery (SRS) is defined to be the alternative of surgery in well-demarcated metastasis, without mass effect by precise beams of radiation with rapid dose fall-off. SRS boost in addition to WBRT in patients with up to three newly diagnosed brain metastases significantly improves intracranial control rates as compared with WBRT alone, while there is no survival benefit with multiple brain metastases (*Mehta MP, Tsao MN, Whelan TJ et al (2005) The ASTRO evidence-based review of the role of SRS for brain metastases. Int J Radiat Oncol Biol Phys 63:37–46*).

SRS dose guidelines have been defined based on minimizing the risk of radiation necrosis, besides size, location, and histology of the lesion. Table 1A.18 shows RTOG guidelines for SRS doses.

Table 1A.18 RTOG SRS dose guidelines

Diameter (cm)	Dose (Gy)
≤2.0	24
2.1–3.0	18
3.1–4.0	15

Sources: Shehata MK, Young B, Reid B et al (2004) Stereotatic radiosurgery of 468 brain metastases < or =2 cm: implications for SRS dose and WBRT. Int J Radiat Oncol Biol Phys 59:87–93; Shaw E, Scott C, Souhami L et al (2000) Single dose radiosurgical treatment of recurrent previously irradiated primary brain tumors and brain metastases: final report of RTOG protocol 90-05. Int J Radiat Oncol Biol Phys 47:291–298

SRS can be delivered via Gamma Knife, linear accelerator (Linac) based systems, or protons (Figure 1A.3). Linac can be adapted or dedicated to deliver SRS within mechanical tolerances with physics quality assurance. In addition, frameless radiosurgery starts to be an option (*Clark GM, Popple RA, Young PE et al (2009) Feasibility of single-isocenter volumetric modulated arc radiosurgery for treatment of multiple brain metastases. Int J Radiat Oncol Biol Phys 76:296–302; Lamba M, Breneman JC, Warnick RE (2009) Evaluation of image-guided positioning for frameless intracranial radiosurgery. Int J Radiat Oncol Biol Phys 74:913–919; Sonke JJ, Rossi M, Wolthaus J et al (2009) Frameless stereotactic body radiotherapy for lung cancer using 4-D cone beam CT guidance. Int J Radiat Oncol Biol Phys 74:567–574*).

Radiation-Induced Adverse Effects in WBRT

WBRT causes acute effects mainly including hair loss, skin erythema, somnolence, fatigue, and distractibility, as well as late effects including mainly impaired memory, dementia (2–5%), and rarely, radiation necrosis, leukoencephalopathy, and cerebral atrophy.

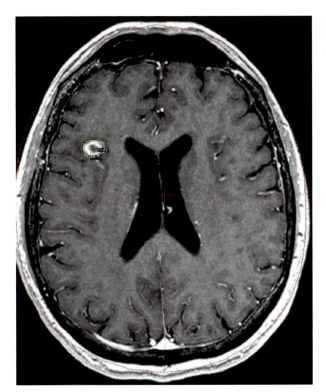

Figure 1A.3 Gamma Knife-based SRS for a right frontal metastasis (20 Gy @ 50%)

Dosimetric parameters correlating with late toxicity are scarce, which are mainly from survivors of childhood brain tumors treated with radiotherapy. Adult prospective studies have shown that partial brain irradiation in the dose range of 50–60 Gy cause minimal to no discernable effect on memory and cognition. Memory, an important neurocognitive function, is considered preserved if hippocampal area is spared. Treated target volume, dose, and conformality index of SRS can potentially affect any late radiation effects. Acute effects of SRS (incidence of 1–2%) are mainly nausea, vomiting, aphasia, motor neuropathy, seizures, swelling, or hemorrhagic stroke and late effects are mainly radiation necrosis (2–3%), radiation associated secondary malignancies, or death (extremely rare).

Baseline neurocognitive impairment at initial diagnosis was particularly noted in patients with brain metastases related to the disease process itself. Balancing attempts to achieve tumor control and toxicities associated with various brain metastasis treatments are important considerations towards preserving neurocognitive function.

1B

Palliative Radiotherapy for Bone Metastases

Alysa Fairchild[1] and Stephen Lutz[2]

Key Points

- Bone is the most common site of cancer metastasis, with an estimated 300,000–400,000 US cancer patients affected by bone metastases (BM) each year.

- While BM may be asymptomatic, they commonly cause significant morbidity and functional impairment due to pain, pathologic fracture, or spinal cord compression (SCC).

- The workup of bone metastases includes a detailed pain history, physical examination, and relevant radiographic studies (plain x-ray, bone scan, computed tomography [CT] scan, magnetic resonance imaging [MRI], or positron-emission photography [PET]). Biopsy should be considered when histology is in question.

- By definition, all patients with bone metastases have stage IV disease, although prognosis varies greatly depending on patient-related (age, performance status, co-morbidities, presences of extraosseous metastases), tumor-related (histology and grade of the primary tumor, tumor marker levels), and treatment-related factors.

- Choice of optimal treatment modality requires interdisciplinary assessment. Options include pharmacologic therapy, radiotherapy (external beam, radionuclides), systemic therapy (bisphosphonates, chemotherapy, hormonal therapy), and surgery (including minimally invasive techniques such as vertebroplasty).

- Several randomized controlled trials (RCTs) have shown that external-beam radiotherapy (EBRT) provides successful, efficient, and cost-effective treatment of BM. Single-fraction RT is as effective as multiple fractions for analgesia, although the evidence for equivalence in prevention of pathologic fracture and SCC is not as conclusive.

- Surgical treatment is most appropriate for patients with impending or established pathologic long-bone fracture, or impending or established SCC, assuming adequate performance status (PS) and life expectancy. RCT evidence suggests that appropriately selected patients with SCC who had timely surgical decompression and postoperative RT have better outcomes, including higher rates of ambulation, compared with EBRT alone.

[1] Alysa Fairchild, BSc, MD, FRCPC
Email: alysa.fairchild@albertahealthservices.ca

[2] Stephen Lutz, MD
Email: slutz@bvhealthsystem.or

J. J. Lu, L. W. Brady (Eds.), *Decision Making in Radiation Oncology*
DOI: 10.1007/978-3-642-13832-4_2, © Springer-Verlag Berlin Heidelberg 2011

Epidemiology and Etiology

Bone metastases (BM) develop in ~30–70% of all cancer patients. Two thirds to three quarters of patients with advanced breast or prostate cancer have BM, while lung, thyroid, and renal cell carcinomas metastasize to bone 30–40% of the time. BM are the most common indication for palliative radiotherapy (RT) (*Chow E, Hird A, Velikova G et al (2009) The European Organisation for Research and Treatment of Cancer Quality of Life Questionnaire for patients with bone metastases: the EORTC QLQ-BM22. Eur J Cancer 45:1146–1152*).

Anatomy

There are 126 bones in the human body, which provide structural support and act as the primary site for hematopoiesis. Bones routinely undergo remodeling over a person's entire life, with the balance between bone destruction and bone formation resulting from the homeostatic interaction between osteoclasts and osteoblasts, respectively.

Metastases can occur in any bone, though they are more common in sites containing red bone marrow: ~70% of BM occur in the axial skeleton (spine, pelvis, ribs, and skull) and 10% in the appendicular skeleton, usually in the proximal ends of long bones.

Pathology

Lytic lesions, such as those that are seen in the setting of multiple myeloma, stimulate the production of factors that promote osteoclast growth and activity (Figure 1B.1). Destruction of cortical bone causes weakening and, in the case of vertebral bodies, may cause collapse:

- ~1% of BM leads to pathologic fracture, with annual fracture rates of 5–20%.
- ~10% of all BM require some form of surgical intervention, with high-risk areas including the femoral neck, subtrochanteric, and intertrochanteric regions.

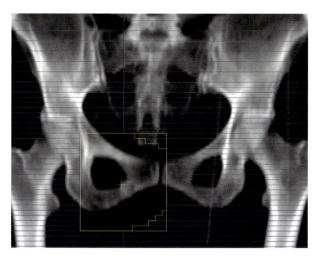

Figure 1B.1 A digitally reconstructed radiograph of a 62-year-old woman with multiple myeloma shows numerous lytic metastases throughout the anterior pelvis. The prominent lesion in the right pubic ramus caused her significant pain, which was successfully palliated with radiotherapy delivered through the portal shown

Conversely, the overstimulation of osteoblasts may cause dense but disorganized and structurally weakened blastic lesions, such as those produced by prostate cancer metastases (Figure 1B.2). Continued tumor infiltration and growth within bone may eventually obliterate the marrow cavity and prevent normal hematopoiesis.

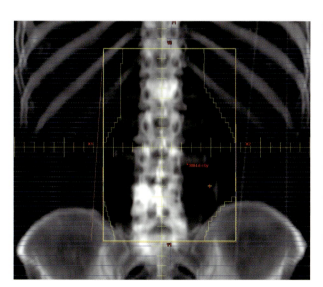

Figure 1B.2 A 60-year-old male presented with back pain, a serum prostate-specific antigen (PSA) of 212 ng/ml, and a biopsy-proven Gleason Score 10 adenocarcinoma of the prostate. He was found to have osteoblastic metastases involving the lumbar spine, with his most painful sites of disease in the spine responding well to radiotherapy. The treated field spans beyond the lateral spinous processes to include areas of metastatic adenopathy

Diagnosis, Staging, and Prognosis

On history, the nature, duration, and intensity of the pain, any alleviating or aggravating factors, motor or sensory changes, and both analgesic use and functional status must be assessed. Appropriate neuromusculoskeletal examination should be performed, including inspection for visible masses, point tenderness, increased pain with movement, cranial nerve palsy, or lower motor neuron neurologic signs. Commonly observed signs and symptoms from BM are illustrated in Table 1B.1. Both bone pain and other associated symptoms may negatively impair their quality of life (QoL). Radiological studies in patients with suspected BM are detailed in Table 1B.2.

Table 1B.1 Signs and symptoms of BM

Type	Description
Bone pain	Up to 75% of cases with BM experience some degree of discomfort
	Classically described as a progressive, continuous, dull, aching pain at rest, which increases in severity and becomes sharp with movement
	Tends to be easily localizable by the patient, with the exception of referred or radiating neuropathic pain or pain due to peripheral nerve root involvement
Other symptoms	Significant symptom burden due to BM may also cause depression, anxiety, sleep disturbances, social isolation, extended or repeat hospital admissions, or disruption in antineoplastic treatment

Table 1B.2 Radiographic workup of bone metastases

Type of Study	Advantages	Limitations
Plain x-rays	■ Fast, simple, inexpensive ■ Quantifies risk of pathologic fracture ■ Reveals lytic lesions	■ Low sensitivity ■ Poor spatial resolution ■ Misses extraosseous tumor
Bone scan	■ Sensitive ■ Relatively cost effective ■ Images entire skeleton	■ 2D spatial resolution only ■ Specificity somewhat low ■ Misses extraosseous tumor ■ False negative for lytic lesions
Computed tomography	■ Quick, sensitive, specific ■ Measures degree of bone destruction ■ May guide planned biopsy or surgery ■ Visualizes internal structures	■ Not as sensitive as MRI is for CNS ■ Somewhat expensive
Magnetic resonance imaging	■ Sensitive, specific, high resolution ■ Gold standard for measuring SCC ■ Shows small lesions, soft tissue disease ■ Benign versus malignant vertebral collapse	■ Cumbersome, expensive, lengthy ■ Access may be limited ■ May cause claustrophobia ■ Contraindicated in some patients
Positron-emission tomography	■ Fairly sensitive ■ Measures activity of cells ■ Scans most of skeleton	■ Expensive, relatively nonspecific ■ Access may be limited ■ Not 100% concordant with bone scan
Biopsy	■ Proves diagnosis in unknown primary ■ Confirms metastatic recurrences	■ May be nondiagnostic ■ Painful ■ Risk of bone fracture ■ May damage adjacent structures

By definition, all patients with BM have stage IV disease. Advances in systemic treatment have improved the overall survival (OS) of many BM patients, although their median survival remains only 30 weeks. Prognostic factors in patients with BM are detailed in Table 1B.3.

Table 1B.3 Prognostics factors for BM

Factor	Description
Disease related	■ Histology: median survival of patients with BM in breast, prostate, and lung cancer are 69, 40, and 13 weeks, respectively ■ Presence of only a limited number of bone metastases and absence of visceral metastases is a favorable factor
Patient related	■ Good performance status ■ Absence of comorbidities
Treatment related	■ Response to treatment especially hormone or chemotherapy

Source: Steenland E, Leer J, van Houwelingen H et al (1999) The effect of a single fraction compared to multiple fractions on painful bone metastases: a global analysis of the Dutch Bone Metastasis Study. Radiother Oncol 52:101–109

Treatment

The goals in the treatment of BM include pain relief, preservation of mobility and function, prevention of future complications, optimized quality of life (QoL), maintenance of skeletal integrity, and minimization of hospitalization. Choice of the optimal treatment modality requires interdisciplinary assessment (Table 1B.4). The treatment of asymptomatic bone metastases may be deferred unless the patient is at risk of a serious adverse outcome such as spinal cord compression or pathologic fracture (Figure 1B.3) (*Janjan N, Lutz S, Bedwinek J et al (2009) Therapeutic guidelines for the treatment of bone metastasis: A report from the American College of Radiology Appropriateness Criteria Expert Panel on Radiation Oncology. J Palliat Med 12:417–423*).

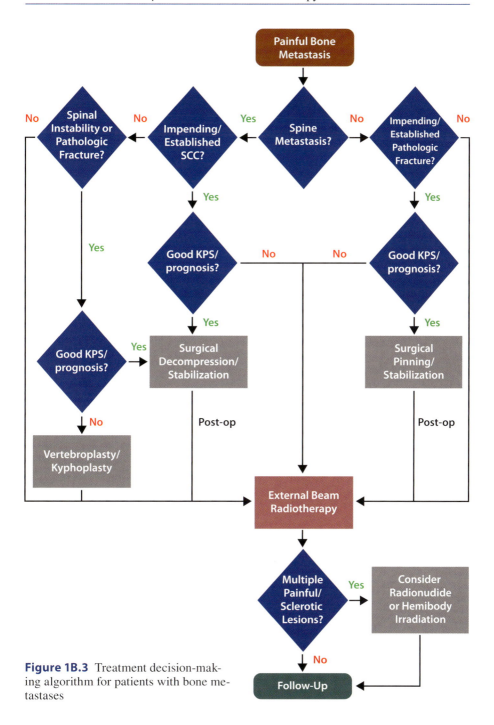

Figure 1B.3 Treatment decision-making algorithm for patients with bone metastases

Table 1B.4 Treatment modalities used for bone metastases

Modality	Description	
Intervention	Indications	Limitations
Systemic treatments		
Pharmacologic therapy	■ Minimal contraindications ■ Addresses multisite pain ■ Can tailor to pain mechanism	■ Side effects must be proactively addressed ■ Require monitoring for titration
Chemotherapy	■ Systemic disease treatment ■ May prolong survival, improve QoL	■ Response rates, duration may be low ■ Side effects are systemic ■ Many agents are expensive ■ Long interval before relief onset
Hormonal therapy	■ Systemic disease treatment ■ May prolong survival, improve QoL	■ Response rates, duration may be low ■ Long interval before relief onset
Bisphosphonates	■ Prevent or delay skeletal events ■ Evidence mounting ■ Treatment of hypercalcemia	■ Expensive ■ Risk of jaw osteonecrosis ■ Must monitor renal function
Radiotherapy		
External-beam radiotherapy	■ Good rate of pain relief ■ Relatively inexpensive ■ Single fraction time efficient ■ Few absolute contraindications	■ Acute effects on adjacent organs ■ Limited re-treatment options
Hemibody irradiation	■ Treats several sites ■ Single fraction time efficient ■ Fast onset of relief ■ Lytic, blastic, and extraosseous lesions	■ Requires premedication ■ Acute GI and hematopoietic side effects ■ Limited data about its use

Table 1B.4 (*continued*)

Modality	Description	
Intervention	**Indications**	**Limitations**
Radionuclides	■ Addresses multisite pain ■ May improve refractory pain ■ Fast onset of relief	■ Side effects (pain flare, blood counts) ■ Require blood count monitoring ■ Expensive, lack of availability ■ Ineffective for lytic metastases
Surgery		
Surgery	■ Spinal cord decompression ■ Prevention or fixation of fracture	■ Requires sufficient prognosis and PS ■ May delay other treatment types ■ Inpatient treatment
Kyphoplasty/ vertebroplasty/ cementoplasty	■ Pain relief, improved mobility ■ Stabilization of lytic lesions ■ Outpatient treatment	■ Data in the metastatic setting scant ■ Side effect risks not fully defined ■ Not for extraosseous disease

QoL: quality of life

Radiation Therapy

Principles and Practice

RT remains the mainstay of treatment for symptomatic BM and can be delivered in various forms including local conventional external-beam RT (EBRT), radionuclides, wide-field (hemibody) irradiation, or highly conformal techniques. The goal of radiation therapy for BM is to provide relief with minimal morbidity, cost, and time commitment. Performance status and degree of systemic disease must be considered prior to treatment.

The application and dose arrangement of RT techniques are detailed in Table 1B.5.

Table 1B.5 Treatment techniques, dose, and volume by clinical circumstance

Type	Description
Spine	■ Inclusion of at least one vertebral body level above and below those affected ■ Prescribed to mid- or posterior vertebral body
Non-spine sites	■ Treat disease responsible for symptoms, not necessarily all visible disease ■ Field arrangement, technique, and energy depend on treatment volume and depth ■ Prescription point based upon field arrangement, such as midplane for parallel opposed fields ■ Treatment volume includes at least a 2-cm margin to gross disease ■ Adjacent joints spared unless their inclusion is necessitated by an appropriate margin or tumor involvement
Post operative (PORT)	■ Fields encompass the surgical bed and implanted hardware with a margin, often treating the entire bone ■ Notice that implanted hardware may shield radiation

Hemibody irradiation	■ Upper
	  ■ Base of skull to below spinal cord and above iliac crest
	  ■ Dose and fractionation: 6 Gy in 1 fraction
	■ Middle
	  ■ Above diaphragm to below pubic symphysis, based on pain
	  ■ Dose and fractionation: 6 Gy in 1fraction
	■ Lower
	  ■ Below spinal cord and above iliac crest to distal femurs
	  ■ Dose and fractionation: 8 Gy in 1 fraction

EBRT Fractionation and Delivery

Approximately 25 randomized clinical trials (RCTs) and three meta-analyses have demonstrated equivalency of single (SF) and multiple-fraction RT for pain relief from uncomplicated BM (Table 1B.6). No consistent differences have been found between doses in rates of pathologic fracture, spinal cord compression, acute toxicity, QoL, time to first improvement in pain, time to complete pain relief, time to pain progression, opioid use, or overall survival. Other advantages of SF include decreased cost and lower risk of acute side effects (*Chow E, Harris K, Fan G et al (2007) Palliative radiotherapy trials for bone metastases: a systematic review. J Clin Oncol 25:1423–1436*).

Table 1B.6 Selected RCTs comparing single versus multiple-fraction EBRT

Study	Patient number, tumor histology	Fractionation	Overall response (%)	Complete response (%)	Acute toxicity (%)	Late toxicity (%)	Re-treatment rate (%)
Radiation Therapy and Oncology Group 97-14[a]	n = 898, breast or prostate cancer	8 Gy per 1 fraction	66%	15%	10%	4%	18%
		30 Gy per 10 fractions	66%	18%	17%	4%	9%
Trans-Tasman Radiation Oncology Group 96-05 (neuropathic pain)[b]	n = 272, various histologies	8 Gy per 1 fraction	53%	26%	5%	5%	29%
		20 Gy per 5 fractions	61%	27%	11%	4%	24%
Prospective randomized multicenter trial on single-fraction radiotherapy versus multiple fractions[c]	n = 376, various histologies	8 Gy per 1 fraction	Equivalent	NR	NR	4%	15%
		30 Gy per 10 fractions	Equivalent	NR	NR	11%	4%
Randomized clinical trial with two palliative radiotherapy regimens in Spain[d]	n = 160, various histologies	8 Gy per 1 fraction	75%	15%	12%	NR	28%
		30 Gy per 10 fractions	86%	13%	18%	NR	2%

Simulation and verification films to document target localization recommended for all EBRT cases (*Chow E, Wu J, Hoskin P et al (2002) International consensus on palliative radiotherapy endpoints for future clinical trials in bone metastases. Radiother Oncol 64:275–280*)

[a] Source: *Hartsell W, Konski A, Scott C et al (2005) Randomized trial of short versus long-course radiotherapy for palliation of painful bone metastases. J Natl Cancer Inst 97:798–804*

[b] Source: *Roos D, Turner S, O'Brien P et al (2005) Randomized trial of 8 Gy in 1 versus 20 Gy in 5 fractions of radiotherapy for neuropathic pain due to bone metastases (Trans-Tasman Radiation Oncology Group, TROG 95.05). Radiother Oncol 75:54–63*

[c] Source: *Kaasa S, Brenne E, Lund J-A et al (2006) Prospective randomized multicentre trial on single fraction radiotherapy (8Gy × 1) versus multiple fractions (3 Gy × 10) in the treatment of painful bone metastases. Radiother Oncol 79:278–284*

[d] Source: *Foro P, Fontanals A, Galceran J et al (2008) Randomized clinical trial with two palliative radiotherapy regimens in painful bone metastases: 30 Gy in 10 fractions compared with 8 Gy in single fraction. Radiother Oncol 89:150–155*

Most authors recommend multiple fractions for primary treatment of a complicated BM for which there is no surgical option, or for postoperative treatment (20–40 Gy over 1–3 weeks). The goals of postoperative radiation therapy (PORT) are to decrease pain, promote bone healing, and minimize the risk of disease progression. PORT is generally initiated within 2–4 weeks of surgery.

Highly conformal therapies such as intensity-modulated RT, CyberKnife, tomotherapy, and extracranial stereotactic radiosurgery (SRS) are being investigated for certain clinical circumstances, such as retreatment of BM near the spinal cord. Prospective cohort and retrospective series suggest 95% local control with up to half reporting some degree of pain relief at follow-up. There are no RCTs on the role of SRS for BM or spinal cord compression (*Sahgal A, Larson DA, Chang EL (2008) Stereotactic body radiosurgery for spinal metastases: a critical review. Int J Radiat Oncol Biol Phys 71:652–665*).

Hemibody Irradiation

Retrospective and prospective phase I and II studies suggest that hemibody irradiation (HBI) provides pain relief in 70–80% of patients with multiple sites of painful metastases (Figure 1B.4). Studies also report decreased opioid use and need for localized external beam radiotherapy. Patients should be premedicated with intravenous fluid, antiemetics, corticosteroids, and analgesics in case of pain flare. Sequential treatment of both upper and lower HBI requires a 6-week gap for recovery of myelosuppression.

Radiation therapy techniques in various situations of BM are summarized in Table 1B.7.

Table 1B.7 Radiation therapy techniques for treating BM

Type	Description
Eligibility criteria	■ Osteoblastic metastasis shown by technetium-99 bone scan ■ Minimum Karnofsky Performance Status of 42.50 ■ Life expectancy >3 months ■ Platelets >100,000, white cell count >3,000, adequate creatinine clearance ■ Painful sites of disease on both sites of the diaphragm ■ At least a 12-week interval between sequential radionuclide injections
Regimens and dosage	■ Strontium-89: 148 mBq (4 mCi) by slow IV injection (over 1–2 min) accompanied by hydration of at least 500 ml ■ Samarium-153: 37 mBq/kg (1mCi/kg) by slow IV injection (1–2 min) accompanied by hydration of at least 500 ml
Outcome	■ Pain relief is expected in 60–80% of patients with breast or prostate cancer, with complete response rates of 5–20% ■ Response usually takes 2–3 weeks ■ Mean duration of pain relief is 3–6 months
Contraindications	■ Impending or established pathologic fracture ■ Spinal cord or nerve root compression ■ Hypercalcemia
Adverse effects	■ Flare reaction occurs in ~10% of patients (anecdotally, patients who experience flare may be more likely to respond) ■ Myelosuppression is usually grade 2 or less, self-limited, with recovery in 8–12 weeks ■ Radionuclides may preclude further systemic chemotherapy or eligibility for clinical trials of systemic therapy

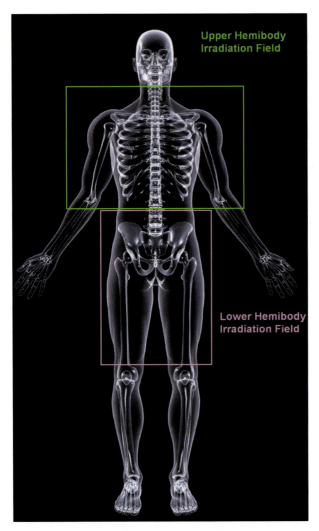

Figure 1B.4 Upper and lower hemibody irradiation fields. Adjoining field edges are located at the umbilicus and below the level of the spinal cord to minimize risk of myelopathy in the case of inadvertent overlap. Some would advocate that a patient cross the arms over the chest to treat the entirety of the upper extremities and to minimize lung dose. The upper field may be extended to cover the entire head or the lower field may be extended to cover the entire lower extremities if the clinical situation should so dictate. (Image copyright © 2000–2010 by Linda Bucklin at www.dreamstime.com)

Radionuclides

Radiopharmaceuticals are intravenously administered as inorganic soluble compounds whose uptake is greater where new reactive bone is being formed, as in the setting of osteoblastic metastases, and therefore mirrors the pattern of uptake seen on a technetium bone scan. Surrounding normal tissue is relatively spared, due to the very short range of the radioactive particles (*Finlay I, Mason M, Shelley M (2005) Radioisotopes for the palliation of metastatic bone cancer: a systematic review. Lancet Oncol 6:392–400*).

Impending Fracture and Risk Prediction

An impending fracture is defined as a bony metastasis that, if not addressed, has a significant likelihood of fracture under normal physiological loads. The most widely known scoring system predicts fracture risk, based on grading of the metastatic site, pain pattern, lesion size, and radiographic appearance. Those whose score indicates a significant risk should be considered for surgical stabilization, if prognosis and performance status justify that level of intervention (*Mirels H (1989) Metastatic disease in long bones. A proposed scoring system for diagnosing impending pathologic fractures. Clin Orthop Relat Res 249:256–264*).

Spinal Cord Compression

Main treatment modalities for impending or established SCC include surgery, followed by postoperative RT (PORT) or RT alone (Table 1B.8).

Table 1B.8 Treatment of impending or established spinal cord compression

Modality	Indication
Surgery	■ Tissue diagnosis required ■ Neurologic deterioration during or after maximal dose radiation therapy ■ Relatively radioresistant tumor ■ Rapid evolution of symptoms or acute onset paraplegia ■ Spinal instability (compression fracture/dislocation/retropulsed bone fragments) ■ Solitary site of compression
EBRT	■ Surgically unapproachable tumor ■ Surrounding bone inadequate to support implanted hardware ■ Medical contraindications to surgery or poor life expectancy ■ Lesions at multiple levels or below conus medullaris ■ Long duration of paraplegia
Chemotherapy	■ Chemosensitive tumors, especially with systemic disease (lymphoma, myeloma)

A prospective randomized trial evaluated patients with non-central nervous system (CNS), non-hematologic, and non-germ cell histology, which caused a single level of spinal cord compress above the conus manifested with at least one neurologic sign or symptom. Patients needed to have an expected OS of >3 months, be paraplegic for <48 h, and had to be surgical candidates. RT was 30 Gy in 10 fractions, either up front or within 14 days of surgery. Combined modality patients had significantly better ambulatory rates (84 versus 57%), retention of continence, maintenance of functional and motor scores, and lower median doses of steroids and analgesics. Nineteen percent of patients who received RT alone regained the ability to walk, versus 62% of paretic patients receiving surgery that was followed by PORT. Survival (126 versus 100 days), and 30-day morbidity were significantly better with initial surgery (*Patchell R, Tibbs P, Regine W et al (2005) Direct decompressive surgical resection in the treatment of spinal cord compression caused by metastatic cancer: a randomised trial. Lancet 366:643–648*).

EBRT for Spinal Cord Compression

RT may be employed in cases of impending spinal cord compression in which surgical intervention is either not indicated or is not feasible. Treatment may provide pain relief rates of 55–60%, maintain ambulatory rates of about 70%, and normal bladder function roughly 90% of the time. These patients generally have a median duration of motor response of 3.5 months and median survival of 4.0 months.

A total dose of 30 Gy in 10 daily fractions of 3 Gy is the most commonly prescribed regimen. The available literature does not provide enough data to suggest the optimal fractionation schedule, although one trial did suggest that a single 8-Gy fraction provided passable results to 16 Gy in 2 fractions (*Maranzano E, Trippa F, Casale M et al (2009) 8-Gy single-dose radiotherapy is effective in metastatic spinal cord compression: results of a phase III randomized multicentre Italian trial. Radiother Oncol 93:174–179*).

Re-irradiation

Re-irradiation is offered in clinical situations in which other modalities, such as surgery or chemotherapy, are either ineffective or not indicated. Many patient-, treatment-, and disease-related factors must be taken into account when considering re-irradiation, including dose, volume, and location of previous RT.

Modalities other than EBRT such as SRS or radiopharmaceuticals might be needed to minimize additional toxicity to surrounding normal tissue. The preferred modality and dose schedule for repeat EBRT for painful BM is unknown, but there is an ongoing international multicenter study looking at this facet. Available data suggest that re-irradiation provides pain relief for 66–70% of patients who previously received a single fraction, and for 33–57% of those who previously received a multifraction course.

It is suggested that 4–6 weeks is the required interval for maximum response after EBRT for BM. Thus, retreatment should be delayed for 6 weeks after the first course of RT to allow adequate assessment of response and resolving of pain flare (*Chow E (2006) A phase III international randomized trial comparing single with multiple fractions for re-irradiation of painful bone metastases: National Cancer Institute of Canada Clinical Trials Group (NCIC CTG) SC 20. Clin Oncol 18:125–128*).

Follow-Up

The follow-up schedule recommended by the International Bone Metastases Consensus Working Party and suggested workups are detailed in Table 1B.9. Determination of response is clinical, thus biochemical or imaging studies are not routinely required in follow-up.

Table 1B.9 Follow-up schedule and examinations recommended by the International Bone Metastases Consensus Working Party

Schedule	Frequency
First follow-up	▪ 2 Weeks after treatment
Months 0–6	▪ Monthly
Months 6+	▪ Every 3–6 months (for long-term survivors)
Examinations	
History and physical	▪ Complete history and physical examination including ▪ Pain score and analgesic use ▪ Recent change in systemic therapy and treatment related toxicities ▪ Skeletal-related events and requirement for surgical intervention
Laboratory/ imaging studies	▪ Usually not required unless clinically indicated

Source: Chow E, Wu J, Hoskin P et al (2002) International consensus on palliative radiotherapy endpoints for future clinical trials in bone metastases. Radiother Oncol 64:275–280

Acute side effects of radiotherapy for BM are generally mild, site-specific, self-limiting, and responsive to therapeutic interventions. Their severity depends on treatment site, volume, and dose. Large treatment fields should be used with caution in patients with severe fatigue or bone marrow dysfunction. Pain flare is a self-limited worsening of pain at the index site within a week of commencing treatment. Its incidence varies from 10 to 44% after EBRT and lasts for a median of 3 days. Some studies have suggested a slight increase in pathologic fracture risk immediately after completion of radiotherapy, while others have shown that re-ossification does occur in an increased fashion in the months after EBRT.

Although the possibility of late side effects should be considered in patients treated for BM, median lifespan is often too short for those risks to manifest (*Chow E, Ling A, Davis L et al (2005) Pain flare following external beam radiotherapy and meaningful change in pain scores in the treatment of bone metastases. Radiother Oncol 75:64–69*).

Section II
Head and Neck Cancers

2

Nasopharyngeal Carcinoma

Jiade J. Lu[1], Lin Kong[2] and Nancy Lee[3]

Key Points

- Nasopharyngeal carcinoma (NPC) is a relatively rare malignancy in Western countries, but it is the most commonly diagnosed head and neck cancer in Southeast Asia.

- Early-stage NPC usually has no specific symptoms. Common signs and symptoms in advanced disease include cervical lymphadenopathy, nasal blockage, a nasal twang, and symptoms associated with distant metastasis such as bone pain.

- Accuracy of clinical diagnosis is based on history and physical examination, laboratory, and imaging studies. Tissue from either primary or cervical lymphadenopathies can be used for pathologic diagnosis.

- Stage at diagnosis is the most important prognostic factor. Long-term overall survival (OS) of patients with stages I–II disease exceeds 80% after conventional radiation, and those of stage III–IVB diseases ~60% after combined chemoradiation therapy. However, cure is unlikely once distant metastasis occurs.

- Commonly observed metastatic sites include lung, bone, and liver. Although direct intracranial extension is common in the late stages, hematogenous metastasis to the brain or other organs/tissues is uncommon.

- Treatment of NPC depends on the stage of the disease. Radiation therapy is the only curative treatment modality. Radiation alone for stages I and II NPC, and combined chemoradiotherapy for stages IIB–IVB diseases is the current standard.

- As compared with conventional radiation therapy, intensity-modulated radiation therapy (IMRT) significantly improves therapeutic ratio and is the standard treatment technique for NPC currently.

- Three-year overall survival, disease-free survival, and local control rates after IMRT or chemo-IMRT approximate 90, 85, and 95%, respectively, for non-metastatic NPC. Treatment-induced grades III or IV adverse effects are rare after IMRT.

- Surgery is the mainstay treatment for recurrence in the neck, and local recurrent foci can be treated with nasopharyngectomy (selected cases) or irradiation.

- Chemotherapy combined with palliative radiation therapy is the mainstay treatment for metastatic or recurrent NPC not suitable for definitive treatment.

[1] Jiade J. Lu, MD, MBA (✉)
Email: mdcljj@nus.edu.sg

[2] Lin Kong, MD
Email: konglinj@gmail.com

[3] Nancy Lee, MD
Email: leen2@mskcc.org

J. J. Lu, L. W. Brady (Eds.), *Decision Making in Radiation Oncology*
DOI: 10.1007/978-3-642-13832-4_3, © Springer-Verlag Berlin Heidelberg 2010

Epidemiology and Etiology

Epidemiology statistics and etiologic factors are presented in Table 2.1. Screening in high-risk people, such as siblings of confirmed nasopharyngeal cancer (NPC) patients, by using physical examination, imaging, or laboratory tests (including nasopharyngoscopy, Epstein-Barr virus [EBV] immunoglobulin [Ig]A titer or DNA, computed tomography [CT], etc.) may facilitate early detection, especially in endemic areas. No effective chemoprevention agent has been confirmed for clinical use.

Table 2.1 Statistics and risk factors of NPC

Type	Description
Statistics	Incidence of NPC varies widely worldwide: 20–50/100,000 per year in southern China, 0.2–0.5/100,000 in North America and other Western countries, 10–15/100,000 in Southeast Asia, Arctic Native People, and northern Africa/Middle East. ~40% of newly diagnosed NPC patients are Chinese
	Age of diagnosis shows a bimodal distribution that peaks at 50–60 years of age, with a small peak among adolescents in the low- to medium-incidence area
	The male:female ratio of NPC is 2–3:1
Etiologic factors	Positive Epstein-Barr (EBV) serology rate is higher with nonkeratinizing or poorly differentiated NPC, versus keratinizing SCC
	Incidence in 1st-degree relatives is 4- to 10-fold that of the control population
	High consumption of salted fish and pickled food was suggested as a risk factor in southern China and Hong Kong
	Industrial chemicals such as formaldehyde and wood dust, trace elements (e.g., nickel), and some Chinese herbs
	The association between smoking and alcohol consumption and NPC is controversial; smoking may increases NPC by 2- to 6-fold

Anatomy

The nasopharynx is a roughly cuboidal structure and is located below the central skull base. Its anterior border is the posterior nasal apertures and septum. Its roof abuts the basisphenoid (sphenoid sinus floor) and slopes posteroinferiorly along the clivus/basiocciput to the upper cervical vertebrae.

The soft palate separates the nasopharynx from the oropharynx inferiorly. The medial pterygoid plate, palatal muscle, torus tubarius, and pharyngeal fossa (i.e., fossa of Rosenmüller) form the lateral wall of nasophaynx (Figure 2.1).

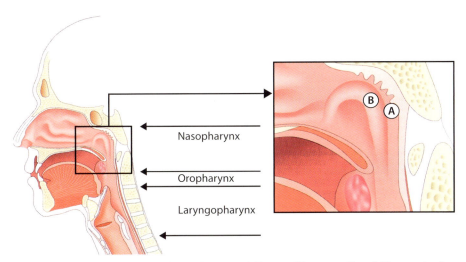

Figure 2.1 The lateral wall of nasopharynx. *A* Fossa of Rosenmüller. *B* Torus tubarius

The parapharyngeal space is located anterior to the styloid process, which extends from the skull base to the level of the angle of the mandible. It lies lateral to the nasopharynx, separating it from the masticator space (Figure 2.2). It contains the deep lobe of the parotid gland, small branches of the mandibular division of CN V, and vascular structures. Between the nasopharyngeal mucosal space and the prevertebral muscles is the retropharyngeal space, within which are the medial and lateral retropharyngeal nodes. The carotid space is located posterior to the parapharyngeal space and forms the posterolateral border of the nasopharynx.

Cervical Lymph Nodes

The classification of the neck lymph nodes (the Robbins Classification) is illustrated in Figure 2.3. Neck nodes of various levels delineated on computed tomography (CT) slides, as well as the consensus guidelines for radiological boundaries of them, are detailed in Figure 2.4 and Table 2.2.

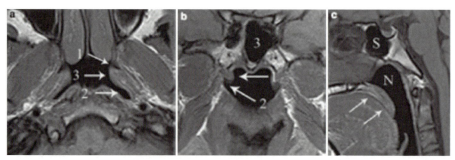

Figure 2.2a–c Normal anatomy of the nasopharynx. **a** Axial T_1-weighted magnetic resonance imaging (MRI) reveals the left Eustachian tube opening (*arrow 1*), fossa of Rosenmüller (*arrow 2*), and torus tubarius (*arrow 3*). **b** Coronal T_1-weighted MRI demonstrates the right torus tubarius (*arrow 1*), Eustachian tube opening (*arrow 2*), and sphenoid sinus (*3*). **c** Sagittal T_1-weighted MRI delineates the nasopharynx (*N*), sphenoid sinus (*S*), and soft palate (*arrows*). (*Adapted from Chong VF, Ong CK. Nasopharyngeal carcinoma. Eur J Radiol 2008; 66:437–447. Used with permission from Elsevier*)

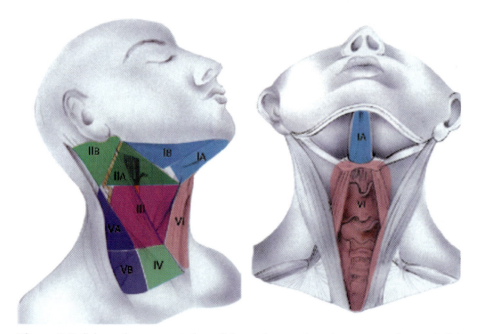

Figure 2.3 Schematic representation of the various neck node groups: submental (*Ia*) and submandibular (*Ib*), upper jugular (*II*), mid jugular (*III*), lower jugular (*IV*), posterior triangle (*V*), and anterior compartments (*VI*)

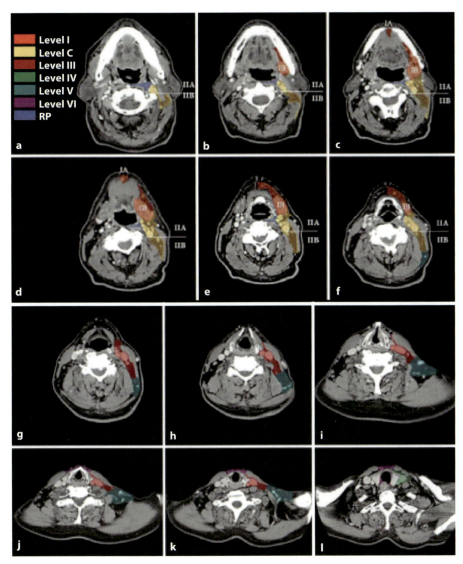

Figure 2.4a–l CTV of neck nodes of various levels delineated on the image of a laryngeal cancer patient with T1N0M0 disease

Table 2.2 Consensus guidelines for the radiological boundaries of the neck node levels

Level	Anatomical boundaries					
	Cranial	Caudal	Anterior	Posterior	Lateral	Medial
Ia	Geniohyoid muscle, plane tangent to basilar edge of mandible	Plane tangent to body of hyoid bone	Symphysis menti, platysma muscle	Body of hyoid bone	Medial edge of anterior belly of digastric muscle	NA[a]
Ib	Mylohyoid muscle, cranial edge of submandibular gland	Plane through central part of hyoid bone	Symphysis menti, platysma muscle		Posterior edge of submandibular gland	Basilar edge/inner side of mandible, platysma muscle, skin
IIa	Caudal edge of lateral process of C1	Caudal edge of body of hyoid bone	Posterior edge of submandibular glands, anterior edge of internal carotid artery; posterior edge of posterior belly of digastric muscle	Posterior border of internal jugular vein	Medial edge of sternocleidomastoid muscle	Medial edge of internal carotid artery, paraspinal (levator scapulae muscle)
IIb	Caudal edge of internal process of C1	Caudal edge of body of hyoid bone	Posterior border of internal jugular vein	Posterior border of sternocleidomastoid muscle	Medial edge of sternocleidomastoid muscle	Medial edge of internal carotid artery, paraspinal (levator scapulae muscle)

IV	Caudal edge of cricoid cartilage	2 cm cranial to sternoclavicular joint	Anteromedial edge of sternocleidomastoid muscle	Posterior edge of sternocleidomastoid muscle	Medial edge of sternocleidomastoid muscle	Internal edge of carotid artery, paraspinal (scalenus) muscle
V	Cranial edge of body of hyoid bone	CT slice encompassing transverse cervical vessels[b]	Posterior edge of sternocleidomastoid muscle	Anterolateral border of trapezius muscle	Platysma muscle, skin	Paraspinal (levator scapulae, splenius capitis) muscle
VI	Caudal edge of body of thyroid cartilage[c]	Sternal manubrium	Skin, platysma muscle	Separation between trachea and esophagus[d]	Medial edges of thyroid gland, skin, and anteromedial edge of sternocleidomastoid	NA
Retropharyngeal	Base of skull	Cranial edge of body of hyoid bone	Fascia under pharyngeal mucosa	Prevertebral muscles (longus colli, longus capitis	Medial edge of internal carotid artery	Midline

[a] Midline structure lying between the medial borders of the anterior bellies of the digastric muscles

[b] For NPC, the reader is now referred to the original description of the American Joint Committee on Cancer (AJCC)/International Union Against Cancer (UICC) 1997 edition of Ho's triangle. In essence, the fatty planes below and around clavicle down to the trapezius muscle

[c] For paratracheal and recurrent nodes, the cranial border is the caudal edge of the cricoid cartilage

[d] For pretracheal nodes, trachea and anterior edge of cricoid cartilage

Source: Grégoire V, Levendag Ang KK et al (2003) P, Ang CT-based delineation of lymph node levels and related CTVs in the node-negative neck: DAHANCA, EORTC, GORTEC, NCIC, RTOG consensus guidelines. Radiother Oncol 69:227–236

Pathology

Malignant neoplasms of the nasopharynx usually arise from the epithelium of the postnasal space. According to the World Health Organization (WHO) classification of NPC, common pathologic types include:
- Keratinizing squamous cell carcinoma: formerly known as WHO type I (squamous cell carcinoma)
- Nonkeratinizing carcinoma, differentiated: formerly known as WHO type II (transitional cell carcinoma)
- Nonkeratinizing carcinoma, undifferentiated: formerly known as WHO type III (lymphoepithelial carcinoma)
- Basaloid squamous cell carcinoma

Nonkeratinizing carcinoma is the most common type of NPC, accounting for ~95% in endemic areas.

Routes of Spread

Local extension, regional (lymphatic), and distant (hematogenous) metastases are the three major routes of spread in NPC (Figure 2.5; Table 2.3).

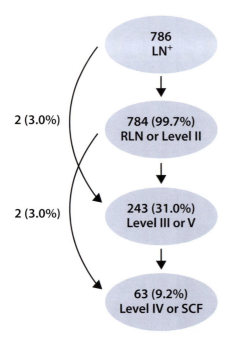

Figure 2.5 The distribution of lymph node metastases and the orderly pattern of spread. *LN*+ positive lymph nodes, *RLN* retropharyngeal lymph nodes, *SCF* supraclavicular fossa

Source: Tang L, Mao Y, Liu L et al (2009) The volume to be irradiated during selective neck irradiation in nasopharyngeal carcinoma: analysis of the spread patterns in lymph nodes by magnetic resonance imaging. Cancer 115:680–688

Table 2.3 Routes of spread in NPC

Type	Description
Local extension	■ Most NPC originate in the lateral pharyngeal recess. The tumors tend to spread submucosally, with early infiltration of the deeper neck spaces ■ **Anteriorly,** NPC often extends into the nasal cavity, and subsequently through the sphenopalatine foramen into the pterygopalatine fossa ■ **Posteriorly,** NPC may infiltrate the retropharyngeal space and the prevertebral muscle of the perivertebral space. In advanced disease, the vertebrae are destroyed, with tumor extension into the spinal cord ■ **Superiorly,** by erosion of the base of skull, sphenoid sinus, and the clivus; or, via the foramen lacerum (located immediately above the fossa of Rosenmüller) into cavernous sinus and the middle cranial fossa; or, via the foramen ovale into the middle cranial fossa, the petrous temporal bone, and the cavernous sinus ■ **Laterally,** extension into the parapharyngeal space through the sinus of Morgagni, leading to invasion of the levator and tensor veli palatini muscles. The medial and lateral pterygoid muscle involvement causes trismus. Extension of tumor in lateral retropharyngeal node may involve carotid space and CN IX–XII ■ **Inferiorly,** NPC may spread along the submucosal plane to the oropharynx; direct involvement of soft palate is uncommon
Regional lymph node metastasis	■ Lymph node involvement is seen in ~90% of cases at diagnosis; ~50% have bilateral neck node spread ■ Level II and retropharyngeal nodes (lateral groups) are considered the first-echelon nodal groups ■ Follows an orderly fashion in the craniocaudal direction and "skip metastasis" in cervical lymph nodes is rare (Figure 2.5) ■ Contralateral cervical nodal metastasis alone is uncommon ■ Mediastinal node spread may occur in patients with supraclavicular adenopathy
Distant metastasis	■ 1–5% of patients present with distant metastasis (DM) at diagnosis; but 20–50% present during the course of the disease ■ Hematogenous metastases usually occur after cervical lymph node (especially lower neck nodes) metastases ■ The most common site of DM is bone, specifically the thoracolumbar spine. Other common regions of DM include lung, liver, superior mediastinal, and hilar lymph nodes ■ Hematogenous spread to spine, lungs, and liver may occur in patients with N0 NPC when disease invades the basal venous sinus

Diagnosis, Staging, and Prognosis

Clinical Presentation

The presenting symptoms and signs of localized NPC can be classified according to the involved regions and structures. Rarely, NPC may present with a paraneoplastic syndrome (Table 2.4). Patients with metastatic disease at diagnosis may also present with symptoms (e.g., bone pain) at metastatic foci.

Table 2.4 Commonly observed signs and symptoms in NPC

Stage	Description
General	■ Cervical mass (usually painless with concurrent inflammatory or infectious process) is the most common presenting symptom ■ ~43% of patients present with unilateral or bilateral cervical mass on examination ■ ~30% patients present with blood-stained nasal discharge, uni- or bilateral nasal obstruction (which may induce a nasal twang), or posterior nasal discharge ■ Unilateral hearing loss is usually caused by middle ear effusion due to blockage of the Eustachian tube; ~a third of NPC patients present with unilateral tinnitus ■ Headache in NPC is usually unilateral and temporoparietal in location, and usually indicates skull base involvement with disease ■ Trismus can occur when pterygoid muscles are involved
Neurological symptoms	■ Usually indicates advanced disease, and CN V and VI are the most commonly involved cranial nerves. Diplopia on lateral gaze is a manifestation of CN VI involvement ■ **Petrosphenoidal syndrome of Jacod** (unilateral trigeminal type neuralgia, unilateral ptosis, complete ophthalmoplegia, and amaurosis) results from CN II–VI by direct intracranial extension of NPC ■ **Villaret's syndrome** (difficulty in swallowing; perversion of taste; problem in salivation; paralysis and atrophy of the trapezius and SCM muscle; unilateral weakness and atrophy of the soft palate or tongue; and hyperesthesia, hypoesthesia, or anesthesia of the mucous membranes of the soft palate, pharynx, and larynx) results from CN IX–XII cervical sympathetic nerve involvement by retropharyngeal lymph node metastasis in the retroparotid space ■ **Horner's syndrome** usually presents in conjunction with deficits of CN IX–XII when cervical sympathetic nerves are also involved

Table 2.4 *(continued)*

Stage	Description
Paraneoplastic syndrome	■ Dermatomyositis may present as the initial manifestation (~1% of cases) ■ The skin lesions consist of distinctive hyperkeratotic, follicular, erythematous papules; the first lesion usually appears on the face and eyelids and they eventually involve the neck, shoulders, and upper extremities ■ Muscular weakness usually follows skin manifestation

Diagnosis and Staging

Figure 2.6 illustrates the diagnostic algorithm for NPC, including suggested examination and tests.

Tumor, Node, and Metastasis Staging

Diagnosis and clinical staging of NPC depends on findings from history and physical examination, imaging, and laboratory tests. The 7th edition of the tumor, node, and metastasis (TNM) staging system of American Joint Committee on Cancer (AJCC) is presented in Tables 2.5 and 2.6.

Table 2.5 AJCC TNM classification of carcinoma of the nasopharynx

Stage	Description
Primary tumor (T)	
TX	Primary tumor cannot be assessed
T0	No evidence of primary tumor
Tis	Carcinoma in situ
T1	Tumor confined to the nasopharynx, or tumor extends to oropharynx and/or nasal cavity without parapharyngeal extension (i.e., posterolateral infiltration of tumor)
T2	Tumor with parapharyngeal extension (i.e., posterolateral infiltration of tumor)
T3	Tumor involves bony structures of skull base and/or paranasal sinuses
T4	Tumor with intracranial extension and/or involvement of cranial nerves, hypopharynx, orbit, or with extension to the infratemporal fossa/masticator space ▶

Table 2.5 *(continued)*

Stage	Description
Regional lymph nodes (N)	
NX	Regional lymph nodes cannot be assessed
N0	No regional lymph node metastasis
N1	Unilateral (including ipsilateral) metastasis in cervical lymph node(s), ≤6 cm in greatest dimension, above the supraclavicular fossa, and/or unilateral or bilateral, retropharyngeal lymph nodes, ≤6 cm in greatest dimension
N2	Bilateral metastasis in cervical lymph node(s), ≤6 cm in greatest dimension, above the supraclavicular fossa
N3a	Metastasis in a lymph node(s) >6 cm in dimension
N3b	Metastasis in a lymph node(s) to the supraclavicular fossa
Distant metastasis (M)	
M0	No distant metastasis
M1	Distant metastasis (including seeding of the peritoneum and positive peritoneal cytology)

Source: Edge SB, Byrd DR, Compton CC et al (2009) American Joint Committee on Cancer, American Cancer Society. AJCC cancer staging manual, 7th edn. Springer, Berlin Heidelberg New York

Table 2.6 Stage grouping of carcinoma of the nasopharynx

Stage Grouping				
	T1	T2	T3	T4
N0	I	II	III	IVA
N1	II	II	III	IVA
N2	III	III	III	IVA
N3	IVB	IVB	IVB	IVB
M1	IVC	IVC	IVC	IVC

Source: Edge SB, Byrd DR, Compton CC et al (2009) American Joint Committee on Cancer, American Cancer Society. AJCC cancer staging manual, 7th edn. Springer, Berlin Heidelberg New York

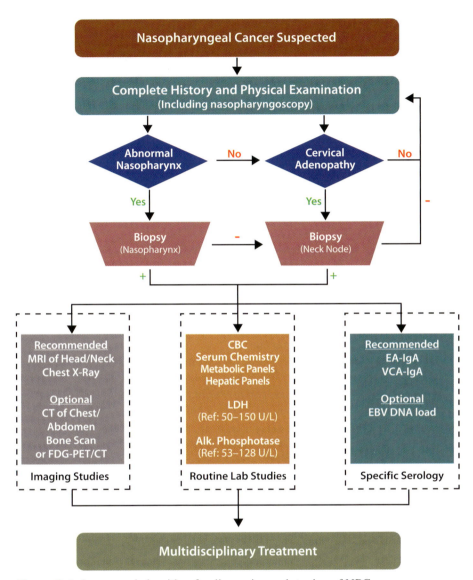

Figure 2.6 A proposed algorithm for diagnosing and staging of NPC

Prognostic Factors

Significant prognostic factors of NPC are detailed in Table 2.7.

Table 2.7 Prognostic factors for NPC

Stage	Description
Disease related	■ **Stage** at diagnosis is the most important prognostic factor: T-category → local control; N-category → neck and distant control
	■ **Tumor volume** at the primary and of neck lymph adenopathy is of prognostic significance
	■ **Squamous cell carcinoma (SCC) pathology** is a poor prognostic factor
	■ **Plasma Epstein-Barr virus (EBV) DNA** (less than versus equal to or greater than 1500 copies/ml) is a significant predictive factor for overall survival (OS) and relapse-free survival (RFS)
	■ **Anti-EBV antibodies** (early antigen [EA]-immunoglobulin [Ig] A, EA-IgG, [viral capsid antigen] VCA-IgG) at diagnosis are **not** prognostically important
Patient related	■ **Age:** younger age
	■ **Gender** and **ethnic background** (for the same pathology) are not prognostically significant
	■ **Performance status, weight loss,** and **anemia** before treatment are not significant in patients treated definitively
Diagnostic or treatment related	■ **Treatment delay** of more than 8 weeks after diagnosis or extended break during radiation therapy (RT) may adversely affect outcome
	■ **Treatment strategy/techniques** (use of chemoradiation and intensity-modulated RT [IMRT]) improves overall treatment outcome as compared with conventional therapy
	■ **Extent of tumor regression** during RT is not prognostically significant

Source: Lin J-C (2009) Prognostic factors in nasopharyngeal cancer. In: Lu JJ, Cooper JS, Lee AW (eds) Nasopharyngeal cancer: multidisciplinary management. Springer, Berlin Heidelberg New York

Treatment

Principles and Practice

Treatment modalities utilized in the treatment of NPC are detailed in Table 2.8. A proposed treatment algorithm based on the best available clinical evidence is presented in Figure 2.7.

Definitive Radiation Therapy with IMRT for Non-metastatic NPC

Radiation therapy alone is the mainstay curative treatment modality for stages I and II NPC. Chemotherapy is not usually indicated. Treatment technique and dose of radiation for early and locoregionally advanced NPC are identical using intensity-modulated radiation therapy (IMRT).

Table 2.8 Treatment modalities for NPC

Stage	Description
Radiation Therapy	
Indications	■ Definitive treatment for non-metastatic NPC ■ Palliative treatment to primary or metastatic foci
Techniques	■ IMRT is the preferred external-beam radiation (EBRT) technique ■ Intracavitary brachytherapy or stereotactic radiosurgery has been used as a boost for residual disease; however, its value in combination with IMRT is unknown ■ Interstitial brachytherapy can be used for local recurrence in selected cases
Chemotherapy	
Indications	■ Concurrent treatment with RT for locoregionally advanced disease ■ Neoadjuvant chemotherapy may further improve outcome, especially local control for advanced T disease ■ The efficacy of adjuvant chemotherapy is unknown ■ Mainstay treatment for metastatic NPC
Medications	■ Cisplatin is the most commonly used cytotoxic agent ■ Cisplatin plus 5-FU has been used as adjuvant regimen ■ The optimal second-line regimen is unknown ■ Gemcitabine, paclitaxel, and cetuximab are being studied
Surgery	
Indications	■ Surgery has limited role in the definitive treatment of NPC ■ Biopsy at the primary or neck adenopathy for diagnosis ■ Neck dissection plays an important role in patients with regional recurrence ■ Nasopharyngectomy can be used in selected patients with limited recurrence in the nasopharynx

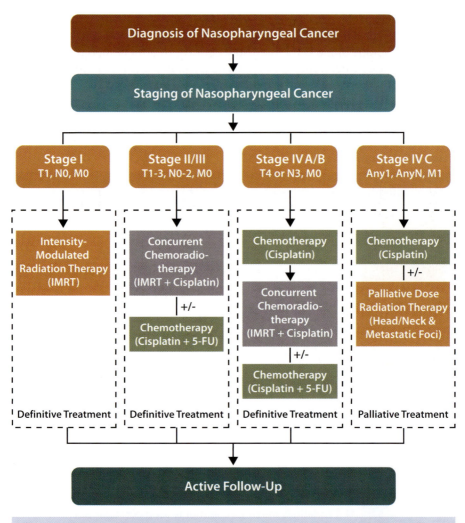

Figure 2.7 A proposed treatment algorithm for nasopharyngeal cancer

Treatment of Locoregionally Advanced Disease (T3, T4, or N⁺)

The efficacy of concurrent chemoradiation therapy has been repeatedly demonstrated in meta-analyses (Table 2.9) and randomized trials (Table 2.10), and is the mainstay treatment strategy for locoregionally advanced NPC. Proposed treatment strategy for locoregionally advanced NPC using IMRT is illustrated in Figure 2.8.

Table 2.9 Clinical evidence for the treatment of locoregionally advanced NPC: meta-analyses

Meta-analysis	Description
Baujat et al	■ Analyzed 1,753 cases of locally advanced NPC in 8 randomized trials to study the efficacy of chemotherapy used with definitive radiation therapy ■ The pooled hazard ratio (HR) of death was 0.82 (95% confidence interval [CI], 0.71–0.94, $p = 0.006$), corresponding to an absolute survival benefit of 6% at 5 years from the use of chemotherapy ■ The pooled HR of tumor failure or death was 0.76 (95% CI, 0.67–0.86, $p < 0.0001$), corresponding to an absolute event-free survival benefit of 10% at 5 years ■ Concurrent chemotherapy provided highest benefit, while no significant benefit in survival was observed by adjuvant chemotherapy

Source: Baujat B, Audry H, Bourhis J et al (2006) Chemotherapy in locally advanced NPC: an individual patient data meta-analysis of eight randomized trials and 1,753 patients. Int J Radiat Oncol Biol Phys 64:47–56

Table 2.10 Clinical evidence for the treatment of locoregionally advanced NPC: randomized trials

Trial	Description
INT 0099 (a.k.a. RTOG 8817)[a]	■ Randomized 147 cases of stage III–IV (1988 AJCC system) NPC to compare RT versus concurrent chemoradiation therapy (CRT) followed by adjuvant chemotherapy ■ RT in 2 arms used identical regimens of 70 Gy in 2 Gy per daily fraction ■ CRT used 3 cycles of cisplatin (100 mg/m² bolus, day 1, weeks 1, 4, and 7); adjuvant chemotherapy used 3 cycles of cisplatin (80 mg/m² bolus, day 1, weeks 11, 15, and 19) plus 5-FU (1 g/m²/24 h infusion, days 1–4, weeks 11, 15, and 19) ■ 3-Year OS (78 versus 47%) and progression-free survival ([PFS] 69 versus 24%) favored CRT arms over RT alone ■ Local control improved with CRT over RT (not reported) ▶

Table 2.10 *(continued)*

Trial	Description
Wee et al (Singapore)[b]	■ Randomized 221 cases of stages II (N[+]), III, and IV (1997 AJCC system) NPC to compare RT (70 Gy in 7 weeks by using conventional RT) versus CRT followed by adjuvant chemotherapy (same RT regimen) ■ CRT used 3 cycles of cisplatin (25 mg/m^2/day, days 1–4 or 30/30/40 mg/m^2/day, days 1–3, weeks 1, 4, 7); adjuvant chemotherapy used 3 cycles of cisplatin (20 mg/m^2/day, days 1–4, weeks 10, 14, and 18) plus 5-FU (1 g/m^2/24 h infusion, days 1–4, weeks 10, 14, and 18) ■ 5-Year OS (80 versus 65%, $p = 0.006$) and disease-free survival ([DFS] 72 versus 53%, $p = 0.02$) favored CRT arms over RT alone
Lin et al (Taiwan)[c]	■ Randomized 284 cases of stages III–IV (1988 AJCC system) NPC to compare RT versus CRT, followed by adjuvant chemotherapy ■ RT in 2 arms used similar regimens of 70–74 Gy in 2 Gy per daily fraction ■ CRT used 2 cycles of cisplatin (20 mg/m^2/day) plus 5-FU (400 mg/m^2/96 h infusion) during weeks 1 and 5 of RT ■ 5-Year OS (72.3 versus 54.2%, $p = 0.0022$), PFS (71.6 versus 53%, $p = 0.0012$), and local control (96.8 versus 92.1%) favored CRT arms over RT alone
Chan et al (Hong Kong)[d]	■ Randomized 350 NPC cases of Ho stages N2–3 or any node ≥4 cm to compare RT (66 Gy followed by a parapharyngeal boost in ~70% of patients) versus CRT (same RT regimen) ■ CRT arm used cisplatin (40 mg/m^2 weekly) ■ 5-Year OS (70.3 versus 58.6%, $p = 0.049$) favored CRT arms over RT alone ■ Subgroup analysis revealed no difference in OS between arms for T1–T2 disease ($p = 0.74$), but a difference between T3–T4 disease ($p = 0.013$) favoring CRT over RT alone
Zhang et al (Guangzhou)[e]	■ Randomized 115 cases of stage III–IV (1997 AJCC system) NPC to compare RT versus CRT ■ RT in both arms used 70–74 Gy with an optional boost of 10 Gy in selected patients ■ CRT used 6 doses of oxaliplatin (70 mg/m^2 weekly) from the 1st day of RT ■ 2-Year OS (100 versus 77%, $p = 0.01$), relapse-free survival ([RFS] 96 versus 83%, $p = 0.02$) and distant metastasis-free survival ([DMFS] 92 versus 80%, $p = 0.02$) favored CRT arms over RT alone ■ No grade 4 toxicity; grade 3 toxicity occurred in 39% CRT-treated patients

Table 2.10 *(continued)*

Trial	Description
Kwong et al (Hong Kong)[f]	■ Randomized 222 cases of T3 or N2–3 or N1 with node >4 cm (Ho staging system) NPC in 2 × 2 setting to compare (1) RT versus CRT and (2) with or without adjuvant chemotherapy ■ RT in both arms used same regimen: >68 Gy, and selected patients received 10-Gy boost ■ CRT used 5-FU prodrug uracil and tegafur in a 4:1 ratio (UFT) 200 mg TID, 7 days/week during RT; adjuvant chemotherapy alternating cisplatin plus 5-FU and vincristine, bleomycin, and methotrexate (VBM) every 3 weeks × 6 cycles ■ 7-Year DFS (66.6 versus 52.4%, $p = 0.016$), DMFS (82.9 versus 68.6%) ($p = 0.014$), and DFS (78.6 versus 68.9%, $p = 0.057$) favored CRT arms over RT alone ■ Local control was not improved by chemotherapy ■ No parameters were improved by adjuvant chemotherapy
Lee et al (Hong Kong)[g]	■ Randomized 348 cases of AJCC (1997) T1–4N2–3M0, World Health Organization (WHO) type 2 and 3 NPC to compare RT versus CRT followed by adjuvant chemotherapy (same RT regimen) ■ CRT used cisplatin 100 mg/m2 on days 1, 22, and 43, followed by cisplatin 80 mg/m2 and 5-FU 1,000 mg/m2/d for 96 h beginning on days 71, 99, and 127 ■ 3-Year failure-free survival ([FFS] 72 versus 62%, $p = 0.027$) as a result of improved locoregional control (92 versus 82%, $p = 0.005$) favored CRT ■ No significant difference in distant metastases ([DM] 76 versus 73%) and OS (78% in both arms) were observed

[a] *Source: Al-Sarraf M, LeBlanc M, Shanker Giri et al (1998) Chemo-radiotherapy versus radiotherapy in patients with advanced NPC. Phase III randomized intergroup study 0099. J Clin Oncol 16:1310–1317*
[b] *Source: Wee J, Tan EH, Tai BC et al (2005) Randomized trial of radiotherapy versus concurrent chemoradiotherapy followed by adjuvant chemotherapy in patients with AJCC/UICC stage III and IV NPC of the endemic variety. J Clin Oncol 23:6730–6738*
[c] *Source: Lin JC, Jan JS, Hsu CY et al (2003) Phase III study of concurrent chemoradiotherapy versus radiotherapy alone for advanced NPC: positive effect on overall and progression-free survival. J Clin Oncol 21:631–637*
[d] *Source: Chan AT, Leung SF, Ngan RK et al (2005) Overall survival after concurrent cisplatin-radiotherapy compared with radiotherapy alone in locoregionally advanced NPC. J Natl Cancer Inst 97:536–539*
[e] *Source: Zhang L, Zhao C, Peng PJ et al (2005) Phase III study comparing standard radiotherapy with or without weekly oxaliplatin in treatment of locoregionally advanced NPC: preliminary results. J Clin Oncol 23:8461–8648*
[f] *Source: Kwong DL, Sham JS, Au GK et al (2008) Long-term results of concurrent and adjuvant chemotherapy for advanced NPC. J Clin Oncol 26:Abstract 6056*
[g] *Source: Lee AW, Lau WH, Tung SY et al (2005) Preliminary results of a randomized study on therapeutic gain by concurrent chemotherapy for regionally-advanced NPC: NPC-9901 Trial by the Hong Kong NPC Study Group. J Clin Oncol 23:6966–6975*

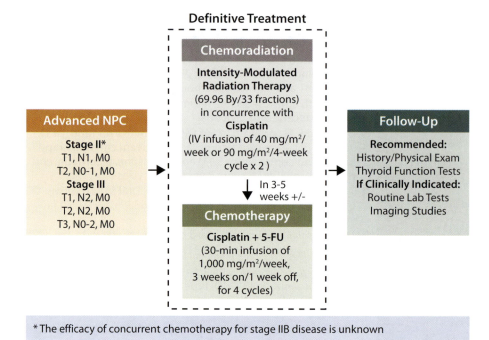

Definitive Treatment

Figure 2.8 Proposed treatment algorithm for stage IIB and III nasopharyngeal carcinoma using IMRT

Neoadjuvant Chemotherapy

The efficacy of neoadjuvant chemotherapy alone prior to radiation therapy has not been demonstrated to improve overall survival (Table 2.11). However, neoadjuvant chemotherapy followed by concurrent chemoradiation therapy can be used in patients with stage III or stage IV disease (Figure 2.9). Neoadjuvant chemotherapy is reasonable for reducing tumor bulk of disease with extensive intracranial extension or bulky cervical adenopathy prior to concurrent chemoradiation therapy.

Table 2.11 Neoadjuvant chemotherapy and radiation for locally advanced NPC: randomized trials

Trial	Description
International NPC study[a]	■ Randomized trial compared RT (conventional) versus neoadjuvant chemotherapy plus RT ■ Randomized 339 cases of regionally advanced NPC (N ≥ 2 by 1987 UICC staging) to RT (70 Gy in 7 weeks by using conventional RT) alone or 3 cycles of chemotherapy with bleomycin/epirubicin/cisplatin plus RT with same regimen ■ 2-Year DFS (54 versus 40%), favored neoadjuvant chemotherapy group ($p < 0.01$) ■ No significant difference in OS was observed

Table 2.11 *(continued)*

Trial	Description
Ma et al (China)[b]	■ Randomized 456 cases of locoregionally advanced NPC to RT alone (70 Gy in 7 weeks by using conventional RT), or 2–3 cycles of cisplatin plus bleomycin plus 5-FU chemotherapy plus RT with same regimen ■ 5-Year OS (63 versus 56%, $p = 0.11$) and distant control (79 versus 75%, $p = 0.40$) rates were not significantly different ■ 5-Year RFS (49 versus 59%, $p = 0.05$) and local control (82 versus 74%) rates favored neoadjuvant chemotherapy group ($p = 0.04$)
AOCOA (Hong Kong, China)[c]	■ Randomized trial compared RT (conventional) versus neoadjuvant chemotherapy plus RT ■ Randomized 334 cases of locoregionally advanced NPC (T3, N ≥ 2, or ≥3 cm by Ho staging) to RT (70 Gy in 7 weeks by using conventional RT) alone or 3 cycles of chemotherapy with epirubicin/cisplatin plus RT with same regimen ■ 3-Year DFS (48 versus 42%,) and OS (78 versus 71%); both demonstrated no significant difference between the groups
Hui et al (Hong Kong)[d]	■ Randomized phase II trial for efficacy of neoadjuvant docetaxel and cisplatin for stage III–IVB NPC ■ 34 versus 31 patients were treated with or without 2 cycles of cisplatin (75 mg/m^2) plus docetaxel (75 mg/m^2) every 3 weeks with neoadjuvant CRT ■ Identical CRT in both arms: chemotherapy used weekly cisplatin (40 mg/m^2) ■ 3-Year OS (94.1 versus 67.7%, $p = 0.012$) favored neoadjuvant over control arm ■ 97% had grades 3–4 neutropenia in neoadjuvant chemotherapy arm

AOCOA: Asian-Oceanian Clinical Oncology Association

[a] *Source: VUMCA I Trial (1996) Preliminary results of a randomized trial comparing neoadjuvant chemotherapy (cisplatin, epirubicin, bleomycin) plus radiotherapy versus radiotherapy alone in stage IV (N2, M0) undifferentiated NPC: a positive effect on progression-free survival. International NPC Study Group. Int J Radiat Oncol Biol Phys 35:463–469*

[b] *Source: Ma J, Mai HQ, Hong MH et al (2001) Results of a prospective randomized trial comparing neoadjuvant chemotherapy plus radiotherapy with radiotherapy alone in patients with locoregionally advanced nasopharyngeal carcinoma. J Clin Oncol 19:1350–1357*

[c] *Source: Chua DT, Sham JS, Choy D et al (1998) Preliminary report of the Asian-Oceanian Clinical Oncology Association randomized trial comparing cisplatin and epirubicin followed by radiotherapy versus radiotherapy alone in the treatment of patients with locoregionally advanced nasopharyngeal carcinoma. Asian-Oceanian Clinical Oncology Association Nasopharynx Cancer Study Group. Cancer 83:2270–2283*

[d] *Source: Hui EP, Ma BB, Leung SF et al (2009) Randomized phase II trial of concurrent cisplatin-RT with or without neoadjuvant docetaxel and cisplatin in advanced NPC. J Clin Oncol 27:242–249*

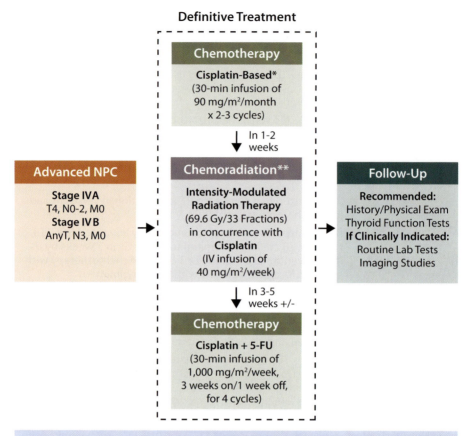

Figure 2.9 A proposed treatment algorithm of definitive treatment of locoregionally advanced NPC with neoadjuvant and concurrent chemotherapy and IMRT

A proposed treatment algorithm for stages IVA–IVB NPC is detailed in Figure 2.9.

Adjuvant Chemotherapy

The value of adjuvant chemotherapy in definitive treatment of locoregionally advanced NPC has not been proven, according to the results of the aforementioned meta-analysis and a number of randomized trials.

Radiation Therapy Techniques

Definitive Radiation Therapy

Although conventional radiation techniques have been used in the treatment of NPC for decades, the superiority of IMRT has been repeatedly demonstrated in both retrospective and prospective studies. Currently, IMRT is the recommended technique for definitive treatment in NPC thus is the focus of the following discussion.

Results of selected experiences in NPC treatment using IMRT are listed in Table 2.12.

Simulation and Target Volume Delineation

A CT scan (3-mm cuts) with intravenous (IV) contrast should be performed from the top of the head to the upper mediastinum. Magnetic resonance imaging (MRI) fusion with planning CT is highly recommended. Setup with thermoplastic mask covering head, neck, and shoulders is illustrated in Figure 2.10.

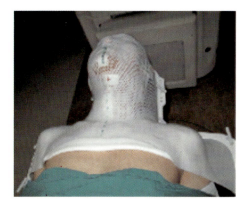

Figure 2.10 Thermoplastic mask system extending from vertex of scalp to shoulders for immobilization of the patient in the treatment of NPC

Table 2.12 Results of selected experiences of IMRT for NPC (studies with ≥30 months follow-up)

Author	No. of patients	Follow-up (months)	Stages III–IVb	Chemo-therapy	LC (years)	RC (years)	DMF (years)	OS (years)
Lee et al[a]	67	31	47 (70%)	50 (75%)	97% (4)	98%	66% (4)	88% (4)
Wolden et al[b]	74	35	57 (77%)	69 (93%)	91% (3)	93% (3)	78% (3)	83% (3)
Tham et al[c]	195	37	123 (63%)	112 (57%)	90% (3)	–	89% (3)	94% (3)
Lin et al[d]	323	30	260 (80%)	295 (91%)[e]	95% (3)	98% (3)	90% (3)	90% (3)

[a] Source: Lee N, Xia P, Quivey JM et al (2002) Intensity-modulated radiotherapy in the treatment of NPC: an update of the UCSF experience. Int J Radiat Oncol Biol Phys 53:12–22

[b] Source: Wolden SL, Chen WC, Pfister DG et al (2006) IMRT for NPC: update of the Memorial Sloan-Kettering experience. Int J Radiat Oncol Biol Phys 64:57–62

[c] Source: Tham IW, Hee SW, Yeo RM et al (2009) Treatment of NPC using IMRT–the NCC Singapore experience. Int J Radiat Oncol Biol Phys 75:1481–1486

[d] Source: Lin S, Pan J, Han L et al (2009) NPC treated with reduced-volume IMRT: report on the 3-year outcome of a prospective series. Int J Radiat Oncol Biol Phys 75:1071–1078

[e] Neoadjuvant with or without concurrent chemotherapy

NPC has a high rate of regional metastases to the cervical lymph nodes. Therefore, radiation to subclinical cervical nodal chains is important in the definitive treatment of NPC.

Gross tumor volume (GTV) at primary (GTV-P) and neck regions (GTV-N), clinical target volumes (CTV-P and -N), and planning target volumes (PTV), as well as organs at risk (OAR), should be delineated (Table 2.13). GTV-P includes all known gross disease determined from CT, MRI, clinical examination, and endoscopic findings. GTV-N are defined as any lymph nodes >1 cm or nodes with necrotic centers.

Table 2.13 Schemes for high-risk CTV-P delineation

Region	RTOG 0615
Minimum margin to GTV-P	10 mm
Nasopharynx	Entire
Sphenoid sinus	Inferior part (entire if involved)
Clivus	Anterior third
Maxillary sinus	5 mm anterior to maxillary mucosa
Nasal cavity	5 mm anterior to posterior nasal aperture
Other structures	Pterygoid fossa, parapharyngeal space, and skull base including foramen ovale and rotundum

GTV-P: gross tumor volume at primary; **CTV-P:** clinical target volume at primary

Source: Lee N, Garden A, Kim J et al (2009) RTOG 0615. A phase II study of concurrent chemoradiotherapy using three-dimensional conformal radiotherapy (3D-CRT) or intensity-modulated radiation therapy (IMRT) plus bevacizumab for local or regionally advanced nasopharyngeal cancer. http://www.rtog.org/member/protocols/0615/0615.pdf. Accessed on July 1, 2010

As lymph node spread in NPC follows an orderly fashion, and "skip metastasis" is uncommon, the necessity of irradiating lower neck nodes in N0 disease should be carefully evaluated. The selection of CTV-P and CTV-N is the most challenging step in IMRT planning for NPC. Table 2.14 provides proposed coverage schemes for CTV in both primary and cervical lymph nodal areas.

Table 2.14 Proposed high-risk CTV-N according to the nodal status in treatment of NPC using IMRT

Nodal classification	Levels to be included in the CTV	
	Ipsilateral neck	Contralateral neck
N0	Retropharyngeal (RP) plus II plus III plus Va	RP plus II plus III plus Va
N1	RP plus Ib plus II plus III plus IV plus V	RP plus Ib[a] plus II plus III plus IV plus V
N2	RP plus Ib plus II plus III plus IV plus V	RP plus Ib plus II plus III plus IV plus V
N3	RP plus Ib plus II plus III plus IV plus V ± adjacent structures based on clinical and radiological findings[b]	RP plus Ib plus II plus III plus IV plus V

Uninvolved lower neck nodes in patients with N0 or N1 disease can be considered low-risk regions

[a]The necessity of encompassing contralateral Ib nodes in patients with N1 NPC is not clear

[b]Inclusion of supraclavicular nodes is suggested in case of lymph node involvement in level IV and Vb

Source: Lu JJ, Gregoire V, Lin S (2009) Selection and delineation of target volumes in IMRT for nasopharyngeal cancer. In: Lu JJ, Cooper JS, Lee AW (eds) Nasopharyngeal cancer: multidisciplinary management. Springer, Berlin Heidelberg New York

Dose and Treatment Delivery

The total dose of IMRT to PTV of gross disease in NPC is ~70 Gy delivered in 33–35 fractions (2–2.2 Gy per daily fraction) (Table 2.15).

Table 2.15 Dose and fractionation in definitive treatment using IMRT for NPC

Fields	Borders
GTV at primary plus adenopathy	Total dose: 70 Gy Fractions: 33–35 Daily dose: 2–2.12 Gy
High-risk PTV	Total dose: 54–60 Gy Fractions: 33–35 Daily dose: 1.6–1.8 Gy
Low-risk PTV	Total dose: 54 Gy Fractions: 33–35 Daily dose: ~1.6 Gy

IMRT dose distributions are more conformal when using the simultaneous in-field boost (SIB) schedule as compared with the two-phase IMRT plan (IMRT to the entire treatment volume, including primary and neck diseases as well as subclinical volumes, followed by IMRT boost to the involved areas). Additionally, SIB enables an escalated dose to be delivered per daily fraction. IMRT delivered using "step-and-shoot," dynamic multileaf collimation (MLC), or helical therapy provide similar clinical outcomes.

Figure 2.11 illustrates typical target volumes and radiation dose distribution of a patient with T2N2M0 NPC with the dose-volume histogram (DVH) of the same plan.

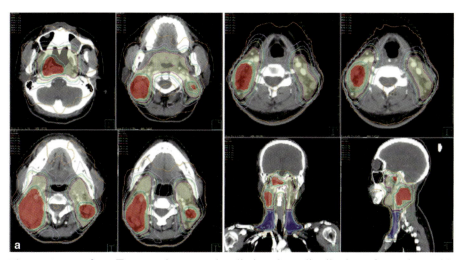

Figure 2.11 a, b a Target volumes and radiation dose distribution of a patient with T2N2M0 NPC, with GTV, CTV, and PTV, delineated according to RTOG 0615 protocol. **b** DVH of the same plan (*Figure 2.11b see next page*)

b

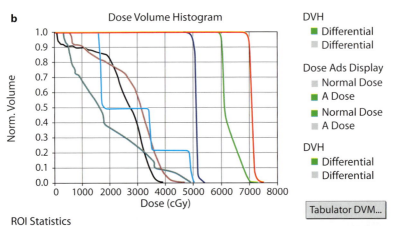

ROI Statistics

Line Type	ROI	Trial	Min	Max	Mean	Std. Cev	% Outside crid	% > Max	Generalized CUD
	Brainstem	Trial_2	497.4	4796.8	2829.2	1030.5	0.00 %	0.00 %	2822.98
	Optic chiasm	Trial_2	1638.4	5047.8	2897.8	1319.7	0.00 %	0.00 %	2969.22
	Optic nerves	Trial_2	318.8	4955.9	1919.2	1304.9	0.00 %	0.00 %	1947.1
	PTV 50.4	Trial_2	3738.8	5476.3	5145.8	73.3	0.00 %	0.00 %	5154.32
	PTV 59.4	Trial_2	5819.7	7375.8	6323.0	300.9	0.00 %	0.00 %	6884.25
	PTV 70	Trial_2	6318.1	7596.3	7138.3	82.6	0.00 %	0.00 %	7148.32
	Spinal cord	Trial_2	81.5	3985.2	2614.2	973.9	0.00 %	0.00 %	2665.90

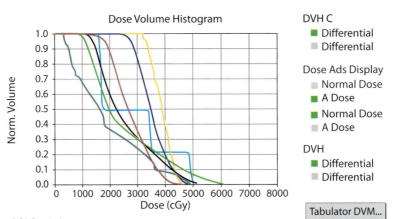

ROI Statistics

Line Type	ROI	Trial	Min	Max	Mean	Std. Cev	% Outside crid	% > Max	Generalized CUD
	Cochlear	Trial_2	3231.4	4662.9	3911.4	388.9	0.00 %	0.00 %	3945.54
	LT parotid	Trial_2	1000.0	5628.5	2570.7	1065.4	0.00 %	0.00 %	2552.52
	Optic nerves	Trial_2	1638.4	5407.3	2897.6	1319.7	0.00 %	0.00 %	2989.52
	Optic chiasm	Trial_2	318.8	4989.3	1919.2	1304.3	0.00 %	0.00 %	1947.1
	RT parotid	Trial_2	838.0	6822.3	2511.4	1348.5	0.00 %	0.00 %	2493.29
	Temporal lobes	Trial_2	2217.4	5502.4	3547.3	540.0	0.00 %	0.00 %	3538.41
	TMJ	Trial_2	336.0	4660.7	2761.8	708.4	0.00 %	0.00 %	2802.25

Normal Tissue Tolerance

OAR in definitive radiation therapy of NPC and their dose limitations are detailed in Table 2.16.

Table 2.16 Recommended dose constraints

OAR	Dose	End point
Brainstem	$D_{max} < 54$ Gy	Permanent neuropathy
Spinal cord	$D_{max} < 50$ Gy	Myelopathy
Optic nerves, chiasm	$D_{max} < 55$ Gy	Optic neuropathy
Brachial plexus	$D_{max} < 66$ Gy	Neuropathy
Retina	Mean dose < 45 Gy	Blindness
Cochlea	Mean dose < 45 Gy	Sensorineural hearing loss
Mandible, transmandibular joint	$D_{max} < 70$ Gy	Joint dysfunction
Parotid glands	Combined mean parotid dose <25 Gy, or at least 1 gland <20 Gy	Permanent xerostomia
Thyroid gland	Mean dose < 45 Gy	Clinical thyroiditis
Larynx[a]	Mean dose < 50 Gy	Aspiration
	$D_{max} < 66$ Gy	Vocal dysfunction
Pharyngeal constrictors[a]	Mean dose < 50 Gy	Dysphagia and aspiration

[a]Constraints apply only if not target structure

Sources: Marks LB, Yorke ED, Jackson, A et al (2010) Use of normal tissue complication probability models in the clinic. Int J Radiat Oncol Biol Phys 76:S10–19; Emami B, Lyman J, Brown A et al (1991) Tolerance of normal tissue to therapeutic irradiation. Int J Radiat Oncol Biol Phys 21:109–122

Follow-Up

Active follow-up after definitive treatment for NPC is recommended. Schedule and suggested examinations for follow-up are detailed in Table 2.17.

Table 2.17 Follow-up schedule and examinations

Schedule	Frequency
Years 0–1	■ Every 1–3 months
Years 1–2	■ Every 2–4 months
Years 3–5	■ Every 4–6 months
Years 5+	■ Annually
Examinations	
History and physical	■ Complete history and physical examination ■ Nasopharyngoscopy ■ Speech, hearing, and swallow evaluation if clinically indicated
Laboratory tests	■ TSH and free T4 (every 6–12 months) ■ Other endocrine tests when clinically indicated ■ EBV DNA monitoring (optional)
Imaging studies	■ MRI of the head and neck (3 months after RT, then annually) ■ Chest X-ray, CT of the thorax/abdomen, bone scan, PET/CT scan is indicated only with clinical signs or symptoms of recurrence

TSH: thyroid-stimulating hormone; **T4:** thyroxine; **PET:** positron-emission tomography

Source: Tham IWK, Lu JJ (2009) Post-treatment follow-up of patients with nasopharyngeal cancer. In: Lu JJ, Cooper JS, Lee AW (eds) Nasopharyngeal cancer: multidisciplinary management. Springer, Berlin Heidelberg New York 2009

Severe, long-term adverse effects secondary to IMRT for NPC such as temporal lobe necrosis, myelitis, cranial nerve palsy, and severe trismus are not common. Dysgeusia (usually resolves in 4–6 months) and mild to moderate xerostomia are the most commonly observed radiation-induced long-term adverse effects.

3

Cancer of the Oral Cavity and Oropharynx

Kenneth S. Hu[1] and Louis B. Harrison[2]

Key Points

- Cancers occurring in both the oral cavity and oropharynx can severely impair appearance and function, including speech, mastication, taste, and swallowing.

- The most common pathology of oral and oropharyngeal cancer is squamous cell carcinoma (SCC).

- Common signs and symptoms in the oral cavity SCC include nonhealing painful ulcer, or ill-fitting denture. In more advanced cases, speech difficulty, dysphagia, otalgia, hypersalivation, and neck mass(es) are common.

- Sore throat and dysphagia are common presenting symptoms of tumors of the tonsils, soft palate, and posterior pharyngeal wall, but not in early tumors of the base of the tongue which often present with asymptomatic lymphadenopathy.

- Tissue from either primary tumor or neck lymphadenopathy is crucial for pathologic diagnosis. Accurate diagnosis and staging are based on history and physical examination, imaging, and laboratory studies.

- Single modality treatment with surgery or radiation therapy is preferred for early-stage oral cavity SCC. Surgery followed by adjuvant therapy or combined chemoradiation is needed for more advanced disease.

- Nonsurgical organ preservation therapy with chemoradiation therapy is preferred for most oropharyngeal cancer cases rather than a primary surgery approach.

- Improvements in imaging, radiation delivery (e.g., altered fractionation and intensity-modulated radiation therapy [IMRT]), and the use of combined chemotherapy and biological therapy have substantially improved treatment outcomes.

[1] Kenneth S. Hu, MD
Email: khu@chpnet.org

[2] Louis B. Harrison, MD
Email: lharrison@chpnet.org

J. J. Lu, L. W. Brady (Eds.), *Decision Making in Radiation Oncology*
DOI: 10.1007/978-3-642-13832-4_4, © Springer-Verlag Berlin Heidelberg 2011

Epidemiology and Etiology

In 2009, approximately 28,500 new cases of oral cavity and oropharyngeal cancer were diagnosed in the USA, and about 6,100 patients died of these cancers. The male-to-female ratio of these diseases is about 2:1, and the average age of diagnosis is 62 (although a third of patients are younger than 55).

Cancers of the oral cavity and oropharynx are most commonly diagnosed in the following sites: tongue (~25%), tonsils (~10–15%), lips (~10–15%), and minor salivary glands (~10–15%). The rest are found in the gums, floor of the mouth, and other sites.

A number of risk factors have been identified for head and neck cancer (Table 3.1). However the benefit of screening in high-risk patients using imaging or laboratory tests is not supported by clinical evidence.

Table 3.1   Risk factors of oral cavity/oropharynx cancer

Type	Description
Patient related	**Age and gender:** predisposition in males for oral cavity cancer patients, especially those who are smokers and older than 50 years. Distinct subset of young, female nonsmokers who have oral tongue cancer without clear etiology
	Lifestyle: cigarette smoking, alcohol, betel nut chewing. Sexual promiscuity and marijuana smoking are associated with human papilloma virus (*HPV*) positivity
Viral factors	For oropharynx patients, **HPV-positive patients** are younger with equal male:female predisposition, while smoking-related oropharynx cancer patients are usually older males
	HPV subtype 16 is involved in >90% of cases, while HPV-18, -32, and -33 are involved in the remainder
	p16 immunohistochemistry testing is an accurate surrogate for HPV infection. HPV subtyping may be done if p16 is positive

Anatomy

The structures composing the oral cavity and oropharynx, as well as their first echelon lymphatic drainage, are detailed in Table 3.2 and Figure 3.1.

Table 3.2 Anatomy of the oral cavity and oropharynx

Structure	Structure	Lymphatic drainage
Oral cavity	■ Lips ■ Hard palate ■ Anterior two thirds of the tongue ■ Alveolar ridge ■ Retromolar trigone ■ Floor of mouth ■ Buccal mucosa	Levels I, II, and III
Oropharynx	■ Soft palate ■ Tonsillar fossa and pillars ■ Base of tongue ■ Posterior and lateral pharyngeal wall between nasopharynx and pharyngoepiglottic fold	Retropharyngeal Levels II, III, and IV

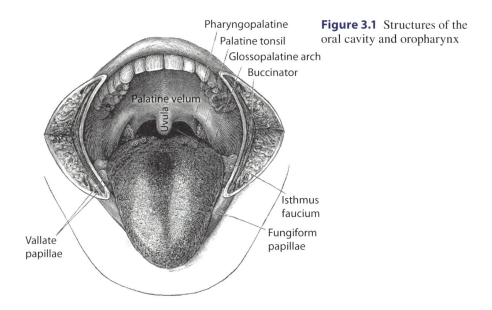

Pharyngopalatine
Palatine tonsil
Glossopalatine arch
Buccinator
Palatine velum
Uvula
Vallate papillae
Isthmus faucium
Fungiform papillae

Figure 3.1 Structures of the oral cavity and oropharynx

Cervical Lymph Nodes

The classification of the neck lymph nodes (the Robbins Classification) is illustrated in Chap. 2, Figure 2.3. Neck nodes of various levels delineated on CT slides, as well as the consensus guidelines for radiological boundaries of them are detailed in Chap. 2, Figure 2.4, and Table 2.2.

Pathology

Squamous cell carcinoma (SCC) accounts for >90% of all oral cavity and oropharyngeal cancers; hence, SCC is the focus of discussion in this chapter. The remaining cancers include minor salivary gland carcinomas, lymphoma, plasmacytoma, sarcoma, and melanoma.

Routes of Spread

Local extension and regional (lymphatic) spread are the most common patterns of spread. Regional spread is predictable and orderly, with first-echelon nodal drainage dependent on location in the oral cavity or oropharynx cancer, the laterality of the tumor, the depth of invasion, and the presence of ipsilateral nodal disease (Table 3.3).

Table 3.3 Routes of spread in oral and oropharyngeal SCC

Type	Description
Local extension	■ Direct invasion of oral cavity cancers into mandible and base of the tongue is possible, while oropharynx cancers may invade the vallecula/larynx, parapharyngeal area into the pterygoid muscles/plates, nasopharynx, and oral cavity (oral tongue and retromolar trigone) ■ Perineural invasion especially along branches of CN V and VII
Regional lymph node metastasis	■ Lymph node involvement is seen in about 30% of oral cavity and 55% of oropharynx cancers ■ Nodal levels I–III and II–IV are the primarily nodal levels at risk for oral cavity and oropharynx, respectively (Table 3.4) ■ Coverage of nodal levels I–V should be considered if nodal disease is present. Retropharyngeal nodes represent a primary echelon nodal drainage for oropharynx cancers. ■ Contralateral nodes are at risk for tumors near midline, advanced T- and N-stage diseases
Distant metastasis	■ In patients with advanced-stage disease, distant metastasis primarily to the lungs is significant in about 20% of patients ■ The most site of hematogenous metastasis is the lung. However, a primary lung cancer should be excluded

Lymph Node Metastasis

Pattern of lymphatic spread depends on the location of the primary (oral cavity versus oropharynx) and clinical nodal status (Table 3.4).

Table 3.4 Lymphatic drainage patterns in oral cavity and oropharynx cancers in a clinically negative or involved neck based on surgical series

Site	Level (%)				
	I	II	III	IV	V
Oropharynx (N⁻) (n = 48)	2%	25%	19%	8%	2%
Oropharynx (N⁺) (n = 165)	14%	71%	42%	28%	9%
Oral (N⁻) (n = 192)	20%	17%	9%	3%	0.5%
Oral (N⁺) (n = 324)	46%	43%	33%	15%	3%

Sources: Shah JP, Candela FC, Poddar AK (1990) Patterns of cervical lymph node metastases from SCC of the oral cavity. Cancer 66:109–113; Shah JP (1990) Patterns of cervical lymph node metastasis from SCC of the upper aerodigestive tract. Am J Surg 160:405–409

Diagnosis, Staging, and Prognosis

Clinical Presentation

Signs and symptoms of oral cavity/oropharynx cancers differ, and they are detailed in Table 3.5. Among newly diagnosed patients with SCC of the oral cavity and oropharynx, ~15% have another cancer in the upper aerodigestive track such as the larynx, esophagus, or lung.

Table 3.5 Commonly observed signs and symptoms in oral cavity/oropharynx cancer

Type	Description
Oral cavity	■ Non-healing ulcer, pain, bleeding, or ill-fitting dentures ■ More advanced lesions may present with speech difficulties, dysphagia, otalgia (referred pain), hypersalivation, and neck mass(es)
Oropharynx	■ **Soft palate tumors:** often present with sore throat and in early-stage due to ready visualization. ■ **Base of tongue cancer:** occult and often diagnosed in later stages, due their remote location and because of the lack of pain fibers at the site. They commonly present with an asymptomatic neck node. However, symptoms may include foreign-body sensation in the throat, otalgia due to referred pain from nerve involvement, dysphagia and changes in voice/articulation due to tongue fixation. ■ **Tonsillar lesions:** may present with pain, sore throat, dysphagia, trismus and ipsilateral neck mass. ■ **Posterior pharyngeal wall lesions:** can present with dysphagia, sore throat and pain

Diagnosis and Staging

Figure 3.2 and Table 3.6 present the suggested workup of SCC of the oral cavity and oropharynx.

Histologic confirmation (fine-needle aspiration [FNA] of a suspected lymph node or open biopsy of the primary disease) is sufficient and critical in determining the histopathology and extent of disease spread to radiologically indeterminate nodes.

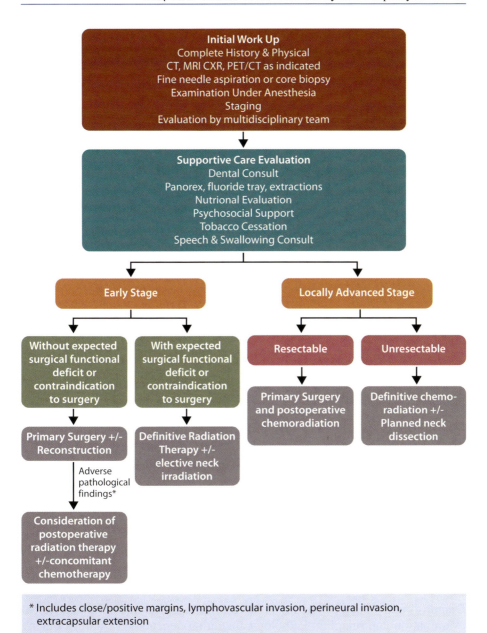

Figure 3.2 Proposed algorithm for workups for suspicious oral cavity lesions. *Pre-irradiation dental evaluation should include Panorex, dental extractions if indicated, and fluoride tray

Table 3.6 Studies for diagnosis and staging of oral cavity and oropharyngeal cancers

Type	Description
Physical examination	■ With special attention to tongue mobility, trismus, extension to nasopharynx, larynx, or hypopharynx ■ Examination of first-echelon nodes (levels I–II for oral cavity and levels II–III in oropharyngeal SCC) is crucial
Endoscopic examination	■ Evaluation of the upper aerodigestive tract is crucial to evaluate the primary site of disease and the presence of synchronous primaries ■ Triple endoscopy including rigid endoscopy of the upper aerodigestive tract, esophagoscopy, and bronchoscopy should be considered.
Laboratory tests	■ Initial lab tests should include a complete blood count, basic blood chemistry, hepatic and metabolic panels ■ Testing for HPV in the biopsy specimen (p16 immunohistochemistry testing) should be considered in oropharynx tumors, especially in patients without significant smoking history
Imaging studies	■ CT scans of the neck and chest are appropriate to evaluate and stage head and neck cancer ■ FDG-PET/CT scan is recommended for diagnosis, staging, and surveillance of head and neck cancer ■ After treatment, PET/CT may be used to monitor for persistent disease in the neck or primary site and is best done 3 months after the end of radiation therapy ■ High false-negative rates are noted in scans done earlier ■ MRI may be useful for delineation of the soft tissue extent of disease, especially in oral cavity patients with dental amalgam or in oropharyngeal cancer patients with trismus.

Tumor, Node, and Metastasis Staging

Diagnosis and clinical staging depends on findings from history and physical examination and imaging. Pathological staging depends on findings during surgical resection and microscopic examination, in addition to those required in clinical staging.

The 7th edition of the tumor, node, and metastasis (TNM) staging systems of American Joint Committee on Cancer (AJCC) for both oral cavity and oropharynx cancers are presented in Tables 3.7 and 3.8.

Table 3.7 AJCC TNM classification of carcinoma of oral cavity and oropharynx

Stage	Description
Primary tumor (T)	
TX	Primary tumor cannot be assessed
T0	No evidence of primary tumor
Tis	Carcinoma in situ
T1	Tumor ≤2 cm in greatest dimension
T2	Tumor >2 cm but ≤4 cm in greatest dimension
T3	Tumor >4 cm in greatest dimension
T4 (lip)	Tumor invades through cortical bone, inferior alveolar nerve, floor of mouth, or skin of face, chin, or nose
T4a (oral cavity)	Tumor invades through cortical bone, into deep (extrinsic) muscle of tongue, maxillary sinus, or skin of face
T4b (oral cavity)	Tumor involves masticator space, pterygoid plates, or skull base, and/or encases internal carotid artery
T4a (oropharynx)	Tumor invades the larynx, deep, extrinsic muscle of tongue/medial pterygoid/hard palate, or mandible
T4b (oropharynx)	Tumor involves lateral pterygoid muscle, pterygoid plates, lateral nasopharynx, skull base, and/or encases internal carotid artery
Regional lymph nodes (N)	
NX	Regional lymph nodes cannot be assessed
N0	No regional lymph node metastasis
N1	Metastasis in a single ipsilateral lymph node, ≤3cm in greatest dimension
N2a	Metastasis in a single ipsilateral lymph node, >3cm but ≤6 cm in greatest dimension
N2b	Metastasis in multiple ipsilateral lymph nodes, none >6 cm in greatest dimension
N2c	Metastasis in bilateral or contralateral lymph nodes, none >6 cm in greatest dimension
N3	Metastasis in a lymph node, >6 cm in greatest dimension
Distant metastasis (M)	
M0	No distant metastasis
M1	Distant metastasis (including seeding of the peritoneum and positive peritoneal cytology)

Source: Edge SB, Byrd DR, Compton CC et al (2009) American Joint Committee on Cancer, American Cancer Society. AJCC cancer staging manual, 7th edn. Springer, Berlin Heidelberg New York

Table 3.8 Stage grouping of carcinoma of oral cavity and oropharynx

Stage Grouping					
	T1	T2	T3	T4a	T4b
N0	I	II	III	IVA	IVB
N1	III	III	III	IVA	IVB
N2	IVA	IVA	IVA	IVA	IVB
N3	IVB	IVB	IVB	IVB	IVB
M1	IVC	IVC	IVC	IVC	IVC

Source: Edge SB, Byrd DR, Compton CC et al (2009) American Joint Committee on Cancer, American Cancer Society. AJCC cancer staging manual, 7th edn. Springer, Berlin Heidelberg New York

Prognosis

Significant prognostic factors of SCC of the oral cavity and oropharynx are detailed in Table 3.9.

Table 3.9 Prognostic factors of SCC of the oral cavity and oropharynx

Type	Description
Disease related	**Stage** at diagnosis is the most important prognostic factor
	In general, the presence of **nodal involvement** decreases survival by half
Patient related	**Male gender and poor performance status** are adverse factors
	Cigarette smoking (>20 pack-years) is associated with poor survival rate
	Oropharyngeal SCC patients who are p16[+] and nonsmokers have a 25–30% improved OS rate compared with heavy smokers (>20 pack-year)
Postoperative Setting	**Extracapsular extension and positive surgical margins** are important predictors of locoregional recurrence and survival

Treatment

Principles and Practice

Surgery is the mainstay treatment modality for SCC of the oral cavity. Locally advanced oral cavity cancer usually requires post-up radiation therapy, with or without concurrent chemotherapy.

Radiation therapy is a mainstay of treatment for oropharyngeal SCC, although surgery can be used in selected cases (Figure 3.3). Locoregionally advanced SCC of the oral cavity or oropharynx usually requires combined chemoradiation therapy.

Treatment modalities and their indications are detailed in Table 3.10.

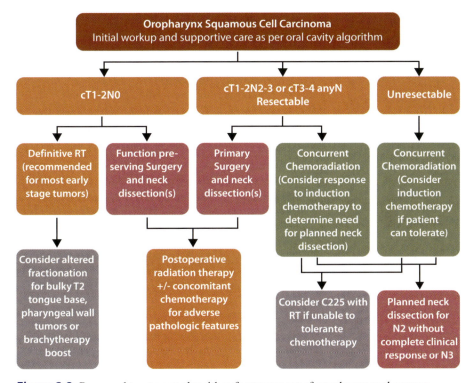

Figure 3.3 Proposed treatment algorithm for treatment of oropharyngeal cancer

Table 3.10 Treatment modalities used in SCC of the oral cavity

Type	Description
Surgery	
Indications	■ Radical resection and selective neck dissection as single modality for stages I and II oral cavity SCC ■ As the primary treatment modality (followed by adjuvant therapy) for stage III and IV (nonmetastatic) oral cavity SCC ■ Surgical reconstruction to optimize functional outcomes including radial forearm free flap reconstruction should be considered
Facts/issues	■ Consider postoperative radiation or chemoradiation in high-risk patients (i.e., positive surgical margins or extracapsular extension [*ECE*]). Intermediate pathologic risk factors include lymphovascular, perineural invasion, level IV nodal involvement, presence of multiple nodes, and close margin and warrant radiation therapy
Radiation therapy	
Indication	■ Adjuvant treatment after complete resection for high-risk patients, with or without chemotherapy ■ Definitive radiation with concurrent chemotherapy is the current standard for unresectable locally advanced disease ■ Palliative treatment to primary or metastatic foci
Techniques	■ External-beam radiation therapy (*EBRT*) using three-dimensional (*3D*)-CRT or IMRT ■ Interstitial brachytherapy if technically available especially in patients treated with definitive radiation ■ In high-risk patients, the entire treatment time from surgery to completion of radiation should be kept to 11 weeks[a]
Chemo-/targeted therapy	
Indications	■ Adjuvant treatment after surgery (with EBRT) → in high risk patients ■ Concurrent with EBRT for definitive treatment ■ Neoadjuvant chemotherapy can be considered in T4–N3 patients prior to concurrent chemoradiation therapy (*CRT*) ■ Mainstay treatment for recurrent disease
Medications	■ Cisplatin is the mainstay chemotherapy agent ■ The addition of Taxotere to cisplatin and fluorouracil ([*5-FU*] *PF*) in neoadjuvant regimen further improves treatment outcome compared to PF neoadjuvant regimen ■ Cetuximab used in patients who cannot tolerate platinum or have platinum refractory recurrent disease

Treatment of Early-Stage Ipsilateral Oropharyngeal SCC

For lateralized T1–2N0–1 oropharynx cancer patients involving the tonsils, ipsilateral radiation therapy is preferred to avoid radiation of the contralateral neck and organs at risk including parotid, submandibular gland, constrictor muscles, and structures important for mastication.

Minimal involvement of the soft palate and tongue base (as defined in Table 3.11) may still be treated unilaterally. However, centralized regions such as base of tongue and soft palate requires usually bilateral neck treatment.

Treatment of T1–2N1–N2a (Intermediate-Stage) Disease

A number of approaches, including altered fractionated radiation alone and radiation with concurrent chemotherapy for radiosensitization, can be used for this group of patients (Table 3.12).

Sources: Ang KK, Trotti A, Brown BW et al (2001) Randomized trial addressing risk features and time factors of surgery plus radiotherapy in advanced head-and-neck cancer. Int J Radiat Oncol Biol Phys. 51:571–578; Cooper JS, Pajak TF, Forastiere AA et al (2004) Postoperative concurrent radiotherapy and chemotherapy for high-risk squamous-cell carcinoma of the head and neck. N Engl J Med 350:1937–1934; Bernier J, Domenge C, Ozsahin M et al (2004) Postoperative irradiation with or without concomitant chemotherapy for locally advanced head and neck cancer. N Engl J Med 350:1945–1952; Ang KK, Trotti A, Brown BW et al (2001) Randomized trial addressing risk features and time factors of surgery plus radiotherapy in advanced head-and-neck cancer. Int J Radiat Oncol Biol Phys 51:571–578; Horiot JC, Le Fur R, N'Guyen T et al (1992) Hyperfractionation versus conventional fractionation in oropharyngeal carcinoma: final analysis of a randomized trial of the EORTC cooperative group of radiotherapy. Radiother Oncol 25:231–241; Posner MR, Hershock DM, Blajman CR et al (2007) Cisplatin and 5-FU alone or with docetaxel in head and neck cancer. N Engl J Med 357:1705–1715

Table 3.11 Clinical evidence supporting ipsilateral radiation therapy in lateralized early-stage SCC of the oropharynx

Trial	Description
Princess Margaret Hospital	■ 228 Patients with tonsillar carcinomas were treated with ipsilateral radiotherapy ■ Eligible patients typically had T1 or T2 tumors (191 T1/2, 30 T3, and 7 T4 cases) with N0 (133 N0, 35 N1, 27 N2–3) diseases ■ Radiation therapy typically used wedged-pair cobalt beams and ipsilateral low anterior neck field to 50 Gy in 4 weeks to the primary volume ■ With a median follow-up of 5.7 years, the 3-year local control, regional control, and cause-specific survival rates were 77, 80, and 76%, respectively ■ Contralateral neck failure occurred in only 3% ■ All patients with T1 or N0 disease had 100% contralateral neck control ■ Patients with a 10% or greater risk of contralateral neck failure included T3 lesions, lesions involving the medial third of the of the soft hemi palate, tumors invading the middle third of the ipsilateral base of tongue and patients with N1 disease

Source: O'Sullivan B, Warde P, Grice B et al (2001) The benefits and pitfalls of ipsilateral radiotherapy in carcinoma of the tonsillar region. Int J Radiat Oncol Biol Phys 51:332–343

Table 3.12 Altered fractionation in the treatment of SCC of head and neck

Trials	Results
EORTC 22791[a]	■ Randomized 356 patients with T2–3N0–1M0 SCC of oropharynx (excluding base of tongue) to either hyperfractionated or conventional radiation therapy ■ Arms included hyperfractionation regimen of 1.15 cGy BID (spaced 4–6 h) to 80.5 Gy over 7 weeks versus conventional fractionation of 1.8–2.0 Gy to 70 Gy over 7–8 weeks ■ With a mean follow-up of about 4 years, hyperfractionation improved 5-year actuarial local regional control as compared with conventional fractionation (59 versus 40%, $p = 0.02$) with a trend toward improved survival (38 versus 29%, $p = 0.08$) ■ T3 tumors benefited from hyperfractionation but not T2 lesions

Table 3.12 *(continued)*

Trials	Results
RTOG 90-03[b]	■ A landmark RTOG trial in which 1,073 patients were randomized to this 4-arm phase III trial Arms included: ■ Conventional fractionation of (*CF*) 70 Gy in 7 weeks ■ Split-course accelerated fractionation (*S-AF*) with 1.6 Gy BID to 67.2 Gy over 6 weeks, with an intentional 2-week break after 38.4 Gy ■ Accelerated radiation by delayed concomitant boost (*DCB*) to 72 Gy in 6 weeks with BID radiation therapy (*RT*) in the last 12 days RT ■ Pure hyperfractionation (*HF*) with 1. 2Gy BID to 81.6 Gy/7 weeks. ■ At 8-year median follow-up, the DCB and HF arms had significantly better locoregional control as compared with CF (48 versus 49 versus 41%), and improved disease-free survival (30 versus 31 vs 21%) ■ No significant difference in distant metastasis ([*DM*]; 27 versus 29 versus 29%) or overall survival ([*OS*] 34 versus 37 versus 30%) were observed
Bonner et al 2006[c]	■ A pivotal phase III trial demonstrated the efficacy of cetuximab (C225), a monoclonal antibody targeting epidermal growth factor receptor (*EGFR*), to radiation ■ Randomized 424 patients with stages III–IV head and neck SCC (64% had oropharyngeal SCC, no oral cavity cancer) to 7 weeks of C225 plus radiation (conventional or altered fractionation) or radiation alone ■ With a median follow-up of 38 months, the C225 plus RT arm was superior to RT alone with respect to 3-year locoregional control (47 versus 34%, $p < 0.01$), 3-year OS (55 versus 45%, $p = 0.05$) and MS (54 versus 28 months, $p = 0.02$) ■ C225 did not significantly increase grades 3 or 4 mucositis, but was associated with increased dermatitis, 34 versus 18% ($p = 0.0003$) and infusion reaction (3%)

[a]*Source: Horiot JC, Le Fur R, N'Guyen T et al (1992) Hyperfractionation versus conventional fractionation in oropharyngeal carcinoma: final analysis of a randomized trial of the EORTC cooperative group of radiotherapy. Radiother Oncol 25:231–241*
[b]*Source: Fu KK, Pajak TF, Trotti A et al (2000) An RTOG phase III randomized study to compare hyperfractionation and two variants of accelerated fractionation to standard fractionation RT for head and neck SCC: first report of RTOG 9003. Int J Radiat Oncol Biol Phys 48:7–16*
[c]*Source: Bonner JA, Harari PM, Giralt J et al (2006) Radiotherapy plus cetuximab for squamous-cell carcinoma of the head and neck. N Engl J Med 354:567–578*

Treatment of Advanced-Stage Disease

Concurrent chemoradiation is the standard treatment for advanced-stage SCC of the oral cavity and oropharynx.

Randomized trials have demonstrated a survival and locoregional control benefit when adding concurrent chemotherapy to altered fractionated radiation therapy as compared with altered fractionated radiation alone (Table 3.13). However, in the setting of concurrent chemoradiation, there is no benefit of altered fractionated radiation over conventional fractionated radiation, except that patients treated with altered fractionated radiation may be planned for fewer cycles of chemotherapy.

Table 3.13 Clinical evidence supporting the use of concurrent chemotherapy and altered fractionated radiation therapy in oropharynx cancer

Trials	Results
FNCLCC-GORTEC (French multicentric randomized trial)[a]	■ 163 patients with unresectable oropharynx ($n = 123$) or hypopharynx ($n = 40$) SCC to either CRT or RT alone ■ RT used hyperfractionated scheme (1.2 Gy BID to 80.4 Gy) in both arms ■ Concurrent cisplatin (100 mg/m^2 on days 1, 22, and 43) plus 5-FU (750 mg/m^2/5 days on day 1, 430 mg/m^2/5 days on days 22 and 43) was used in the experimental arm ■ Actuarial 2-year local control (*LC*), disease-free (*DFS*), and OS rates were better in the patients receiving concurrent chemoradiation: 59 versus 27.5% ($p = 0.0003$), 48.2 versus 25.2% ($p = 0.002$), and 37.8 versus 20.1% ($p = 0.038$), respectively ■ The addition of chemotherapy substantially increased acute mucositis, hematologic toxicity, and feeding tube dependence
German multicentric randomized trial[b]	■ A 2 x 2 study of 246 stages III–IV oropharyngeal ($n = 178$) and hypopharyngeal cancer ($n = 62$) patients to address the benefit of chemotherapy with accelerated radiation by delayed concomitant boost ■ All patients were treated with delayed concomitant boost (69.6 Gy/5.5 weeks) ■ Patients were randomized to carboplatin (70 mg/m^2) plus 5-FU (600 mg/m^2/day for 5 days) on weeks 1 and 5 of RT, then randomized again to receive G-CSF or not ■ With a median follow-up of 22 months, the 1- and 2-year rates of LC were 69 and 51% after CRT as compared with 58 and 45% after RT ($p = 0.14$) ■ Patients receiving granulocyte colony-stimulating factor receptor (*G-CSF*) had reduced locoregional control (55 versus 38%, $p = 0.0072$) and decreased mucositis ($p = 0.06$), raising the issue of possible tumor radioprotection with G-CSF ■ The addition of chemotherapy substantially increased acute mucositis, hematologic toxicity, and feeding tube dependence

Treatment of T4b or N3 Disease

Treatment generally should follow the concurrent chemoradiation therapy strategy. However, in cases where concurrent chemoradiation alone may be suboptimal for very advanced primary or nodal disease, induction chemotherapy may be considered (Table 3.14).

Table 3.14 Induction chemotherapy for advanced head and neck SCC and supporting clinical evidence

Randomized trials	Description
EORTC #24971[a]	■ Randomized 358 locally advanced head and neck SCC patients to receive TPF (docetaxel plus cisplatin plus 5-FU) or PF (cisplatin plus 5-FU), followed by conventional or altered fractionated radiation ■ TPF regimen used was 75 mg/m^2 day 1, 750 mg/m^2 continuous infusion on days 1–5, respectively) or PF (100 mg/m^2 day 1, 1,000 mg/m^2 continuous infusion on days 1–5) ■ With a median follow-up of 51 months, the TPF arm demonstrated superior response rate (68 versus 54%, $p = 0.007$), and increased 3-year OS (36.5 versus 23.9%) ■ Patients who received TPF had less grades 3-4 toxicity and fewer toxic deaths (3.7 versus 7.8%) compared with those receiving PF, due to the reduced doses of platinum and 5FU in the TPF regimen
Posner et al 2007[b]	■ Randomized 494 cases to 3 cycles of induction chemotherapy with docetaxel 75 mg/m^2, cisplatin 100 mg/m^2, and 5-FU 1,000 mg/m^2 (TPF) or 3 cycles of PF (100 mg/m^2, 1,000 mg/m^2), followed by concurrent chemoradiation ■ Radiation and current chemotherapy used 70 Gy/7 weeks and weekly carboplatin (AUC 1.5) ■ At a median follow-up of 42 months, 3-year OS (62 versus 48%, $p = 0.0058$) and PFS (49 versus 37%, $p = 0.004$) favored TPF compared to PF

Patients should have excellent performance status and significant efforts to minimize any treatment break between induction chemotherapy, and subsequent radiation must be emphasized

[a]*Source: Vermorken JB, Remenar E, van Herpen C et al (2007) Cisplatin, 5-FU, and docetaxel in unresectable head and neck cancer. N Engl J Med 357:1695–1704*
[b]*Source: Posner MR, Hershock DM, Blajman CR et al (2007) Cisplatin and 5-FU alone or with docetaxel in head and neck cancer. N Engl J Med 357:1705–1715*

---

[a]*Source: Bensadoun RJ, Bénézery K, Dassonville O et al (2006) French multicenter phase III randomized study testing concurrent twice-a-day RT and cisplatin/5-FU chemotherapy (BiRCF) in unresectable pharyngeal carcinoma: results at 2 years (FN-CLCC-GORTEC). Int J Radiat Oncol Biol Phys 64:983–094*
[b]*Source: Staar S, Rudat V, Stuetzer H et al (2001) Intensified hyperfractionated accelerated radiotherapy limits the additional benefit of simultaneous chemotherapy--results of a multicentric randomized German trial in advanced head-and-neck cancer. Int J Radiat Oncol Biol Phys 50:1161–1171*

Adjuvant Chemoradiation Therapy

For patients with high-risk SCC of the oral cavity or oropharynx, adjuvant chemoradiation therapy has been studied in Radiation Therapy Oncology Group (RTOG) and European Organization for Research and Treatment of Cancer (EORTC) randomized clinical trials (Figure 3.4; Table 3.15). Both groups showed that the addition of concurrent chemotherapy improved locoregional control and disease-free survival (Table 3.16).

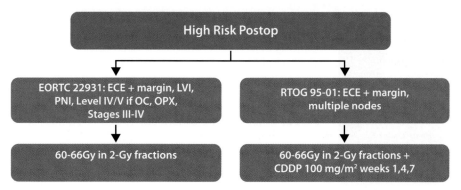

Figure 3.4 Schema of EORTC 22931 and RTOG 95-01 randomized trials. *CDDP* cisplatin, *LVI* lymphovascular invasion, *PNI* perineural invasion, *OC* oral cavity, *OPX* oropharynx

Table 3.15 Characteristics of patients and radiation therapy of RTOG 9501 and EORTC 22931 trials

Parameter	Trial	
	RTOG 9501	EORTC 22931
Patients (*n*)	459	334
Subsites[a] (%)	42%/27%/21%/10%	30%/26%/22%/20%
T3–4 disease (%)	61%	66%
N2–3 disease (%)	94%	57%
With ECE and/or positive margins[b] (%)	59%	70%
Radiation dose of 66 Gy (%)	13%	91%

[a] Disease type: oropharynx/oral cavity/larynx/hypopharynx
[b] Both trials considered ECE and positive surgical margin as high-risk factors

Sources: Cooper JS, Pajak TF, Forastiere AA et al (2004) Postoperative concurrent radiotherapy and chemotherapy for high-risk squamous-cell carcinoma of the head and neck. N Engl J Med 350:1937–1934; Bernier J, Domenge C, Ozsahin M et al (2004) Postoperative irradiation with or without concomitant chemotherapy for locally advanced head and neck cancer. N Engl J Med 350:1945–1952

Table 3.16 Comparison of outcomes from the RTOG 95-01 and EORTC 22931

Outcome	RTOG 9501	EORTC 22931
	3-Year	5-Year
Median follow-up	46 Months	60 Months
LRF	22 versus 33% (*p* = 0.01)	18 versus 31% (*p* = 0.007)
DFS	47 versus 36% (*p* = 0.04)	47 versus 36% (*p* = 0.04)
OS	56 versus 47% (*p* = 0.09)	53 versus 40% (*p* = 0.02)
DM	20 versus 23% (*p* = 0.46)	21 versus 24% (*p* = 0.61)
Grades 3–4 acute toxicities	77 versus 34% (*p* < 0.0001)	44 versus 21% (*p* = 0.001)
All late toxicities	21 versus 17% (*p* = 0.29)	38 versus 41% (*p* = 0.25)

LRF: locoregional failure

Radiation Therapy Techniques

Radiation fields should encompass the tumor bed plus regional lymph nodal areas.

Conventional Radiation Therapy Techniques

Simulation and Field Setup

A shoulder pull-board helps to separate the shoulders from the head to minimize skin folds and to extend the larynx away from the oral cavity/oropharynx. Setup with a thermoplastic mask covering head, neck, and shoulders is illustrated in Chap. 2, Figure 2.10.

Palpable neck disease should be outlined with wire. For tongue cancers, a bite block may be used to depress the tongue down and away from the palate, allowing easier avoidance of the palate and preventing a bolus effect from closure of the mouth. For base-of-tongue cancers, a bite block may be used to push back the tongue to allow sparing of the anterior oral cavity.

Bolus should be considered in postoperatively treated patients to ensure skin coverage. A computed tomography (CT) scan (3-mm cuts) with intravenous (IV) contrast should be performed from the top of head to the upper mediastinum.

Typical Target Volume Delineation and Field Setup

The target volume of the parallel-opposed fields should include the primary with margin plus draining lymph nodes of the upper neck, with a high match above the arytenoids for oropharynx and oral cavity lesions, using a split isocenter technique (Figure 3.5).

Field setup using the conventional technique is detailed in Table 3.17. Attention should be given that the match line does not cut through involved lymph node(s).

Dose and Treatment Delivery

Radiation doses to PTVs of various risk are detailed in Table 3.17.

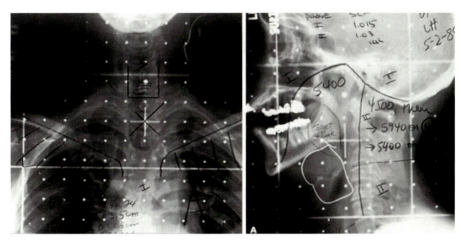

Figure 3.5 2D technique used for definitive treatment of locoregionally advanced tonsillar SCC with left-sided lymphadenopathy (wired). The entire upper neck was first treated to 45 Gy in 25 fractions, then 9 Gy in 5 fractions to the anterior ("off-cord"), using opposed lateral photon fields. The left and right posterior neck electron fields were matched to the anterior off-cord fields and were treated to 59.4 and 54 Gy, respectively. A single anterior lower neck field (with a spinal cord block) was used to treat the lower neck and supraclavicular lymph nodes

Table 3.17 Conventional treatment for oral cavity or oropharyngeal SCC

Field	Borders and doses
Initial opposed lateral fields[a]	■ Superior: skull base ■ Inferior: bottom of hyoid bone and match with lower anterior neck field (half-beam block) ■ Anterior (oral cavity): mentum for oral cavity ■ Anterior (oropharynx): 2 cm behind mentum to cover Ib nodes ■ Posterior: spinous process ■ Dose to 40–45 Gy
Off-cord cone-down lateral fields for elective areas	■ Superior: same as initial portal ■ Inferior: same as initial portal ■ Anterior: same as initial portal ■ Posterior: middle of vertebral bodies[b] ■ Dose to a total of 50–54 Gy with initial opposed lateral fields
Electron post-neck E-strips	■ Use shape of initial photon field involving posterior neck to match with off cord field in the middle of vertebral bodies ■ N⁻ elective: doses of 50–54 Gy ■ N⁺ boost: dose to 70 Gy ▶

Table 3.17 *(continued)*

Field	Borders and doses
Final cone down	■ 2-cm margin to GTV via lateral fields ■ Coverage of nodal station at high risk with electron (en face) or unilateral anterior/posterior(AP)/PA to lower neck ■ T1–2 disease: dose to 66–70 Gy ■ T3–4 disease: dose to 70 Gy ■ Adenopathy: dose to 70 Gy
Low anterior neck field	■ Superior: bottom of hyoid bone and match with upper neck lateral fields (with a spinal cord/vocal cord block) ■ Inferior: inferior edge of the clavicular head ■ Lateral: Two thirds of the clavicle or 2 cm lateral to adenopathy (which ever more lateral)

[a]Retropharyngeal lymph nodes up to the skull base should be covered in oropharyngeal SCC

[b]For posterior pharyngeal wall lesions or retropharyngeal nodes, moving the posterior border from the middle to the posterior edge of the vertebral body improves local control

Postoperative Radiation

Simulation and setup are as described above (Table 3.17). The upper (opposed lateral) and lower (anterior) neck fields should match above the arytenoids for both diseases.

A typical dose and fractionation schedule would be 63–66 Gy to high risk areas, 57.6–59.4 Gy to intermediate regions of the neck (1.8 Gy per fraction), and 50–54 Gy to low-risk areas. The low anterior neck region is treated to a dose of 50 Gy.

The stoma (when present) often is boosted with electrons to 60 Gy.

Ipsilateral Radiation Therapy Technique

The techniques used in a case of early-stage tonsillar SCC treated with ipsilateral radiation alone are presented in Figure 3.6.

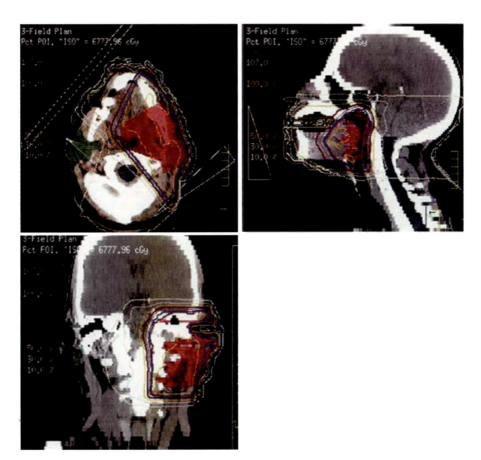

Figure 3.6 A case of lateralized early stage tonsil SCC (T2N0M0) treated with unilateral radiation therapy (three-field plan involved wedged pair) with curative intention. A low-weighted, right anterior oblique field, to help cover the tongue extension without overdosing the spinal cord, was used. The PTV is contoured. The primary site, extension along the soft palate, extension into the base of tongue, upper neck nodes, and retropharyngeal nodes are all included. An axial, sagittal, and coronal dose distribution shows that the PTV is well covered. The salivary gland tissue of the contralateral neck, especially the parotid gland, is well protected

Intensity-Modulated Radiation Therapy

Compared to conventional technique, intensity-modulated radiation therapy (IMRT) presents the opportunity to minimize dose to the normal organs at risk (OAR) – salivary glands, constrictor muscles, cochlea, visual pathways and pterygoid muscles – with superior conformality around the tumor bed and nodal drainage areas.

The clinical outcomes of selected series on IMRT for oral/oropharyngeal SCC are presented in Table 3.18. IMRT should be considered particularly for tumors near the spinal cord (e.g., posterior pharyngeal wall tumor) or for those where significant parotid sparing can be attained (e.g., patients with negative contralateral neck nodes).

Table 3.18 Treatment outcome of selected series of oropharyngeal SCC treated with IMRT

Series	Patient no. (%)[a]	Median follow-up (months)	LRC
Chao et al[b]	52 (54%)	26	79%
RTOG 0022[c]	133 (60%)	32	84%
Yao et al[d]	90 (71%)	29	96% (LC)
De Arruda et al[e]	48 (100%)	18	98% (LC)
Lawson et al[f]	34 (100% base of tongue)	20	90% (LC)

LRC: locoregional control

[a]Percentage of oropharyngeal SCC

[b] *Source: Chao KS, Ozyigit G, Blanco AI et al (2004) IMRT for oropharyngeal carcinoma: impact of tumor volume. Int J Radiat Oncol Biol Phys 59:43–50*

[c] *Source: Eisbruch A, Harris J, Garden AS et al (2010) Multi-institutional trial of accelerated hypofractionated IMRT for early-stage oropharyngeal cancer. Int J Radiat Oncol Biol Phys 7:1333–1338*

[d]*Source: Yao M, Dornfeld KJ, Buatti JM et al (2005) IMRT for head-and-neck SCC – the University of Iowa experience. Int J Radiat Oncol Biol Phys 63:410–421*

[e] *Source: de Arruda FF, Puri DR, Zhung J et al (2006) IMRT for the treatment of oropharyngeal carcinoma: the Memorial Sloan-Kettering Cancer Center experience. Int J Radiat Oncol Biol Phys 64:363–373*

[f] *Source: Lawson JD, Otto K, Chen A et al (2008) Concurrent platinum-based chemotherapy and simultaneous modulated accelerated RT for locally advanced SCC of the tongue base. Head Neck 30:327–335*

Simulation and Target Volume Delineation

The patient should be immobilized and the neck extended as described above. Positron-emission tomography (PET)/CT or magnetic resonance (MRI) can be fused with the treatment-planning CT to help in gross target volume (GTV) delineation. High-risk clinical target volumes (CTV) for areas of gross disease are to be outlined as well as intermediate- and/or low -risk CTV. OAR should be delineated. Dose objectives and tolerance should then be declared.

An isocenter should be selected to treat the primary and upper neck nodes for oropharyngeal cancers, with a lower border matched to a low anterior neck field (either above or below arytenoids depends on nodal status) to treat the lower cervical and supraclavicular node.

However, an extended single field treating the primary and all regional nodes should be considered for patients with extensive lymphadenopathy involving multiple nodal levels.

Definitions of target volumes are detailed in Table 3.19.

Table 3.19 General definitions of target volumes in the treatment of oral and oropharyngeal SCC

Target volumes	Definitions
GTV	■ Gross tumor on imaging studies
CTV	■ High risk: GTV ■ Intermediate risk: areas with high likelihood of nodal disease or tumor spread ■ Low risk: elective nodal treatment
PTV	■ CTV plus 3–5 mm

Care must be taken not to underdose regional nodes near the parotid as well as to evaluate dose at the match line (if used). If a patient has a clinically negative neck, the superior border of regional node delineation can end at the bottom of the C1 transverse process, sparing significant parotid tissue.

Sources: Grégoire V, Coche E, Cosnard G et al (2000) Selection and delineation of lymph node target volumes in head and neck conformal radiotherapy. Proposal for standardizing terminology and procedure based on the surgical experience. Radiother Oncol 56:135-150; Grégoire V, Levendag P, Ang KK et al (2003) CT-based delineation of lymph node levels and related CTVs in the node-negative neck: DAHANCA, EORTC, GORTEC, NCIC,RTOG consensus guidelines. Radiother Oncol 69:227-236

Dose Recommendations and Treatment Delivery

A total dose of 66–70 Gy in 30–33 fractions using simultaneous integrated boost (SIB) technique with 7–14 coplanar fields can be used according to the shape of PTV:
■ High-risk PTV: 70 Gy to high-risk CTV
■ Intermediate-risk PTV: 59.4 Gy
■ Low-risk elective PTV: 50–54 Gy

The RTOG oropharyngeal cancer treatment protocol (without concurrent chemotherapy) with the SIB technique recommends the following schedule over 30 fractions:
■ High-risk PTV: 66 Gy to high-risk CTV
■ Intermediate-risk PTV: 60 Gy
■ Low-risk elective PTV: 54 Gy

Dose Constraints

Prescription isodose should cover at least 95% of the planned target volume (PTV); no more than 20% should receive >110% of the prescribed dose; no more than 1% should receive <93% of the prescribed dose; no more than 1% of normal tissues outside the PTV should receive >110% the prescribed dose. The dose constraints for OARs are detailed in Chap. 6, Table 6.13.

Sample IMRT plans and dose–volume histograms for treatment of oropharyngeal cancer (base of tongue) are illustrated in Figures 3.7 (both cases treated to ~60 Gy with IMRT, followed by brachytherapy boost).

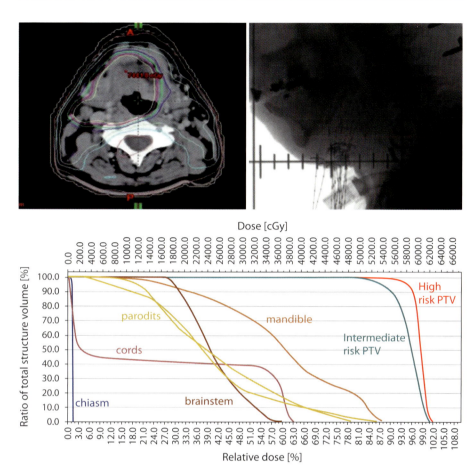

Figure 3.7 Example of 62-year-old male patient with a T2N2bM0 base-of-tongue carcinoma treated with combined EBRT and concurrent chemotherapy, brachytherapy implant, and planned neck dissection. EBRT was delivered with IMRT with a reduced dose of 59.4 Gy to the involved primary site and nodes, followed by 20-Gy brachytherapy boost. The bottom of the figure presents the dose–volume histogram demonstrating dose distribution from the IMRT course

Normal Tissue Tolerance

Normal OAR in radiation therapy in oral cavity and oropharynx cancer, in both adjuvant and definitive settings, include parotid, mandible, constrictors, brachial plexus, and spinal cord. The dose constraints of the OARS are detailed in Chap. 6, Table 6.13.

Follow-Up

Close follow-up of patients is required especially during the first 2 years of treatment, during which locoregional failure is most likely to occur.

Suggested follow-up schedules and examinations are illustrated in Table 3.20.

Table 3.20 Follow-up schedule and examinations

Schedule	Frequency
First follow-up	■ 1–2 weeks after radiation therapy
Years 0–1	■ Every 1–2 months
Years 2–3	■ Every 2–3 months
Years 4–5	■ Every 4–6 months
Years 5+	■ Annually
Examinations	
History and physical	■ Complete history and physical examination ■ Flexible endoscopy ■ Indirect mirror examination
Laboratory tests	■ TSH every 6 months the first 3 years, then annually
Imaging studies	■ PET/CT at 3 months after definitive treatment, then 3–6 months the first year ■ CT of the neck every 3–6 months, years 1–2, then annually ■ CT of the chest or chest x-ray annually during the first 5 years

Source: Hu K, Harrison L (2008) Cancer of oral cavity and oropharynx. In: JJ Lu, LW Brady (eds) Radiation oncology: an evidence-based approach. Springer, Berlin Heidelberg New York

Prevention of chronic toxicities such as dental caries, neck fibrosis, trismus, and swallowing dysfunction is important during this time.

Of those who are cured of oral or oropharyngeal cancer, 10–20% will develop a secondary primary tumor (SPT) in the aerodigestive track. The risk of developed a SPT may be decreased by half if patients cease smoking or consuming alcohol.

4

Cancer of the Major Salivary Glands

Hiram Gay[1] and Surjeet Pohar[2]

Key Points

- Salivary malignancies are rare and make up less than 0.3% of all malignancies and 6% of head and neck cancers.

- About 60–70% of the total stimulated salivary production is derived from the parotids.

- Approximately 80% of all salivary gland neoplasms originate in the parotid gland.

- Primary salivary gland tumors are a morphologically diverse group of tumors.

- There are prognostic indices for predicting the risk of lymph node involvement in salivary gland tumors.

- Signs and symptoms of salivary gland cancer depend on the location of the primary tumor.

- Prognostic factors for overall survival include T classification, skin invasion, bone invasion, sex, and age.

- For locoregional control, several studies have shown tumor size (pathologic T stage), pathologic N stage, tumor grade (high versus not high), use of adjuvant radiotherapy, bone invasion, and close or positive margins to be significant.

- Surgery remains the mainstay of diagnosis and treatment.

- Radiotherapy has a key role in preventing locoregional recurrences in high-risk patients.

- In inoperable and recurrent tumors, fast neutron therapy has shown higher rates of local control, as compared with photon therapy in retrospective and prospective studies.

[1] Hiram Gay, MD (✉)
Email: hgay@radonc.wustl.edu

[2] Surjeet Pohar, MD
Email: spohar@netzero.net

J. J. Lu, L. W. Brady (Eds.), *Decision Making in Radiation Oncology*
DOI: 10.1007/978-3-642-13832-4_5, © Springer-Verlag Berlin Heidelberg 2010

Epidemiology and Etiology

Salivary malignancies are rare and involve less than 0.3% of all malignancies, and 6% of head and neck cancers. The age-adjusted incidence rate for 2006 was 1.4 per 100,000 in the Surveillance, Epidemiology, and End Results (SEER) Program US database. In Western countries, approximately 65% of all salivary gland tumors are benign, and 35% are malignant. The international variation in the incidence of salivary gland carcinoma is relatively small, and the incidence rate has remained stable from 1992 to 2006. Approximately 80% of all salivary gland neoplasms originate in the parotid gland.

A number of risk factors have been identified for salivary gland cancer (Table 4.1). However, screening in high-risk populations is not supported by clinical evidence.

Table 4.1 Risk factors for salivary gland cancer

Stage	Description
Patient-related	**Age and gender:** The male-to-female ratio for malignant salivary gland tumors is 0.6. The average ages of presentation for mucoepidermoid carcinoma, adenoid cystic carcinoma, and polymorphous low-grade adenocarcinoma are 49, 59, and 61 years, respectively
	Lifestyle: Cigarette smoking has a strong association with Warthin's tumor, a benign tumor of the parotid gland
	Occupational: Hairdressers, rubber manufacturing, exposure to metal in the plumbing industry and nickel compounds, and woodworking in the automobile industry
	Ethnic: Inuit men and women have the highest incidence rate of salivary gland cancer in the world, primarily from an excess of lymphoepithelial carcinomas
Environmental	**Ionizing radiation (including ^{131}I):** risk factor mostly for mucoepidermoid carcinomas and Warthin's tumors. An increased risk has also been observed for adenocarcinomas among Hodgkin lymphoma survivors. Risk increases as the radiation exposure age decreases
	Epstein-Barr virus: lymphoepithelial carcinomas

Anatomy

The major salivary glands are the parotid, submandibular, and sublingual (Figures 4.1, 4.2, and 4.3; Table 4.2). Major salivary gland malignancies originate in the parotid gland, submandibular, and sublingual glands about 80, 15, and 5% of the time, respectively.

Resting (unstimulated) salivary production is done primarily by the submandibular, sublingual, and minor salivary glands. About 60–70% of the total stimulated salivary production is derived from the parotids.

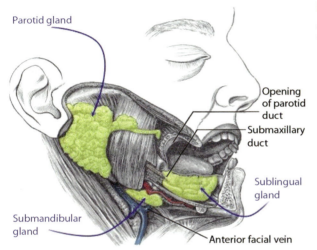

Figure 4.1 Major salivary glands: parotid, submandibular, and sublingual

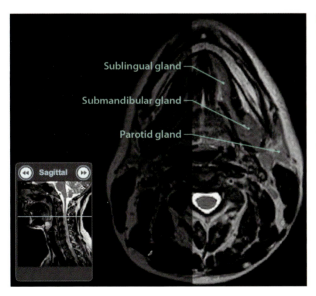

Figure 4.2 MRI axial view of the major salivary glands: parotid, submandibular, and sublingual. Sagittal image shows level of the axial slice

Source: Micheau A, Hoa D. e-Anatomy (http://www.imaios.com)

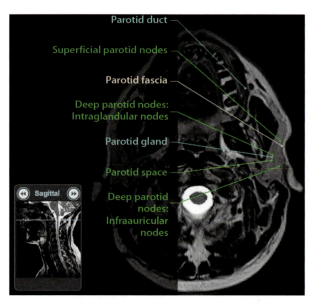

Figure 4.3 MRI axial view of the parotid gland. Note the opening of the parotid duct lateral to the second molar. The sagittal image shows the level of the axial slice

Source: Micheau A, Hoa D. e-Anatomy (http://www.imaios.com)

Table 4.2 Characteristics of major salivary glands

Stage	Description
Parotid	■ Each paired gland occupies the gap between the ramus of the mandible and the styloid process of the temporal bone, and has an irregular shape ■ The largest of the three major salivary glands ■ Each parotid gland drains into the oral cavity through Stensen's duct, which is about 7 cm long, and opens opposite the second upper molar tooth (Figure 4.3) ■ Major structures within the gland: facial, great auricular, and auriculotemporal nerves; external carotid artery and terminal branches, posterior facial vein; and lymph nodes, which number from 1 to more than 20 ■ The gland is almost purely serous
Submandibular	■ Lie along the body of the mandible ■ Each paired submandibular gland drains into the oral cavity through Wharton's duct, which is about 5 cm long ■ The gland is mixed serous (~90%) and mucus
Sublingual	■ Each paired, almond-shaped gland lies between the mandible and the genioglossus muscle in the floor of the mouth ■ The smallest and most deeply situated major salivary gland ■ Each sublingual gland has 8–20 excretory ducts that either drain directly into the oral cavity or eventually join Wharton's duct ■ The gland is mixed, but predominantly mucus in type

Pathology

Primary salivary gland tumors are a morphologically diverse group of tumors. The World Health Organization (WHO) 2005 classification of parotid cancers lists 24 malignant epithelial histopathological classifications (Table 4.3). About 25% of parotid, 40% of submandibular, and 75% of sublingual gland tumors are malignant.

Table 4.3 WHO 2005 classification of malignant salivary epithelial tumors

Tumor type	Tumor type
Mucoepidermoid carcinoma	Polymorphous low-grade adenocarcinoma
Adenoid cystic carcinoma	Carcinoma ex pleomorphic adenoma
Acinic cell carcinoma	Adenocarcinoma, not otherwise specified
Cystadenocarcinoma	Epithelial–myoepithelial carcinom
Basal cell adenocarcinoma	Clear cell carcinoma, not otherwise specified
Myoepithelial carcinoma	Lymphoepithelial carcinoma
Salivary duct carcinoma	Low-grade cribriform cystadenocarcinoma
Mucinous adenocarcinoma	Sebaceous lymphadenocarcinoma
Squamous cell carcinoma	Metastasizing pleomorphic adenoma
Small cell carcinoma	Sebaceous carcinoma
Large cell carcinoma	Oncocytic carcinoma
Carcinosarcoma	Sialoblastoma

The biologic behavior varies among the different classifications, with some having higher incidences of perineural invasion.

In the UK, mucoepidermoid carcinoma is the most common malignant diagnosis (33%), followed by adenoid cystic carcinoma (24%), polymorphous low-grade adenocarcinoma (11%), carcinoma ex pleomorphic adenoma (9%), acinic cell carcinoma (7%), and adenocarcinoma not otherwise specified (5%).

Malignant lymphoma and metastatic disease represent about 9% of major salivary gland tumors. The primary diagnosis of squamous cell carcinoma of the parotid gland is rare. However, skin cancer frequently metastasizes to the parotid.

Routes of Spread

Local extension, perineural spread, regional (lymphatic) and distant (hematogenous) metastases are the four major routes of spread in salivary cancer (Table 4.4).

Table 4.4 Routes of spread in salivary gland cancer

Stage	Description

Local extension	■ Parotid tumors :
	   ■ Direct involvement of the parotid gland, facial, or auriculotemporal nerve
	   ■ Deep-lobe tumors invade the parapharyngeal space and base of the skull, and compromise cranial nerves
	 ■ Direct extension to the skin, bone, and muscles

Regional lymph node metastases	■ Lymph node involvement as shown in Figure 4.4 and predicted in Table 4.4 ■ Lymphatic drainage depends on the origin of the primary disease ■ Squamous cell carcinoma arising in the auricle has about a 10% metastatic rate to the parotid and deep cervical chain
Distant metastases	■ Depends on histologic type ■ Mucoepidermoid tumor: tends to metastasize to lung, liver, bone, and brain ■ Adenoid cystic carcinoma has 25–55% rates of distant metastases to lung, bone, brain, and liver ■ Carcinoma ex pleomorphic adenoma can spread to lung, bone (spine), abdomen, and central nervous system ■ Acinic cell tends to spread to lung ■ Polymorphous low-grade adenocarcinomas rarely metastasize

Lymph Node Metastasis

Figure 4.4 shows the percent risk of levels I–V positive neck nodes according to tumor site. Table 4.5 aids in predicting the risk of nodal metastases based on T stage, histological type, and location of the primary tumor. There is also a prognostic index for predicting lymph node metastases in minor salivary gland cancer. *(Source: Lloyd S, Yu JB, Ross DA et al (2010) A prognostic index for predicting lymph node metastasis in minor salivary gland cancer. Int J Radiat Oncol Biol Phys 76:169–175).*

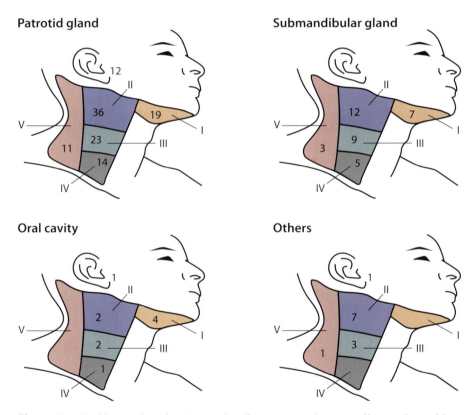

Figure 4.4 Positive neck nodes (percent) at first presentation according to site and level (I–V).

Source: Terhaard CHJ, Lubsen H, Rasch CRN et al (2005) The role of radiotherapy in the treatment of malignant salivary gland tumors. Int J Radiat Oncol Biol Phys 61:103– 111 (Figure 1 in original article). Used with permission from Elsevier Science, Inc.

Table 4.5 Risk of positive neck nodes according to summation of scores and site

Summation: T score[a] plus histological type score[b]	Parotid gland (%)	Submandibular gland (%)	Oral cavity (%)	Other locations (%)
2	4%	0%	4%	0%
3	12%	33%	13%	29%
4	25%	57%	19%	56%
5	33%	60%	–	–
6	38%	50%	–	–

[a]T score: T1 = 1, T2 = 2, T3–4 = 3

[b]Histological type score: acinic/adenoid cystic/carcinoma ex pleomorphic adenoma = 1, mucoepidermoid carcinoma = 2, squamous cell/undifferentiated carcinoma = 3

Source: Terhaard CHJ, Lubsen H, Rasch CRN et al (2005) The role of radiotherapy in the treatment of malignant salivary gland tumors. Int J Radiat Oncol Biol Phys 61:103–111 (cited as Table 4 in original article). Used with permission from Elsevier Science, Inc.

Diagnosis, Staging, and Prognosis

Clinical Presentation

Stage distribution was localized, regional, and distant in 45, 31, and 16% of patients, respectively, according to the 2000–2006 US SEER database.

Signs and symptoms of salivary gland cancer depend on the location of the primary tumor. Commonly observed symptoms include an asymptomatic mass in the gland; other symptoms are detailed in Table 4.6.

Table 4.6 Commonly observed signs and symptoms of salivary gland cancer

Stage	Description
Mucoepidermoid carcinoma	■ Solitary, firm, fixed mass ■ Pain, otorrhea, paraesthesia, dysphagia, trismus, facial paralysis, and bleeding may occur
Adenoid cystic	■ Slow-growing mass ■ Pain and facial paresthesia develop frequently because of a high incidence of nerve invasion
Polymorphous low-grade adenocarcinoma	■ Firm, painless swelling involving the mucosa of the hard and soft palates (is often found at their junction) ■ Discomfort, bleeding, telangiectasia, or ulceration of the overlying mucosa may occasionally occur
Carcinoma ex pleomorphic adenoma	■ Painless, long-standing mass, with rapid growth over the prior months ■ 1/3 of patients may experience facial paralysis ■ Pain and skin fixation may occur
Acinic cell carcinoma	■ Slow-growing, mobile mass in the parotid gland ■ 1/3 experience vague and intermittent pain ■ 5–10% experience facial paralysis
Adenocarcinoma NOS	■ Solitary, painless mass ■ 20% experience pain and facial weakness

Diagnosis and Staging

Figure 4.5 illustrates the diagnostic procedures of salivary cancer, including suggested examination and tests.

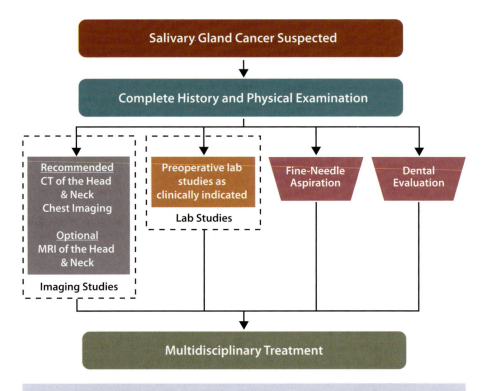

Figure 4.5 A proposed algorithm for diagnosis and staging salivary gland cancer

Tumor, Node, and Metastasis Staging

Diagnosis and clinical staging depends on findings from history and physical examination, imaging, and lab tests. Pathological staging depends on findings during surgical resection and pathological examination, in addition to those required in clinical staging.

The 7th edition of the tumor, node, and metastasis (TNM) staging system and groupings of the American Joint Committee on Cancer (AJCC) for malignant tumors of the major salivary glands is presented in Tables 4.7 and 4.8.

Table 4.7 AJCC TNM classification of malignant tumors of the major salivary glands

Stage	Description
Primary tumor (T)	
TX	Primary tumor cannot be assessed
T0	No evidence of primary tumor
T1	Tumor ≤2 cm in greatest dimension without extraparenchymal extension (i.e., clinical or macroscopic evidence of soft tissue invasion)
T2	Tumor >2 cm but ≤4 cm in greatest dimension without extraparenchymal extension
T3	Tumor >4 cm in greatest dimension and/or extraparenchymal extension
T4a	Moderately advanced disease: Tumor invades skin, mandible, ear canal, and/or facial nerve
T4b	Very advanced disease: Tumor invades skull base and/or pterygoid plates and/or encases carotid artery
Regional lymph nodes (N)	
NX	Regional lymph nodes cannot be assessed
N0	No regional lymph node metastasis
N1	Metastasis in a single ipsilateral lymph node, ≤3 cm in greatest dimension
N2a	Metastasis in a single ipsilateral lymph node, >3 cm but ≤6 cm in greatest dimension
N2b	Metastasis in multiple ipsilateral lymph nodes, none >6 cm in greatest dimension
N2c	Metastasis in bilateral or contralateral lymph nodes, none >6 cm in greatest dimension
N3	Metastasis in a lymph node, >6 cm in greatest dimension
Distant metastasis (M)	
M0	No distant metastasis
M1	Distant metastasis

Source: Edge SB, Byrd DR, Compton CC et al (2009) American Joint Committee on Cancer, American Cancer Society. AJCC cancer staging manual, 7th edn. Springer, Berlin Heidelberg New York

Table 4.8 Stage grouping of malignant tumors of the major salivary glands

Stage Grouping					
	T1	T2	T3	T4a	T4b
N0	I	II	III	IVA	IVB
N1	III	III	III	IVA	IVB
N2	IVA	IVA	IVA	IVA	IVB
N3	IVB	IVB	IVB	IVB	IVB
M1	IVC	IVC	IVC	IVC	IVC

Source: Edge SB, Byrd DR, Compton CC et al (2009) American Joint Committee on Cancer, American Cancer Society. AJCC cancer staging manual, 7th edn. Springer, Berlin Heidelberg New York

Prognoses

Prognostic factors for overall survival include T classification, skin invasion, bone invasion, sex, and age (Table 4.9). In the SEER US database, the 5-year overall survival from 1999 to 2005 for this heterogeneous group of tumors was 73.9%.

For locoregional control, several studies have shown tumor size (pathologic T classification), pathologic N classification, site, tumor grade (high versus not high), use of adjuvant radiation therapy (RT), bone invasion, and close or positive margins to be significant.

Table 4.9 Overall survival according to treatment, based on retrospective series

Years	Localized disease	
	Surgery (%)	Surgery plus RT (%)
5	55–77%	55–78%
10	47–63%	40–67%

Treatment

Principles and Practice

Surgery remains the mainstay of diagnosis and treatment (Table 4.10). However, radiotherapy plays a key role in preventing locoregional recurrence in
high-risk patients. There is little evidence regarding the use of chemotherapy
in salivary gland tumors.

Table 4.10 Treatment modalities used in salivary gland cancer

Stage	Description
Surgery	

Indications	■ Treatment of choice that provides valuable pathologic information
	■ For parotid tumors, surgical options include total and superficial parotidectomy:
	  ■ Total parotidectomy is performed if the deep lobe is involved
	  ■ Superficial parotidectomy is usually feasible in T1–T2 superficial parotid lobe tumors without facial nerve invasion

Facts	■ Temporary facial palsy after parotid surgery varies between 10 and 65%, recovery may take months, and permanent paralysis is usually <3% ■ Current thought is that the facial nerve should be preserved unless it is grossly involved with tumor
RT	
Indications	■ Adjuvant treatment in high-risk patients ■ Definitive treatment only in unresectable patients ■ Palliative treatment to primary or metastatic foci
Techniques	■ Photon RT using 3D-CRT or IMRT ■ Fast neutron radiotherapy
Chemo-/targeted therapy	
Indication	■ Metastatic disease
Medications	■ CAP regimen: **c**yclophosphamide (500 mg/m^2), doxorubicin (Adriamycin; 50 mg/m$^2)$, and cisplatin (Platinol; 50 mg/m^2) on first day of a 28-day regimen ■ Paclitaxel 200 mg/m^2 every 21 days (**no response in adenoid cystic carcinoma**) ■ Targeted therapy may prove useful in the future as some histologies express EGFR, C-kit, and/or HER-2

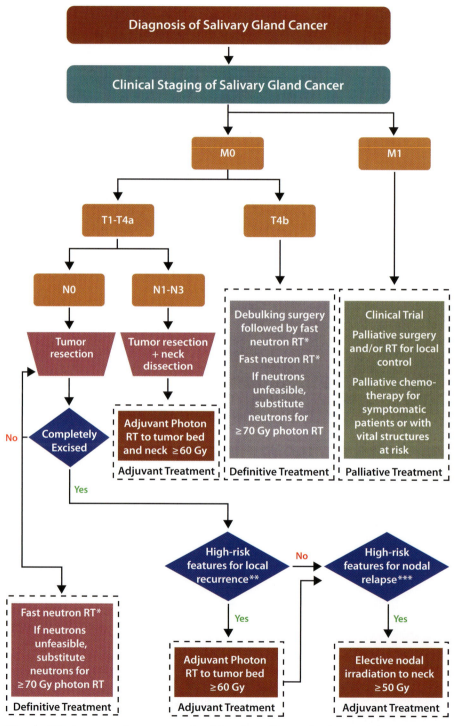

Figure 4.6 A proposed treatment algorithm for salivary gland cancer (*see next page for comments*)

*   Histologic types where neutron therapy is appropriate include squamous cell carcinoma, adenoid cystic carcinoma, mucoepidermoid carcinoma, adenocarcinoma NOS, and acinic cell carcinoma

**   High-risk features for local recurrence include T3–T4, <5 mm margins, incomplete resection, bone invasion, perineural invasion, major nerve involvement, highhistologic grade/intermediate-grade mucoepidermoid, and pathologic lymph node metastases. Retrospective evidence supports adjuvant treatment for adenoid cystic carcinoma and carcinoma ex pleomorphic adenoma, based on histology alone. Histologic types with a higher propensity for perineural invasion include adenoid cystic carcinoma, polymorhous low-grade adenocarcinoma, epithelial–myoepithelial carcinoma, squamous cell carcinoma, large cell carcinoma, and basal cell adenocarcinoma

*** High-risk features for nodal relapse in the clinical N0 neck include squamous cell carcinoma, undifferentiated carcinoma, adenocarcinoma, mucoepidermoid carcinoma (especially intermediate and high grade), tumors >4 cm in size, and high-grade tumors. Table 4.4 can also be used to estimate the risk of nodal relapse based on T stage, histological type, and tumor location. Adenoid cystic and acinic cell usually have a low risk of nodal failure

Figure 4.6 presents proposed treatments based on the best available clinical evidence.

Adjuvant Treatment

Clinical evidence for adjuvant (meaning postoperative) malignant salivary gland tumor RT is presented and illustrated in Table 4.11.

Table 4.11 Treatment strategies for adjuvant malignant salivary gland tumor RT, and supporting clinical evidence

Retrospective study	Description

Dutch Head and Neck Cooperative Group (NWHHT)[a]	■ Retrospective analysis of 538 patients: 386 surgery plus adjuvant RT, 112 surgery alone, 40 definitive RT
	■ Adjuvant RT improved 10-year local control significantly, as compared with surgery alone in:
	  ■ T3–T4 tumors (84 versus 18%)
	  ■ Close (<5 mm) resection (95 versus 55%)
	  ■ Incomplete resection (82 versus 44%)
	  ■ Bone invasion (86 versus 54%)
	  ■ Perineural invasion (88 versus 60%)
	■ Adjuvant RT significantly improved the regional control in the pathologically N+ (pN+) neck (86 versus 62% for surgery alone). A marginal dose–response was seen, in favor of a dose >46 Gy
	■ Definitive RT showed a clear dose–response relationship. Five-year local control was 50% with a dose of 66–70 Gy

University of California, San Francisco (UCSF)[b]	■ Retrospective analysis of 207 patients treated with surgery alone
	■ 5- and 10-year estimates of locoregional control were 86 and 74%, respectively
	■ A Cox proportional hazard model identified the following predictors of locoregional recurrence:
	  ■ Pathologic lymph node metastasis (hazard ratio [HR] of 4.8, $p = 0.001$)
	  ■ High histologic grade (HR of 4.2, $p = 0.003$)
	  ■ Positive margins (HR of 2.6, $p = 0.3$)
	  ■ T3–T4 disease (HR of 2.0; $p = 0.04$)
	■ Authors conclude adjuvant RT should be considered for patients with the above characteristics

Table 4.11 *(continued)*

Retrospective study	Description
University of Florida[c]	■ Retrospective analysis of 101 patients with **adenoid cystic carcinoma** of the head and neck treated with RT, or surgery plus adjuvant RT ■ 5- and 10-year rates of local control were RT alone, 56 and 43%; surgery plus adjuvant RT, 94 and 91% ■ T stage ($p = 0.0101$) and treatment group ($p = 0.0008$) significantly influenced local control ■ Authors conclude the optimal treatment for patients with adenoid cystic carcinoma is surgery plus adjuvant RT

UCSF[d]	■ Retrospective analysis of 140 patients with **adenoid cystic carcinoma** of the head and neck treated with surgery or surgery plus adjuvant RT
	
	■ A Cox proportional hazards model identified these independent predictors of local recurrence:
	  ■ T4 disease ($p = 0.0001$)
	  ■ Perineural invasion ($p = 0.008$)
	  ■ Omission of adjuvant RT ($p = 0.007$)
	  ■ Major nerve involvement ($p = 0.02$)

UCSF[e]	■ Retrospective analysis of 63 patients treated with definitive surgery ± adjuvant RT for **carcinoma ex pleomorphic adenoma** of the parotid gland ■ Adjuvant RT significantly improved the 5-year local control from 49 to 75% ($p = 0.005$) and survival among patients without evidence of cervical lymph node metastasis ($p = 0.01$) ■ Authors conclude surgery succeeded by adjuvant RT should be considered the standard of care for patients with carcinoma ex pleomorphic adenoma

[a]*Source: Terhaard CHJ, Lubsen H, Rasch CRN et al (2005) The role of radiotherapy in the treatment of malignant salivary gland tumors. Int J Radiat Oncol Biol Phys 61:103–111*
[b]*Source: Chen AM, Granchi PJ, Garcia J et al (2007) Local-regional recurrence after surgery without postoperative irradiation for carcinomas of the major salivary glands: implications for adjuvant therapy. Int J Radiat Oncol Biol Phys 67:982–987*
[c]*Source: Mendenhall WM, Morris CG, Amdur RJ et al (2004) Radiotherapy alone or combined with surgery for adenoid cystic carcinoma of the head and neck. Head Neck 26:154–162*
[d]*Source: Chen AM, Bucci MK, Weinberg V et al (2006) Adenoid cystic carcinoma of the head and neck treated by surgery with or without postoperative radiation therapy: prognostic features of recurrence. Int J Radiat Oncol Biol Phys 66:152–159*
[e]*Source: Chen AM, Garcia J, Bucci MK et al (2007) The role of postoperative radiation therapy in carcinoma ex pleomorphic adenoma of the parotid gland. Int J Radiat Oncol Biol Phys 67:138–143*

Definitive Treatment

Definitive RT should only be pursued in unresectable cases, patients unfit for surgery, or when the patient refuses surgery. The local control rate of malignant parotid tumors with photon RT alone is ~30%, and with fast neutron therapy is ~60%. Clinical evidence for definitive malignant salivary gland tumor RT is presented in Table 4.12. Fast neutron therapy has demonstrated higher rates of local control, as compared with photon therapy in both retrospective studies (Table 4.12; the prospective Radiation Therapy Oncology Group (RTOG)–Medical Research Council (MRC) Cooperative Randomized Study, discussed below). The increased risk of complications with neutron therapy, lack of availability, and failure to demonstrate a survival benefit (partly due to a distant pattern of failure) have hindered its success despite its superior local control over photons.

Table 4.12 Treatment strategies for definitive malignant salivary gland tumor RT and supporting clinical evidence

Retrospective study	Description
University of Washington[a]	■ Retrospective analysis of 279 patients treated with curative-intent fast neutron RT ■ 6-year actuarial locoregional control rate was 59% ■ Statistically significant improved locoregional control for tumor size ≤4 cm, lack of base of skull invasion, prior surgical resection, and no previous RT ■ The 6-year actuarial rate of development of grade 3 or 4 long-term toxicity was 10%
Huber et al[b]	■ Retrospective analysis of 75 patients with inoperable, recurrent, or incompletely resected **adenoid cystic carcinoma** treated with neutrons, photons, or both ■ 5-year local control was 75% for neutrons, and 32% for both mixed beam and photon ■ The local control advantage for neutrons did not result in improved survival, due to distant metastases occurring in 39% of patients ■ Severe late-grade 3 and 4 toxicity tended to be more prevalent with neutrons (19%) than with mixed beam (10%) and photons (4%)

[a] *Source: Douglas JG, Koh WJ, Austin-Seymour M et al (2003) Treatment of salivary gland neoplasms with fast neutron radiotherapy. Arch Otolaryngol Head Neck Surg 129:944–948*
[b] *Source: Huber PE, Debus J, Latz D et al (2001) Radiotherapy for advanced adenoid cystic carcinoma: neutrons, photons or mixed beam? Radiother Oncol 59:161–167*

Elective Neck Irradiation

Elective neck irradiation (ENI) effectively prevents nodal relapses and it should be used for select patients at high risk for regional failure. Clinical evidence for ENI in malignant salivary gland tumors is presented and illustrated in Table 4.13. (Table 4.5 and Figure 4.4 are useful in planning and determining the necessity of ENI.)

Table 4.13 Treatment strategies for ENI in malignant salivary gland tumors and supporting clinical evidence

Retrospective study	Description

UCSF	■ Retrospective analysis of 251 patients with clinically N0 carcinomas of the salivary glands treated with surgery (58%) or surgery plus RT (42%)
	 ■ Median dose to the neck was 50 Gy (range of 40 to 66 Gy), with 15% receiving 60 Gy or more
	 ■ 69% received ipsilateral and 31% received bilateral RT
	 ■ The use of ENI reduced the 10-year nodal failure rate from 26 to 0% ($p = 0.0001$)
	 ■ The highest crude rates of nodal relapse among those treated without ENI were found in patients with:
	   ■ Squamous cell carcinoma (67%)
	   ■ Undifferentiated carcinoma (50%)
	   ■ Adenocarcinoma (34%)
	   ■ Mucoepidermoid carcinoma (29%)
	 ■ No nodal failures were observed among patients with adenoid cystic or acinic cell histology with or without ENI

Source: Chen AM, Garcia J, Lee NY et al (2007) Patterns of nodal relapse after surgery and postoperative radiation therapy for carcinomas of the major and minor salivary glands: what is the role of elective neck irradiation? Int J Radiat Oncol Biol Phys 67:988–994

Treatment of Inoperable Primary or Recurrent Malignant Salivary Gland Tumors

Based on the RTOG–MRC randomized controlled trial, fast neutron radiotherapy appears to be the treatment of choice for patients with inoperable primary of recurrent malignant salivary gland tumors (Table 4.14).

Table 4.14 Clinical evidence for the treatment of inoperable primary or recurrent salivary gland tumors

Trial	Description
RTOG–MRC cooperative randomized study	■ Randomized 17 patients to receive neutrons and 15 to receive photons
	■ Photon/electron control arm received 70 Gy/7.5 weeks or 55 Gy/4 weeks
	■ Neutron arm received 16.5–22 Gy_{ny} in 12 fractions over 4 weeks
	■ At 10 years, there was a significant improvement in locoregional control for neutrons versus the control arm (56 versus 17%). No significant improvement in overall survival (15 versus 25%)
	■ Authors concluded fast neutron radiotherapy appears to be the treatment of choice for patients with inoperable primary of recurrent malignant salivary gland tumors

Source: Laramore GE, Krall JM, Griffin TW et al (1993) Neutron versus photon irradiation for unresectable salivary gland tumors: final report of an RTOG–MRC randomized clinical trial. Radiation Therapy Oncology Group, Medical Research Council. Int J Radiat Oncol Biol Phys 27:235–240

Metastatic Salivary Gland Cancer

Even in the setting of metastatic disease, achieving local control with surgical and/or radiation techniques could positively affect a patient's quality of life. Palliative chemotherapy should be reserved for patients with progressive disease that is causing symptoms or threatening vital structures. The objective response rates to chemotherapy are modest, ranging from 15 to 50%, and lasting from 6 to 9 months.

The CAP regimen – which entails cyclophosphamide (500 mg/m^2), doxorubicin (Adriamycin; 50 mg/m^2), and cisplatin (Platinol; 50 mg/m^2) on the first day of a 28-day regimen – is one of the multidrug regimens with higher activities. Paclitaxel (no response in adenoid cystic carcinoma), vinorelbine, and mitoxantrone are reasonable choices as single agents.

Radiation Therapy Techniques

Simulation

Patients must have an immobilization device (e.g., Aquaplast mask) made prior to a treatment-planning computed tomography (CT) scan. The treatment-planning CT scan should be performed with intravenous (i.v.) contrast so that the major vessels of the neck are easily visualized. CT slice thickness should be 0.3 cm. Organs at risk (OARs) (listed in Table 4.15) should be delineated.

Table 4.15 Radiotherapy indications, targets, and dose for parotid gland malignancies

Indication(s)	Target(s)	Dose(s)[a]
Adjuvant, tumor bed[b]	Superior: zygomatic arch or higher Anterior: anterior edge of masseter muscle Inferior: thyroid notch Posterior: behind mastoid process Lateral: 3 mm beneath skin Medial: oral cavity	Photons: ≥60 Gy Suggest: – margins: 60 Gy + margins: 66 Gy
Adjuvant, nodes[b]	Levels I, II, and III Any other levels involved based on pathology or imaging Consider covering levels IV and/or V if four or more lymph nodes are positive Neck RT is usually ipsilateral, but may be bilateral depending on nodal pattern	Photons: ≥60 Gy Suggest: 60 Gy Extracapsular extension: 66 Gy
Adjuvant, perineural, or major nerve involvement	In addition to the covering the tumor bed (and nodes if indicated), cover the cranial nerve pathways to the base of skull	Photons: ≥60 Gy Suggest: 64–66 Gy
Definitive, unresected tumor or gross residual[c]	Gross tumor volume as well as normal-appearing gland	Preferably neutrons Photons: ≥70 Gy
Definitive, unresected nodes or gross residual	Levels I, II, and III Any other levels involved based on pathology or imaging Consider covering levels IV and/or V if four or more lymph nodes are positive Neck RT is usually ipsilateral, but may be bilateral depending on nodal pattern	Preferably neutrons Photons: ≥70 Gy

Table 4.15 *(continued)*

Indication(s)	Target(s)	Dose(s)[a]
Elective neck irradiation	Levels I, II, and III, ipsilateral	Photons: ≥ 50 Gy Suggest: 50 Gy

See Figure 4.6 4.2 for the adjuvant and ENI criteria; also refer to Figure 4.4 and Table 4.5

[a] Photons at 1.8–2 Gy/day

[b] Based on presurgical imaging, surgical scar, operative and pathology reports, and/or postoperative imaging findings

[c] Based on imaging and physical examination findings

Field Arrangements (Parotid Gland Tumors)

Two traditional radiation therapy techniques for parotid gland tumors include unilateral anterior and posterior wedge pair fields using 4- to 6-MV photons or ^{60}Co, and 12- to 16- MeV electron (80% of dose) in combination with 4- to 6-MV or ^{60}Co photons (20% of dose).

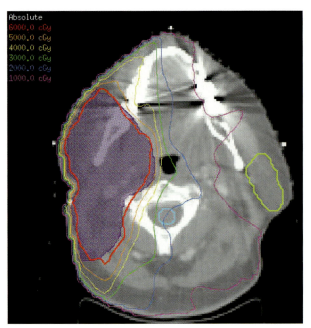

Figure 4.7 IMRT plan for a patient with acinic cell carcinoma of the right parotid. Six coplanar fields ipsilateral to the tumor were used, 340, 306, 277, 244, 224, and 180° to spare the temporal lobe, spinal cord, and contralateral parotid among other critical structures. The prescribed dose was 6,000 cGy at 200 cGy per fraction. The spinal cord is outlined in cyan and the contralateral parotid in light green. The PTV is highlighted as a purple color wash. The red, orange, yellow, green, blue, and magenta isodoses correspond to 60, 50, 40, 30, 20, and 10 Gy, respectively

Intensity-modulated radiation therapy (IMRT; Figure 4.7) reduces the dose to critical normal tissues, especially the cochlea (Figure 4.8) and oral cavity, when compared with three-dimensional conformal radiotherapy (3D-CRT) and conventional RT. A proposed five-field class solution IMRT technique has the following beam arrangement: 15, 55, 125, 165, and 270° (0° representing a direct anterior beam and 180° ipsilateral to the tumor) *(Bragg CM, Conway J, Robinson MH (2002) The role of intensity-modulated radiotherapy in the treatment of parotid tumors. Int J Radiat Oncol Biol Phys. 52:729–738).*

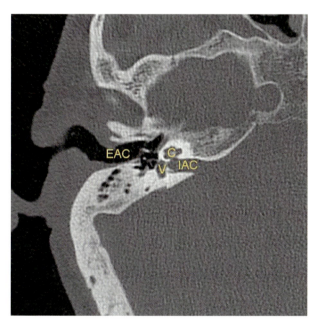

Figure 4.8 Axial *CT* image through the skull base. *EAC* external acoustic canal, *C* cochlea, *V* vestibule, *IAC* internal auditory canal

Source: Niranjan Bhandare AJ, Eisbruch A, Pan CC et al (2010) Radiation therapy and hearing loss. Int J Radiat Oncol Biol Phys 76:S50–S57. Used with permission from Elsevier Science, Inc.

Normal Tissue Tolerance

OARs in RT of parotid cancer include the uninvolved parotid and subman-dibular gland(s), cochlea, temporal lobe of the brain, spinal cord, and other head and neck structures (Table 4.16).

Table 4.16 Dose limitation of OARs in RT for upper abdominal malignancies

OAR	Dose limitation(s)
Cochlea	Mean dose ≤45 Gy (or more conservatively ≤35 Gy) to minimize the risk of sensorineural hearing loss
Parotid, uninvolved	Mean dose <20 Gy (note: not 26 Gy) or as low as possible to uninvolved gland
Submandibular, uninvolved	Mean dose <35 Gy or as low as possible
Brain, temporal lobe	$D_{max} < 60$ Gy Risk of brain necrosis increases significantly with fractions >2 Gy (avoid hot spots) and twice-daily treatment
Brainstem	$D_{max} < 54$ Gy
Spinal cord	$D_{max} < 50$ Gy
Optic nerve, chiasm	$D_{max} < 55$ Gy

D_{max}: maximum dose

Source: Bentzen SM, Constine LS, Deasy JO et al (2010) Quantitative analyses of normal tissue effects in the clinic (QUANTEC): an introduction to the scientific issues. Int J Radiat Oncol Biol Phys 76:S3–S9

Follow-Up

Schedule and suggested examinations during follow-up are presented in Table 4.17.

Radiation-induced adverse effects include partial xerostomia, trismus, conductive or sensorineural hearing loss, bone necrosis, otomastoiditis, dry-eye syndrome, nasolacrimal duct obstruction, cataract, temporal lobe necrosis, and retinopathy.

Table 4.17 Follow-up schedule and examinations

Schedule	Frequency
First follow-up	■ 4–6 weeks after RT
Year 1	■ Every 1–3 months
Year 2	■ Every 2–4 months
Years 3–5	■ Every 4–6 months
Years 5+	■ Every 6–12 months
Examinations	
History and physical	■ Complete history and physical examination
Laboratory tests	■ TSH every 6–12 months if neck irradiated
Imaging studies	■ Chest imaging if clinically indicated

TSH: thyroid-stimulating hormone

5

Cancer of Larynx and Hypopharynx

Jay S. Cooper[1]

Key Points

- Cancers of the larynx and pharynx account for approximately 25,000 new malignancies per year in the USA.
- The most common predisposing factors are smoking cigarettes and drinking alcohol.
- These tumors arise from the mucosal linings and are predominantly squamous cell carcinomas.
- Cancers of the larynx and hypopharynx spread primarily by local extension, less often by lymphatic channels, and uncommonly by vascular channels. When lymphatic spread occurs, levels II and III are the most common locations of disease.
- Early-stage cancers of the larynx and hypopharynx are most likely to be clinically suspected when patients present with hoarseness and difficulty swallowing, respectively.
- Staging is important to facilitate comparison between patient groups and as a guide to prognosis.
- Treatment is better triaged based on the following factors
  - Tumors incapable of regional metastasis
  - Small lesions capable of regional metastasis
  - Advanced lesions suitable for organ conservation
  - Advanced lesions beyond organ conservation: operable vs. inoperable
- Surgery, radiation therapy, and chemotherapy (particularly cisplatin) all have roles to play in the management of cancers of the larynx and hypopharynx, with the specific modality or combination of modalities for a particular patient dependent on the extent of that patient's tumor.
- Outcomes vary widely, depending on the type and extent of tumor: as high as 95% cure for T1 glottic tumors to as low as 20% 2-year survival for advanced inoperable hypopharyngeal tumors.

[1] Jay S. Cooper, MD (✉)
Email: jcooper@maimonidesmed.org

J. J. Lu, L. W. Brady (Eds.), *Decision Making in Radiation Oncology*
DOI: 10.1007/978-3-642-13832-4_6, © Springer-Verlag Berlin Heidelberg 2010

Epidemiology and Etiology

In 2009, approximately 12,290 new laryngeal cancers and 12,610 pharyngeal cancers were diagnosed in the United States, with men being affected approximately four times as frequently as were women. Tumors at these sites accounted for approximately 5,890 deaths (3,660 from laryngeal cancers and 2,230 from pharyngeal cancers), but fortunately, with modern care the death rate from laryngeal cancer in men has dropped from 2.97 (per 100,000) in 1990 to 2.24 (per 100,000) in 2005.

A number of risk factors have been identified for laryngeal/hypopharyngeal cancer (Table 5.1).

Table 5.1 Risk factors for laryngeal/hypopharyngeal cancers

Stage	Description
Patient-related factors	**Age and gender:** most often after age 55. Male-to-female ratio is approximately 4:1
	Lifestyle: cigarette, cigar, and pipe smoking (2–25× increase) and heavy alcohol consumption (2–6× increase) each increase the risk. The combination is synergistic (40–100× increase). Poor nutrition has also been implicated as a factor
	Race: African-Americans are more likely to be affected
	Past medical history: A previous head and neck malignancy correlates with increased risk because of the so-called field effect of carcinogens
	Genetically acquired: Fanconi anemia and dyskeratosis congenita, conditions that lead to aplastic anemia, are associated an increased risk
	Weakened immunity: decreased immunity – as in AIDS or after organ transplant – has been associated with a greater risk of developing head and neck cancers
Environmental factors	**Industrial chemicals:** exposure to sulfuric acid mist, nickel or wood dust, or asbestos reportedly increases the risk of laryngeal cancer

Anatomy

The larynx and hypopharynx, in aggregate, form a complex, mucosally lined, tubular structure that serves as a conduit for air (the larynx) and food (the hypopharynx). The larynx has three major divisions: the supraglottic (superior to the glottis), the glottis (the vocal cords), and the subglottis (inferior to the glottis). The supraglottis, the largest of the divisions, itself is composed of the epiglottis, the aryepiglottic folds, the arytenoids, the ventricles, and the ventricular bands (also known as the false cords). The larynx is supported by nine cartilages: the larger (singular) epiglottic, thyroid, cricoid, and the smaller (paired) arytenoid, cuneiform and corniculate. The hypopharynx also has three major divisions: the pyriform sinuses, the pharyngeal walls, and the postcricoid region. All of the mucosal structures can be assessed by laryngoscopy, and the cartilages can be assessed by computed tomography (CT) and/or magnetic resonance imaging (MRI) (Figure 5.1).

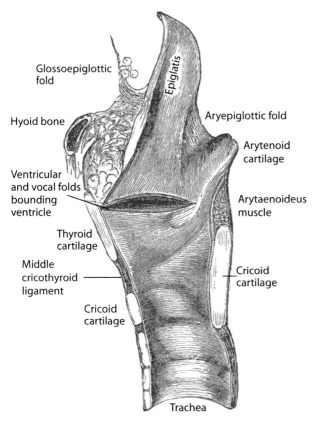

Figure 5.1 Anatomy of the larynx and hypopharynx

Glossoepiglottic fold

Epiglatis

Hyoid bone

Aryepiglottic fold

Arytenoid cartilage

Ventricular and vocal folds bounding ventricle

Arytaenoideus muscle

Thyroid cartilage

Middle cricothyroid ligament

Cricoid cartilage

Cricoid cartilage

Trachea

Diagnosis, Staging, Triage, and Prognosis

Clinical Presentation

The signs and symptoms produced by laryngeal and hypopharyngeal cancers depend on the exact location and extent of the primary tumor. Commonly observed changes are detailed in Table 5.5.

Table 5.5 Commonly observed signs and symptoms in laryngeal and/or hypopharyngeal cancer

Stage	Description
Early laryngeal	■ Hoarseness ■ Change in voice quality
Early hypopharyngeal	■ Difficulty swallowing ■ Cervical adenopathy
Advanced laryngeal and/or hypopharyngeal	■ Hoarseness ■ Difficulty swallowing ■ Cervical adenopathy ■ Weight loss ■ Throat pain/referred pain in the ear(s) ■ Airway obstruction

Staging

Diagnosis and clinical staging depends on findings from history and physical examination, imaging, and lab tests. Pathological staging depends on findings from surgical resection and histologic examination, in addition to those required in clinical staging. Because only some laryngeal and hypopharyngeal tumors are resected, all should have a clinical stage assigned, and only some should (in addition) have a pathologic stage assigned.

The American Joint Committee on Cancer (AJCC) tumor, node, and metastasis (TNM) staging systems and groupings, 7th edition, for both laryngeal and hypopharyngeal cancers are presented in Tables 5.6 and 5.7.

Table 5.6 AJCC TNM classification of carcinoma of the larynx and hypopharynx

Stage	Description
Primary tumor (T)	
TX	Primary tumor cannot be assessed
T0	No evidence of primary tumor
Tis	Carcinoma in situ
Supraglottis	
T1	Tumor limited to 1 subsite of supraglottis, with normal vocal cord mobility
T2	Tumor invades mucosa of more than 1 adjacent subsite of supraglottis or glottis or region outside the supraglottis, without fixation of the larynx
T3	Tumor limited to larynx with vocal cord fixation and/or invades any of the following: postcricoid area, preepiglottic space, paraglottic space, and/or inner cortex of thyroid cartilage
T4a	Moderately advanced local disease: Tumor invades through the thyroid cartilage and/or invades tissues beyond the larynx
T4b	Very advanced local disease: Tumor invades prevertebral space, encases carotid artery, or invades mediastinal structures
Glottis	
T1a	Tumor limited to 1 vocal cord (may involve anterior or posterior commissure) with normal mobility
T1b	Tumor involves both vocal cords (may involve anterior or posterior commissure) with normal mobility
T2	Tumor extends to supraglottis and/or subglottis, and/or with impaired vocal cord mobility
T3	Tumor limited to the larynx with vocal cord fixation and/or invasion of paraglottic space, an/or inner cortex of the thyroid cartilage
T4a	Moderately advanced local disease: Tumor penetrates the outer cortex of the thyroid cartilage and/or invades tissues beyond the larynx
T4b	Very advanced local disease: Tumor invades prevertebral space, encases carotid artery, or involves mediastinal structures
Subglottis	
T1	Tumor limited to the subglottis
T2	Tumor extends to vocal cord(s) with normal or impaired mobility
T3	Tumor limited to larynx with vocal cord fixation
T4a	Moderately advanced local disease: Tumor invades cricoid or thyroid cartilage and/or invades tissues beyond the larynx
T4b	Very advanced local disease: Tumor invades prevertebral space, encases carotid artery, or involves mediastinal structures ▶

Table 5.6 *(continued)*

Stage	Description
Hypopharynx	
T1	Tumor limited to 1 subsite of hypopharynx and/or ≤2 cm in greatest dimension
T2	Tumor invades more than 1 subsite of hypopharynx or an adjacent site, or measures >2 cm but ≤4 cm in greatest dimension
T3	Tumor >4 cm in greatest dimension or with fixation of hemilarynx or extension to esophagus
T4a	Moderately advanced local disease: Tumor invades thyroid/cricoid cartilage, hyoid bone, thyroid gland, or central compartment soft tissue includes prelaryngeal strap muscles and subcutaneous fat
T4b	Very advanced local disease: Tumor invades prevertebral fascia, encases carotid artery, or involves mediastinal structures
Regional lymph nodes (N)	
NX	Regional lymph nodes cannot be assessed
N0	No regional lymph node metastasis
N1	Metastasis in a single ipsilateral lymph node, ≤3 cm in greatest dimension
N2a	Metastasis in a single ipsilateral lymph node, >3 cm but ≤6 cm in greatest dimension
N2b	Metastasis in multiple ipsilateral lymph nodes, none >6 cm in greatest dimension
N2c	Metastasis in bilateral or contralateral lymph nodes, none >6 cm in greatest dimension
N3	Metastasis in a lymph node, >6 cm in greatest dimension
Distant metastasis (M)	
M0	No distant metastasis
M1	Distant metastasis

Triage

Staging is a mechanism that permits assortment of tumors into groups having similar prognosis and therefore facilitates comparison of the outcome of therapy in different trials, settings, patient cohorts, etc. (Figure 5.2). Staging does not necessarily translate directly into appropriate therapy. For practical purposes, potentially curable laryngeal and hypopharyngeal cancers can be grouped into five cohorts based on the nature of the therapy they ideally should receive.

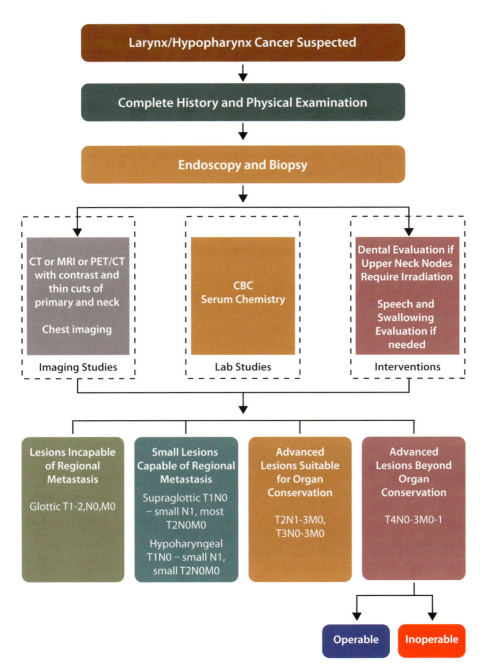

Figure 5.2 A proposed algorithm for diagnosis and triage of laryngeal and hypopharyngeal cancer

Prognosis

The outcome of treatment of cancers of the larynx and hypopharynx varies substantially, from excellent to poor. The most important prognostic factors include the extent/stage at diagnosis, the exact site of origin of disease, and the patient's performance status/ability to tolerate the desired therapy (Table 5.8). Advanced lesions not suited for organ conservation, but suitable for surgery for cure, do not have a worse outcome than have less extensive lesions treated to conserve the larynx. However, inoperable lesions, beyond organ conservation, have a substantially worse prognosis.

Treatment

Localized Lesions Incapable of Regional Metastasis

Principles and Practice

Limited-extent SCC of the glottis (i.e., T1 or T2, N0) do not spread to regional lymph nodes and are effectively treated by radiation therapy to the primary tumor alone or, in select circumstances, by surgery (Figure 5.3). A single modality of treatment should suffice. Radiation therapy is generally the preferred option, based on better subsequent voice quality (Table 5.9). However, no high-level evidence exists to select between treatment options (Table 5.10).

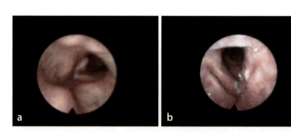

Figure 5.3 a, b Appearance of early glottic cancer:
a T1a glottic cancer
and **b** T1b glottic cancer

Table 5.8 Outcome of treatment

5-Year:	Lesions incapable of regional metastasis	Small lesions capable of regional metastasis	Advanced lesions suitable for organ conservation	Resectable nondisseminated advanced lesions beyond organ conservation	Unresectable nondisseminated advanced lesions beyond organ conservation
	Radiation therapy (%)	Radiation therapy (%)	CERT (%)	Surgery + radiation or CERT (%)	CERT (%)
Local control	85–95 (T1) 70–85 (T2)	85–95 (T1) 65–85 (T2)	35–75	~75	30–50 at 2–3 years
Overall survival	75–95	60–65	25–55	~40	20–35 at 2–3 years

CERT: chemotherapy-enhanced radiation therapy, i.e., the addition of a drug to radiation therapy with the intent of enhancing the biologic effect of radiation rather than eradicating micrometastatic disease

Table 5.9 Treatment modalities used for early glottic cancer

Radiation therapy	
Indication	■ Suitable for virtually all lesions
Techniques	■ Small opposed portals (e.g., 5 × 5 or 6 × 6 cm) treating the primary tumor but not regional nodes ■ 63 Gy in 28 fractions of 2.25 Gy once daily for 5.6 weeks ■ Tissue compensation usually necessary ■ Twice-daily therapy may be beneficial for T2 lesions[a]; 79.2 Gy in 66 fractions of 1.2 twice daily for 6.6 weeks
Laser resection	
Indications	■ Lesions of the free edge of the vocal cord ■ Approximately 50% of T1a lesions are potentially suitable[b]
Technique	■ Transoral endoscopic CO_2 laser

[a] *Sources: Garden AS, Morrison WH, Ang KK et al (1995) Hyperfractionated radiation in the treatment of squamous cell carcinomas of the head and neck: a comparison of two fractionation schedules. Int J Radiat Oncol Biol Phys 31:493–502; Trotti A, Pajak T, Emami B et al (2006) A randomized trial of hyperfractionation versus standard fractionation in T2 squamous cell carcinoma of the vocal cord. Int J Radiat Oncol Biol Phys 66:S15*
[b] *Source: Sjögren EV, Langeveld TP, Baatenburg de Jong RJ (2008) Clinical outcome of T1 glottic carcinoma since the introduction of endoscopic CO2 laser surgery as treatment option. Head Neck 30:1167–1174*

Radiation Therapy Techniques

Simulation and Target Volume Delineation

Irradiation of the primary tumor plus a small margin suffices, without treatment of regional lymph nodes. Generally, the portals extend from the hyoid to the bottom of the cricoid cartilage, and flash the skin to the anterior aspect of the vertebral body (Figure 5.4). Typically, 5 × 5 to 6 × 6 cm laterally and parallelly opposed 4- to 6-MV photon-beam fields are used, although patients with short necks may need the beams to be aimed in an oblique, wedged-pair fashion with compensation. Care must be taken to have the target volume remain within the treatment portals as the patient swallows, displacing the larynx cephalad.

A CT simulation (with thin cuts) permits localization of the glottis, the tumor, and may even identify the biopsy site. Simulation should be performed in the treatment position, mindful of movement of the glottis on swallowing to ensure that the tumor remains in the treatment portals. For far-anteriorly placed lesions, a thin bolus may be needed over the front of the neck to as-

Table 5.10 Supporting clinical evidence

Randomized trial	Description
For T1 tumors: none[a]	■ There are no prospective, randomized, large-scale phase III trials upon which to make an evidence-based choice ■ Numerous retrospective trials appear to demonstrate similar local control rates between radiation therapy and laser surgery ■ Patient-specific (rather than tumor-specific) factors may favor one form of treatment over another
For T2 tumors: RTOG 9512[b]	■ Random 250 patients who had T2N0 glottic cancer; stratified by T2a versus T2b ■ Compared HFX (79.2 Gy in 66 fractions of 1.2 Gy given twice per day) to SFX (70 Gy in 35 fractions given once per day) ■ Hoped to detect a 55% reduction in the yearly hazard rate for local failure ■ The 5-year local control rates were HFX = 79 versus SFX = 70%, $p = 0.11$ (i.e., a 35% decrease in the hazard rate) ■ The 5-year overall survival rates were HFX = 73 versus SFX = 62%, $p = 0.19$

RTOG 9512: Radiation Therapy Oncology Group trial 9512; **HFX:** hyperfractionation; **SFX:** standard *fractionation*

[a] *Source: Kadish SP (2005) Can I treat this small larynx lesion with radiation alone? Update on the radiation management of early (T1 and T2) glottic cancer. Otolaryngol Clin North Am 38:1–9, vii*
[b] *Source: Trotti A, Pajak T, Emami B et al (2006) A randomized trial of hyperfractionation versus standard fractionation in T2 squamous cell carcinoma of the vocal cord. Int J Radiat Oncol Biol Phys 66:S15*

sure the delivery of full dose to the entire lesion, particularly if a 6-MV beam is used.

Dose and Treatment Delivery

In recent years, a dose of 63 Gy in 28 fractions of 2.25 Gy over 5.6 weeks has become very popular. In one prospective randomized, single-institution trial, 180 patients who had T1N0M0 glottic cancers were treated with either 2.25 Gy or 2.0 Gy per fraction. The 5-year local control rates significantly favored the group that had received 2.25 Gy (92 versus 77%); however, the cause-specific survival rates were similar (100 and 97%). Based on numerous retrospective series, doses of less than 2.0 Gy generally should not be

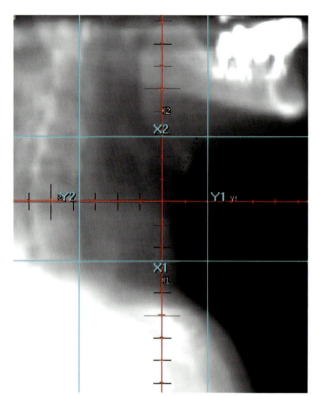

Figure 5.4 Lateral opposed portal borders for early glottic cancer

used; however, total doses of 60 Gy (if only subclinical disease remains after biopsy) to 66 Gy at daily increments of 2.0–2.25 Gy are reasonable.

Localized Lesions Capable of Regional Metastasis

Principles and Practice

Limited-extent SCC of the supraglottic larynx (T1N0-small N1 and most T2N0; Figure 5.5) or hypopharynx (T1N0–1 and small T2N0; Figure 5.6) have such a sufficiently high rate of spread to regional lymph nodes that the nodes need to be addressed as to whether the tumor is treated by radiation therapy or surgery. As a single modality of treatment should suffice, radiation often is the less morbid option (Tables 5.11 and 5.12).

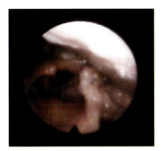

Figure 5.5 T2 supraglottic cancer

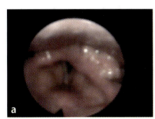 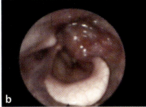

Figure 5.6 a, b Non-bulky **a** and bulky **b** T2 hypopharyngeal cancers

Table 5.11 Treatment modalities used for early supraglottic or hypopharyngeal cancer

Stage	Description
Radiation therapy	
Indications	■ Suitable for most lesions; choice of therapy may be more influenced by patient factors than lesion itself ■ Radiation therapy is preferred therapy if size/extent/location of the tumor would require a total laryngectomy to repair the surgical defect
Techniques	■ For small supraglottic lesions, include the primary tumor plus the upper and mid-cervical (levels 2 and 3) nodes ■ For more extensive supraglottic lesions (e.g., the lesion presented in Figure 5.6 b), also include low, anterior cervical (level 4) nodes ■ If N1 anterior cervical disease is present, the posterior cervical (level 5) nodes should be electively treated ■ For hypopharyngeal tumors, include levels II–V plus the retropharyngeal nodes
Surgical resection	
Indication	■ Akin to radiation therapy, suitable for most lesions; choice of therapy may be more influenced by patient factors than lesion itself
Technique	■ Partial pharyngectomy plus at least ipsilateral neck dissection

Table 5.12 Supporting clinical evidence

Stage	Description
For early laryngeal tumors[a]	■ 18 T1 and 109 T2 supraglottic cancers treated by radiation therapy ■ All patients followed at least 2 years; 91% followed at least 5 years ■ The local control rate was 100% for T1 and 85% for T2 ■ The disease-specific survival rate was 100% for stage I disease and 93% for stage II
For early hypopharyngeal tumors[b]	■ 39 Stage I and 76 stage II hypopharyngeal tumors treated by radiation therapy in 10 institutions between 1990 and 2001 ■ The 5-year local control rate was 87% for T1 (although 18% required additional surgery) and 74% for T2. All patients retained their pretreatment voice ■ The 5-year disease-specific survival rate was 95.8% for T1 disease and 70.1% for T2
For T2 hypopharyngeal tumors[c]	■ Altered fractionation schemes can be beneficial ■ T2 hypopharyngeal tumors were eligible for RTOG 9003, which showed a local control advantage for concomitant boost and HFX regimens

[a] *Source: Hinerman RW, Mendenhall WM, Amdur RJ et al (2002) Carcinoma of the supraglottic larynx: treatment results with radiotherapy alone or with planned neck dissection. Head Neck 24:456–467*
[b] *Source: Nakamura K, Shioyama Y, Kawashima M et al (2006) Multi-institutional analysis of early squamous cell carcinoma of the hypopharynx treated with radical radiotherapy. Int J Radiat Oncol Biol Phys 65:1045–1050*
[c] *Source: Fu KK, Pajak TF, Trotti A et al (2000) A Radiation Therapy Oncology Group (RTOG) phase III randomized study to compare hyperfractionation and two variants of accelerated fractionation to standard fractionation radiotherapy for head and neck squamous cell carcinomas: first report of RTOG 9003. Int J Radiat Oncol Biol Phys 48:7–16*

Radiation Therapy Techniques

Simulation and Target Volume Delineation

Because of the anatomy involved, laterally and parallelly opposed portals are usually sufficient for treatment (Figures 5.7 and 5.8). Intensity-modulated radiotherapy (IMRT) techniques do not offer the same advantage in these sites as they do elsewhere.

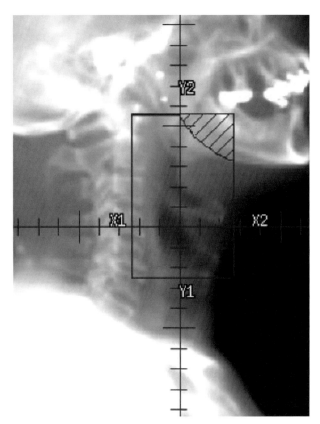

Figure 5.7 Lateral opposed portal borders for early supraglottic cancer

Dose and Treatment Delivery

For T1 supraglottic lesions, a dose of 66 Gy in 33 fractions of 2 Gy daily/6.6 weeks usually suffices. For T2 supraglottic and T1 hypopharyngeal cancers, 70 Gy in 35 fractions of 2 Gy daily/7 weeks is more appropriate. For T2 hypopharyngeal cancers, the accelerated fractionation with concomitant boost technique, as was used in the Radiation Therapy Oncology Group (RTOG) Trial 9003, is recommended. This technique initially delivers 32.4 Gy in 18 fractions of 1.8 Gy/day, 5 days/week over 3.6 weeks. Because accelerated repopulation of residual tumor cells is believed to be a clinical problem at this point in therapy, treatment is subsequently accelerated and given twice daily. In the morning, the large field is continued for an additional 21.6 Gy in 12 fractions of 1.8 Gy each (appropriately shielding the spinal cord and treating the posterior cervical nodes with electron beams after 45 Gy) and no less than 6 h later, a small boost field (encompassing the initial primary tumor and any grossly involved nodes plus a 1- to 1.5-cm margin) is added to deliver 18.0 Gy in 12 fractions of 1.5 Gy each. Consequently, the total dose is 72.0 Gy in 42 fractions over 6 weeks.

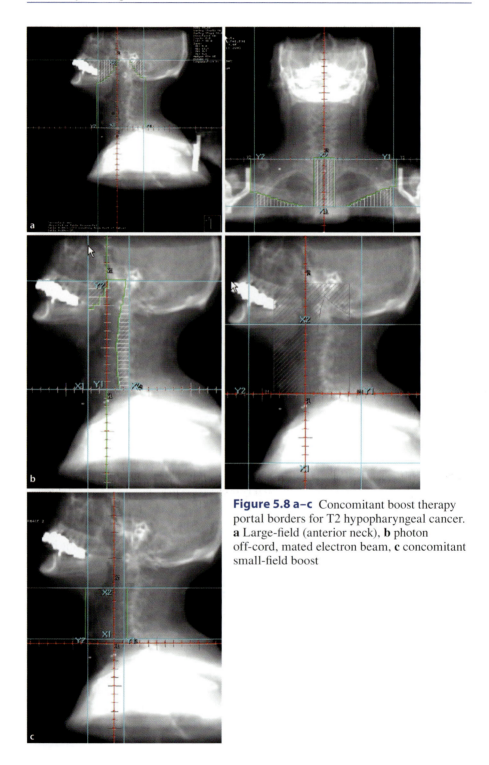

Figure 5.8 a–c Concomitant boost therapy portal borders for T2 hypopharyngeal cancer. **a** Large-field (anterior neck), **b** photon off-cord, mated electron beam, **c** concomitant small-field boost

Advanced Lesions Suitable for Organ Preservation

Principles and Practice

Moderately advanced lesions (T3 and early T4; Figure 5.9) that were traditionally treated by laryngectomy (with or without pharyngectomy) and postoperative radiation therapy are now known to be potentially suitable for larynx-sparing therapies (Tables 5.13 and 5.14). When mated with close posttreatment observation and salvage surgery when needed, survival is not compromised; however, not all lesions suitable for organ preservation arise in patients who are equally suitable for such therapy. Patients who are unreliable, patients who intend to continuing smoking during treatment, and hypersensitive patients who cannot tolerate the likely discomfort of chemotherapy-enhanced radiation therapy may be better served by surgery that removes all gross disease and postoperative radiation therapy delivered as attendance and tolerance permit.

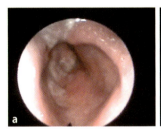 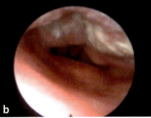

Figure 5.9 a, b Appearance of moderately advanced cancer. **a** T3 larynx cancer and **b** T3 hypopharynx cancer

Table 5.13 Treatment modalities used for organ preservation

Stage	Description
Indications	■ Suitable for advanced lesions that have not penetrated cartilage ■ Vocal cord fixation is not a contraindication
Radiation therapy techniques	■ The primary tumor and clinically involved nodes should receive 70 Gy in 35 fractions of 2 Gy each over 7 weeks ■ All anterior and posterior cervical and supraclavicular nodes that appear to be clinically uninvolved are at risk for subclinical involvement and need to receive a minimum of 50 Gy
Chemotherapy technique	■ Intravenous cisplatin, 100 mg/m^2 on days 1, 22, and 43 of radiotherapy

Source: Forastiere AA, Goepfert H, Maor M et al (2003) Concurrent chemotherapy and radiotherapy for organ preservation in advanced laryngeal cancer. N Engl J Med 349:2091–2098

Table 5.14 Supporting clinical evidence

Randomized trials	Description
Department of Veterans Affairs larynx trial[a]	■ Randomized the care of 332 patients who had stage III or IV laryngeal cancer; median follow-up of 33 months ■ Compared 3 cycles of induction cisplatin plus fluorouracil chemotherapy and then radiotherapy, versus laryngectomy and postoperative radiotherapy ■ 2-Year survival rate was 68% in both treatment groups ($p = 0.98$) ■ There were more local recurrences ($p = 0.0005$) and fewer distant metastases ($p = 0.016$) in the induction chemotherapy group than in the other group ■ In the induction chemotherapy plus radiation therapy group, at 2 years 64% of all patients retained their larynxes, and 64% were free of disease
EORTC 24891[b]	■ Randomized the care of 202 patients who had carcinoma of the pyriform sinus, stages II–IV (but not N2C); median follow-up of 51 months ■ Compared 3 cycles of induction cisplatin chemotherapy and then radiotherapy, versus laryngectomy and postoperative radiotherapy ■ The median duration of survival of 44 months in the induction-chemotherapy arm and 25 months in the immediate-surgery arm (hazard ratio = 0.86) the investigators considered equivalent ■ In the group that received induction chemotherapy plus radiation therapy, at 3 years 42% had retained their larynxes ■ Local and regional recurrence was similar in both groups; however, there were fewer distant recurrences in the induction-chemotherapy arm (25 versus 36%, $p = 0.041$)
RTOG 9111[c]	■ Randomized the care of 520 patients who would otherwise have required laryngectomy for cure; median follow-up of 3.8 years ■ Compared induction cisplatin plus fluorouracil and then radiotherapy, to radiotherapy with concurrent administration of cisplatin to radiotherapy alone ■ Primary endpoint of preservation of the larynx significantly favored concurrent therapy: at 2 years 88% had intact larynxes after radiotherapy with concurrent cisplatin versus 75% with induction chemotherapy then radiotherapy ($p = 0.005$), versus 70% with radiotherapy alone ($p < 0.001$) ■ Secondary endpoint of locoregional control significantly favored concurrent therapy: 78% after radiotherapy with concurrent cisplatin versus 61% with induction chemotherapy and then radiotherapy versus 56% with radiotherapy alone ■ Overall survival was similar in all 3 groups

EORTC 24891: European Organization for Research and Treatment of Cancer Trial 24891

Radiation Therapy Techniques

Simulation and Target Volume Delineation
See Figure 5.10.

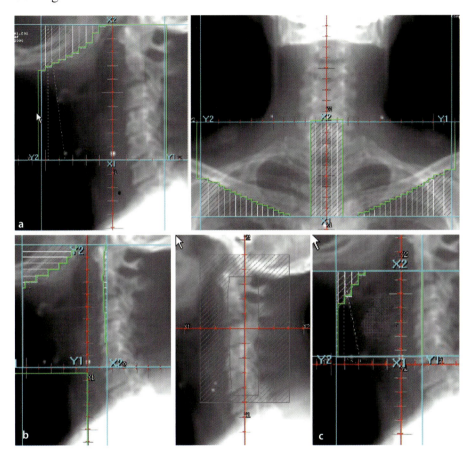

Figure 5.10 a–c Portal borders for T3 larynx cancer treated for laryngeal preservation. **a** Initial laterals initial anterior neck, **b** off-cord lateral mated e-beam, **c** cone down

[a]*Source: Wolf GT, Hong WK, Fisher SG et al (1991) Induction chemotherapy plus radiation compared with surgery plus radiation in patients with advanced laryngeal cancer. The Department of Veterans Affairs Laryngeal Cancer Study Group. N Engl J Med 324:1685–1690*

[b]*Source: Lefebvre JL, Chevalier D, Luboinski B et al (1996) Larynx preservation in pyriform sinus cancer: preliminary results of a European Organization for Research and Treatment of Cancer phase III trial. EORTC Head and Neck Cancer Cooperative Group. J Natl Cancer Inst 88:890–899*

[c]*Source: Forastiere AA, Goepfert H, Maor M et al (2003) Concurrent chemotherapy and radiotherapy for organ preservation in advanced laryngeal cancer. N Engl J Med 349:2091–2098*

Dose and Treatment Delivery

RTOG 9111 has become the gold standard for larynx-preserving therapies, and the details of radiation and chemotherapy (summarized in Table 5.13) described in that protocol have become the guidelines for treatment of this cohort of patients.

Resectable Advanced Lesions Not Suitable for Organ Preservation

Principles and Practice

Organ conservation is not merely about preserving anatomy. Once function is irreparably lost, there is little benefit to preserving anatomy. In addition, some patients are better served by definitive surgery followed by adjuvant irradiation because of (1) co-morbidities or lifestyles that make chemotherapy enhanced radiation therapy particularly toxic (e.g., a severe collagen-vascular disease or refusal to stop incessant smoking), (2) lifestyles that might make chemotherapy enhanced radiation therapy less likely to be effective (e.g., unreliable patients who have a history of not completing medical therapies) and/or (3) patients who emotionally would prefer to have surgery ("I need to have the cancer taken out as quickly as possible"). Often, the integrity of the cartilages is the best surrogate of non-surgical curability; once a cartilage is destroyed, surgery followed by adjuvant radiation therapy generally is considered essential (Figure 5.11 and Table 5.15). Furthermore, if the resected specimen reveals microscopic amounts of tumor at the mucosal surgical margin and/or if metastatic disease in a regional lymph node has transgressed the capsule (extracapsular extension of disease), two randomized phase III studies show that local-regional control can be improved by adding cisplatin chemotherapy concurrent with post-operative radiation therapy (Tables 5.15 and 5.16).

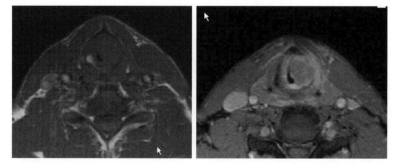

Figure 5.11 Advanced lesion not suitable for organ preservation

Table 5.15 Treatment modalities used for advanced operable laryngeal and hypopharyngeal cancer (beyond laryngeal preservation)

Stage	Description
Radiation therapy	
Indication	Postoperative therapy for all lesions of this extent
Technique	60–66 Gy to operative bed and draining nodes
Chemotherapy	
Indications	Microscopically involved mucosal margins Extracapsular extension of nodal disease
Technique	Intravenous cisplatin, 100 mg/m^2 on days 1, 22, and 43 of radiotherapy treatment

Radiation Therapy Techniques

Target Volume Delineation, Dose, and Treatment Delivery

The primary tumor site, all nodal beds at risk of harboring subclinical disease, and the entire operative bed should be included in the treatment portals. For laryngeal tumors, the upper border includes the nodes in the upper jugular region, whereas for hypopharyngeal primaries (or laryngeal tumors that invade the hypopharynx), the upper border is placed at the base of the skull to include the retropharyngeal nodes. Both ipsilateral and contralateral posterior nodes are included in the treatment portals if there are histologically involved nodes in the anterior chain.

Areas of initial gross disease, any area that has a high-risk feature, and any area that has been dissected (and has an altered vascular supply) should receive 60–66 Gy in 2-Gy-daily increments. Areas that are not dissected and considered at relatively low risk can receive 50–54 Gy.

Unresectable Advanced Lesions Not Suitable for Organ Preservation

Principles and Practice

Unresectable lesions that are detected in patients with no evidence of hematogenous dissemination of disease and who are otherwise in good general condition can be approached with curative-intent, chemotherapy-enhanced radiation therapy. Such therapy can be delivered with once-daily radiation (as described above for organ preservation) or with an altered fractionation regimen; however, less effective control of disease should be expected. For very fit patients, the philosophy supporting induction chemotherapy succeeded by

Table 5.16 Supporting clinical evidence

Randomized trial	Description
RTOG 9501[a]	■ 459 patients who, after definitive surgery, had histologic evidence of invasion of 2 or more regional lymph nodes and/or extracapsular extension of nodal disease and/or microscopically involved mucosal margins of resection; median follow-up of 45.9 months ■ Randomized to radiotherapy alone (60–66 Gy in 30–33 fractions over 6–6.6 weeks) versus identical treatment plus concurrent cisplatin (100 mg/m^2 of body-surface area intravenously on days 1, 22, and 43) ■ Primary endpoint of locoregional control favored concurrent therapy: at 2 years 82% (with chemotherapy) versus 72% (no chemotherapy), $p = 0.01$ ■ Secondary endpoints of disease-free survival also favored concurrent therapy ($p = 0.04$), but overall survival was not significantly different ($p = 0.19$)
EORTC 22931[b]	■ 334 patients who, after definitive surgery, had histologic evidence of extranodal spread, positive resection margins, perineural involvement, or vascular tumor embolism; median follow-up of 60 months ■ Randomized to radiotherapy alone (66 Gy in 33 fractions over 6.6 weeks) versus identical treatment plus concurrent cisplatin (100 mg/m^2 of body-surface area intravenously on days 1, 22, and 43) ■ Primary endpoint of disease-free survival favored concurrent therapy: at 5 years 47% (with chemotherapy) versus 36% (no chemotherapy), $p = 0.04$ ■ Secondary endpoints of overall survival ($p = 0.02$) and locoregional control ($p = 0.007$) both significantly favored concurrent therapy
Combined analysis[c]	■ Pooled the data sets from RTOG 9501 and EORTC 22931 to analyze the effect of possible predictors of benefit from chemotherapy ■ ECE and/or microscopically involved surgical margins were the only risk factors for which the influence of CERT was significant in both trials ■ By itself, having 2 or more lymph nodes invaded by tumor did not predict benefit from chemotherapy

ECE: extracapsular extension

[a] *Source: Cooper JS, Pajak TF, Forastiere AA et al (2004) Postoperative concurrent radiation therapy and chemotherapy in high-risk squamous cell carcinoma of the head and neck: The RTOG 9501/Intergroup phase III trial. N Engl J Med 350:1937–1944*
[b] *Source: Bernier J, Domenge C, Ozsahin M et al (2004) Postoperative irradiation with or without concomitant chemotherapy for locally advanced head and neck cancer. N Engl J Med 350:1945–1952*
[c] *Source: Bernier J, Cooper JS, Pajak TF et al (2005) Defining risk levels in locally advanced head and neck cancers: a comparative analysis of concurrent postoperative radiation plus chemotherapy trials of the EORTC (#22931) and RTOG (#9501). Head Neck 27:843–850*

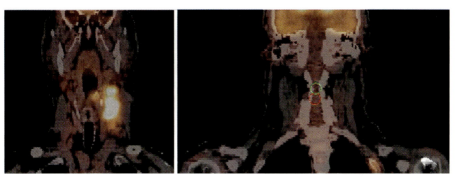

Figure 5.12 Appearance of more advanced disease. T2N3M1, stage IVC hypopharyngeal cancer (left rib metastasis)

chemotherapy-enhanced radiation therapy is appealing, but trials that rigorously compare this approach to the more standard chemotherapy-enhanced radiation therapy are ongoing.

For patients who already have distant dissemination of disease, the intent of treatment must be confined to palliation. Consequently, the intensity of treatment should be tailored to the anticipated survival of the patient with the hope of controlling distressing locoregional signs or symptoms of disease for the duration of the patient's remaining lifetime. In light of the subjectivity of such judgments, there are few objective guidelines in the literature. For patients who have only one or two non–life-threatening lesions, such as a bone metastasis, particularly for patients who have a good response to systemic chemotherapy, radiation therapy that approaches the intensity of definitive treatment may be appropriate. With more advanced metastatic disease (Figure 5.12) in an otherwise "healthy" symptomatic patient, the author tends to favor a split-course regimen (e.g., 30 Gy in 2 weeks and then a 2-week rest, followed by another 30 Gy in 2 weeks to a smaller field [that never overlaps the spinal cord]). For patients whose life expectancy is likely to be only a few months, a very brief (episodic as necessary) technique like "Quad Shot" (Tables 5.17 and 5.18) should suffice.

Table 5.17 Treatment modalities used for far-advanced disease

Stage	Description
Curative intent	
Indication	■ Unresectable advanced lesions not suitable for organ preservation in otherwise healthy patients
Techniques	■ Concurrent chemotherapy-enhanced radiation therapy ■ Possible role for induction therapy then concurrent chemotherapy-enhanced radiation therapy
Palliative intent	
Indications	■ M1 disease ■ Poor general condition ■ Unwillingness/inability to tolerate potentially curative treatment
Techniques	■ Split-course radiation therapy ■ Quad Shot radiation

Table 5.18 Supporting clinical evidence

Randomized trial	Description
For M0 tumors[a]	■ Multi-institutional phase III trial including 295 patients who had unresectable, nondisseminated, head and neck cancer (approximately 28% larynx/hypopharynx) ■ Randomly assigned to "standard" radiation therapy alone (70 Gy at 2 Gy/day) versus identical radiation therapy plus concurrent bolus cisplatin (on days 1, 22, and 43) versus split-course radiation therapy plus bolus cisplatin and continuous-infusion fluorouracil ■ Treatment with radiation therapy plus concurrent bolus cisplatin was associated with significantly improved survival, at the cost of increased toxicity. The 3-year projected overall survival for such treatment was 37%
For M0 tumors[b]	■ 166 patients who had locally advanced (74% operable and 26% inoperable) laryngeal and hypopharyngeal cancers ■ Randomly assigned to treatment with docetaxel (Taxotere), cisplatin (Platinol) and 5-fluorouracil (TPF) induction then chemoradiotherapy versus cisplatin and fluorouracil (PF) then chemoradiotherapy ■ For inoperable tumors, the 2-year overall survival rate was 55% with TPF and 41% with PF ■ For inoperable tumors, the 2-year progression-free survival rate was 42% with TPF, and 30% with PF

Table 5.18 *(continued)*

Randomized trial	Description
For M1 disease[c]	■ 30 patients who had advanced head and neck cancer, nearly all stage IV, 20/30 having a performance score of 2–3
	■ Quad Shot = 14 Gy in 4 fractions, given twice a day at least 6 h apart over 2 consecutive days, and repeated up to twice more every 4 weeks
	■ 53% objective response rate (complete response, 2; partial response, 4)
	■ Median progression free survival 3.1 months; median overall survival 5.7 months
	■ 44% of patients had a measurable improvement in quality of life

[a] *Source: Adelstein DJ, Li Y, Adams GL et al (2003) An intergroup phase III comparison of standard radiation therapy and two schedules of concurrent chemoradiotherapy in patients with unresectable squamous cell head and neck cancer. J Clin Oncol 21:92–98*
[b] *Source: Posner MR, Norris CM, Wirth LJ et al (2009) Sequential therapy for the locally advanced larynx and hypopharynx cancer subgroup in TAX 324: survival, surgery, and organ preservation. Ann Oncol 20:921–927*
[c] *Source: Corry J, Peters LJ, Costa ID et al (2005) The "QUAD SHOT" – a phase II study of palliative radiotherapy for incurable head and neck cancer. Radiother Oncol 77:137–142*

Radiation Therapy Techniques

Target Volume Delineation, Dose, and Treatment Delivery

For patients being treated with chemotherapy-enhanced, curative-intent radiation therapy, the fields and doses are the same as would be used for laryngeal preservation.

For patients who have incurable disease, the fields should be tailored to encompass the known disease, but need not include all sites of potential spread and should not impart normal tissue toxicity if at all avoidable. For patients who are expected to live several months, the author has been generally pleased with the results of split-course therapy as an appropriate compromise, providing enough therapy to hold the locoregional manifestations of tumor in relative check, without unduly consuming the patient's remaining time. For patients who have an even worse prognosis, the Quad Shot technique offers a more appropriate compromise.

Normal Tissue Tolerance

Relatively few critical structures need to be irradiated for the treatment of laryngeal or hypopharyngeal malignancies (Table 5.19).

Table 5.19 Dose-limitation guidelines in radiation therapy of laryngeal and hypopharyngeal malignancies

Organs at risk	Dose limitation (Gy)
Spinal cord	45
Brachial plexus	60
Mandible	70
Posterior neck	<35 (a strip of normal tissue should be left to facilitate lymphatic drainage)

Follow-Up

The vast majority of laryngeal and hypopharyngeal tumors recur within 3 years if they are destined to recur (save for a T1 glottic tumor, which can take up to 5 years to recur). This relatively rapid pattern of recurrence justifies relatively close follow-up in the first few years after treatment. Thereafter, the risk of second (independent, i.e., not recurrent) malignant tumors arising in the head and neck region because of the so-called field effect of carcinogens justifies long-term follow-up. A schedule of suggested follow-up (for non-T1 glottic tumors) is presented in Table 5.20.

Table 5.20 Follow-up schedule and examinations

Schedule	Frequency
First follow-up	■ 2 weeks after radiation therapy (have the acute reactions peaked; is intervention required?)
Years 0–1	■ Every month
Years 1–2	■ Every 2 months
Years 2–3	■ Every 3 months
Years 3+	■ Every 6 months

6 Squamous Cell Carcinoma of Unknown Head and Neck Primary

Ivan W.K. Tham[1]

Key Points

- Squamous cell carcinoma of unknown head and neck primary is a relatively rare condition in which the primary is not diagnosed after standard investigations including panendoscopy and imaging studies.

- Diagnosis of the condition is usually by fine-needle aspiration cytology, with immunohistochemistry or virology studies for further classification of the tumor in some cases.

- The nodal classification of the tumor, node, and metastasis (TNM) staging system for head and neck tumors (excluding nasopharynx and thyroid) is used for staging.

- The prognosis is broadly similar to that of patients with known primary tumor sites in the head and neck region. The main adverse prognostic factor is advanced nodal disease.

- Radical treatment is multidisciplinary, and usually involves surgery, radiation therapy, or the combination of the two.

- Follow-up is recommended to detect new second primary tumors, local or distant recurrences, and to monitor for potential late side effects.

Epidemiology and Etiology

Carcinomas with an unknown primary site (CUP) are tumors that present with lymph node or distant metastases when standard investigations fail to localize a primary site. It is a heterogeneous group of malignancies, which accounts for a minority (0.5–10%) of all tumors. Improvements in imaging technology and immunopathology have further decreased the incidence. Squamous cell carcinomas (SCC) of unknown head and neck primary form a small subset of CUP, with unique features (described in Table 6.1.)

[1] Ivan WK Tham, MD (✉)
Email: ivan_wk_tham@nuhs.edu.sg

J. J. Lu, L. W. Brady (Eds.), *Decision Making in Radiation Oncology*
DOI: 10.1007/978-3-642-13832-4_7, © Springer-Verlag Berlin Heidelberg 2010

Table 6.1 Epidemiology and etiology of SCC of unknown head and neck primary

Stage	Description
Epidemiology	■ Cervical lymph node metastases of SCC from an occult primary make up 2–5% of all CUP patients ■ About 2–9% of head and neck cancer patients present with neck lymph adenopathy with unknown primary site
Etiology	■ Risk factors similar to those of head and neck SCC with known primary sites ■ Main environmental factors including tobacco and alcohol use ■ Viral infection with HPV or EBV also plays a role

CUP: carcinoma with an unknown primary site; **HPV:** human papilloma virus; **EBV:** Epstein-Barr virus

Anatomy

Any neck level may be involved, although large retrospective studies suggest that cervical neck levels II and III are the levels most commonly affected (Figure 6.1).

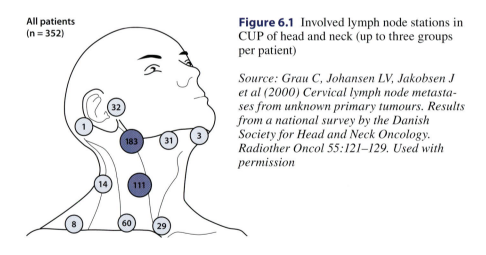

All patients
(n = 352)

Figure 6.1 Involved lymph node stations in CUP of head and neck (up to three groups per patient)

Source: Grau C, Johansen LV, Jakobsen J et al (2000) Cervical lymph node metastases from unknown primary tumours. Results from a national survey by the Danish Society for Head and Neck Oncology. Radiother Oncol 55:121–129. Used with permission

Table 6.2 Pathology of cervical lymph node metastases from an unknown primary tumor

Stage	Description
SCC	■ Most common histological subtype ■ Presence of nonkeratinizing SCC or detection of HPV type 16 may predict for oropharyngeal origin of the primary ■ HPV detection methods include in situ hybridization or IHC for p16 overexpression
Adenocarcinoma	■ Second most common histology subtype ■ May originate from salivary gland, thyroid, or parathyroid primary cancers ■ Often associated with a primary lesion below the clavicles
Undifferentiated carcinoma	■ Patients from regions endemic for NPC may require further evaluation for EBV, by serology, IHC, or circulating EBV DNA viral loads using real-time polymerase chain reaction
Poorly differentiated carcinoma	■ IHC may differentiate melanoma, lymphoma, or neuroendocrine tumors, which have different prognoses and treatment approaches

SCC: squamous cell carcinoma; **IHC:** immunohistochemistry; **NPC:** nasopharyngeal carcinoma; **EBV:** Epstein-Barr virus

Pathology

Table 6.2 summarizes the key points of the histological subtypes commonly diagnosed.

Three explanations have been proposed for the inability to detect the occult primary tumor, despite modern pathology and radiographic techniques:

■ The primary tumor may have involuted spontaneously and is no longer detectable, despite the presence of metastatic disease.

■ The malignant phenotype of the primary tumor favors metastatic biologic behavior over local tumor growth.

■ Current imaging technology lacks the resolution to detect tumors smaller than 5–10 mm in size.

Routes of Spread

In evaluating metastatic SCC to cervical lymph nodes, the occult primary is eventually detected in about half of the cohort, with a predominance of tonsillar fossa and base-of-tongue lesions (Table 6.3). In regions endemic for nasopharyngeal carcinoma (NPC), the rate of diagnosis of primary lesions arising from the nasopharynx is significantly higher.

Table 6.3 Site distribution of primary lesions detected

Primary site	Number of patients	Percent
Tonsillar fossa	59	45%
Base of tongue	58	44%
Pyriform sinus	10	8%
Posterior pharyngeal wall	3	2%
Nasopharynx	1	1%
Supraglottic larynx	1	1%
Total	132	100%

Source: Cianchetti M, Mancuso AA, Amdur RJ et al (2009) Diagnostic evaluation of squamous cell carcinoma metastatic to cervical lymph nodes from an unknown head and neck primary site. Laryngoscope 119:2348–2354

Table 6.4 summarizes data from three large, recently reported series, all of which demonstrate that the majority present with advanced nodal disease.

Table 6.4 Distribution of AJCC/TNM nodal classification

Nodal classification	Number of patients	Percent
N1	64	14%
N2a	128	28%
N2b	93	20%
N2c	19	4%
N3	153	33%
Total	457	100%

AJCC: American Joint Cancer Committee; **TNM:** tumor, node, and metastasis

Sources: Erkal HS, Mendenhall WM, Amdur RJ et al (2001) Squamous cell carcinomas metastatic to cervical lymph nodes from an unknown head-and-neck mucosal site treated with radiation therapy alone or in combination with neck dissection. Int J Radiat Oncol Biol Phys 50:55–63; Grau C, Johansen LV, Jakobsen J et al (2000) Cervical lymph node metastases from unknown primary tumours. Results from a national survey by the Danish Society for Head and Neck Oncology. Radiother Oncol 55:121–129; Patel RS, Clark J, Wyten R et al (2007) Squamous cell carcinoma from an unknown head and neck primary site: a "selective treatment" approach. Arch Otolaryngol Head Neck Surg 133:1282–1287

Diagnosis, Staging, and Prognosis

Clinical Presentation and Diagnosis

Most patients present with neck lumps for investigation. Figure 6.2 summarizes the procedures recommended in the evaluation of a patient.

Fluorodeoxyglucose–positron-emission tomography (FDG-PET) is often utilized in the evaluation of SCC of unknown primary. The main limitation of FDG-PET appears to be low specificity, with suggested reasons including physiological uptake in the tonsils, reactive lymph nodes, or the muscles of mastication. The tonsil also has a low specificity and a high false-positive rate, whereas sensitivity is low at the base of tongue. Other imaging characteristics are shown in Table 6.5.

Table 6.5 Characteristics of FDG-PET imaging

Parameters	Percent
Detection rate of tumors not apparent with conventional workup	25%
Detection rate of regional metastases not previously apparent	16%
Detection rate of distant metastases not previously apparent	11%
Rate of change of treatment strategy after scan	25%
Sensitivity	88%
Specificity	75%
Overall accuracy	79%

FDG-PET: fluorodeoxyglucose–positron-emission tomography

Source: Rusthoven KE, Koshy M, Paulino AC (2004) The role of fluorodeoxyglucose positron emission tomography in cervical lymph node metastases from an unknown primary tumor. Cancer 101:2641–2649

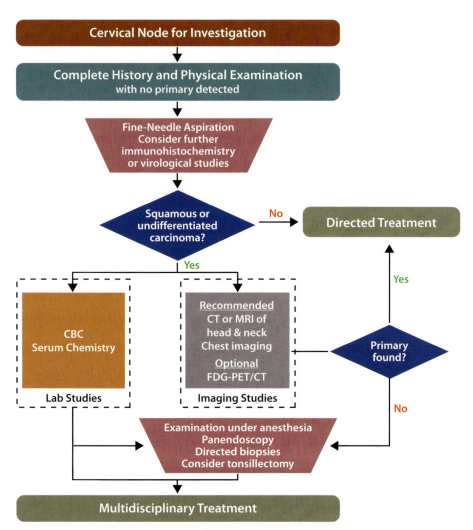

Figure 6.2 Proposed algorithm for diagnosis and staging of cervical lymph node metastases from an unknown primary tumor

Staging

The nodal classification of the tumor, node, and metastasis (TNM) staging systems and groupings of the American Joint Committee on Cancer (AJCC) (7th edition) for head and neck tumors (excluding nasopharynx and thyroid) is utilized, which is described in detail in Chapters 4 and 5.

Prognostic Factors

The reported survival and tumor outcomes vary considerably among studies, suggesting heterogeneity in patient, tumor, and/or treatment characteristics. The commonly reported outcomes are listed in Table 6.6, with known adverse prognostic factors listed in Table 6.7.

Table 6.6 Summary of reported outcomes

Outcome	5-year estimate (%)
Cause/disease-specific survival	48–67%
Overall survival	36–56%
Neck tumor control	51–78%
Emergence of occult primary or mucosal disease	13–19%

- Fine-needle aspiration (FNA) is preferred over core or open biopsy to obtain tissue diagnosis in the first instance, because it is minimally invasive and will not interfere with subsequent treatment
- Cytology most commonly reveals SCC or poorly differentiated carcinoma, but may demonst rate a nonsquamous malignancy, such as adenocarcinoma, lymphoma, thyroid malignancy or melanoma
- Thyroglobulin staining may be useful for adenocarcinoma or anaplastic carcinoma diagnoses
- Additional tests for human papilloma virus (HPV) and Epstein-Barr virus (EBV) may be offered selectively. Detection of HPV suggests an oropharyngeal primary site; EBV positivity points to a nasopharyngeal primary
- Unilateral or bilateral tonsillectomy often offered because the primary is often localized in the tonsils, sampling error is high, and morbidity of the procedure is relatively low
- Repeat panendoscopy does not improve diagnostic yield

Table 6.7 Adverse prognostic factors for SCC of unknown head and neck primary

Stage	Description
Disease related	■ Advanced N classification ■ Extracapsular spread ■ Poorly differentiated disease ■ Low-neck or supraclavicular nodes ■ Subsequent emergence of primary tumor
Treatment related	■ Single modality treatment versus combined modality (i.e., surgery and radiotherapy) ■ Unilateral neck versus pan-mucosal comprehensive RT

Treatment

Principles and Practice

Various strategies – mainly involving surgery or radiation therapy (RT) – have been reported (Table 6.8). However, most published studies are retrospective and based on institutional treatment protocols spanning years or decades. A commonly used approach is ipsilateral neck dissection, followed by adjuvant RT to the likely mucosal primary sites and bilateral neck. Alternatively, concurrent chemoradiation therapy or RT to the ipsilateral neck alone for unilateral neck involvement can be considered.

Radiation Volume

The evidence presented in Table 6.9 demonstrates a trend of improved outcome with comprehensive RT to mucosa and bilateral neck, over ipsilateral neck RT alone. In general, morbidity was poorly reported. Some authors suggest that comprehensive RT may be reserved for patients with poor prognostic features, e.g., advanced nodal disease, extracapsular spread, or high-grade disease, to optimize the therapeutic ratio. In a few patients, a second primary tumor may emerge subsequently, which would not have been treated by the initial RT. Retreatment would then be more feasible for patients treated originally with limited ipsilateral neck RT, as compared with those who had comprehensive RT.

Table 6.8 Treatment modalities

Stage	Description
Surgery	
Indications	■ Comprehensive neck dissection ■ Neck dissection may be performed alone, planned after RT, or as salvage
Facts/issues	■ Crude rate of primary tumor emergence after surgery alone is 25%, with median nodal recurrence rate of 34% ■ May be adequate for pN1 neck disease without extracapsular spread
Radiation Therapy	
Indications	■ Definitive treatment or adjuvant to surgery ■ Salvage of locoregional failure after surgery ■ Palliative treatment to locoregional or distant metastatic sites
Techniques	■ Comprehensive RT to bilateral neck and putative primary mucosal sites ■ Limited locoregional treatment to ipsilateral neck ■ Individualized treatment for metastatic disease
Chemotherapy	
Indications	■ Definitive treatment as induction therapy prior to RT or chemoradiation ■ Adjuvant concurrent chemoradiation ■ Palliative treatment
Medications	■ Platinum-based regimens most commonly used with concurrent chemoradiation ■ Taxane-based regimens often used for induction therapy

Table 6.9 Results of comprehensive versus limited RT

Endpoint	Median results	
	Unilateral RT	**Comprehensive RT**
Mucosal primary emergence rate	8 (5–44%)	10 (2–13%)
Neck relapse rate	52 (31–63%)	19 (8–49%)
Distant metastases rate	38%	19 (11–23%)
5-Year overall survival rate	37 (22–41%)	50 (34–63%)

Source: Nieder C, Gregoire V, Ang KK (2001) Cervical lymph node metastases from occult squamous cell carcinoma: cut down a tree to get an apple? Int J Radiat Oncol Biol Phys 50:727–733

Comprehensive RT Utilizing Three-Dimensional Conformal Radiotherapy or Intensity-Modulated RT

Recent reports (Table 6.10) suggest reduced toxicity or improved outcomes with more conformal RT techniques.

Table 6.10 Supporting evidence for use of 3D-CRT or IMRT in SCC of unknown head and neck primary

Study	Materials and methods	Results and conclusion
Bhide et al[a]	■ Plan comparison of conventional RT versus IMRT for 6 patients undergoing total-mucosal RT	■ Improved dose homogeneity with IMRT ■ Reduced mean contralateral parotid dose for IMRT (23 Gy) versus conventional RT (51 Gy)
Klem et al[b]	■ Single-center retrospective review of 21 patients receiving radical or adjuvant IMRT to total mucosa and bilateral neck	■ 2-Year regional progression-free survival of 90% ■ After 9 months, all patients had grade 1 xerostomia or better
Ligey et al[c]	■ Retrospective review of 95 patients receiving 2D-RT, 3D-CRT, or IMRT to unilateral or bilateral neck	■ Use of 3D-CRT or IMRT improved locoregional control and overall survival

IMRT: intensity-modulated RT

[a]*Source: Bhide S, Clark C, Harrington K, Nutting CM (2007) Intensity-modulated radiotherapy improves target coverage and parotid gland sparing when delivering total mucosal irradiation in patients with squamous cell carcinoma of head and neck of unknown primary site. Med Dosim 32:188–195*

[b]*Source: Klem ML, Mechalakos JG, Wolden SL et al (2008) Intensity-modulated radiotherapy for head and neck cancer of unknown primary: toxicity and preliminary efficacy. Int J Radiat Oncol Biol Phys 70:1100–1107*

[c]*Source: Ligey A, Gentil J, Créhange G et al (2009) Impact of target volumes and radiation technique on loco-regional control and survival for patients with unilateral cervical lymph node metastases from an unknown primary. Radiother Oncol 93:483–487*

Role of Chemotherapy

While the benefit of chemotherapy has not been demonstrated in this particular patient cohort, extrapolation from meta-analyses and phase III trials for head and neck SCC suggest a role for concurrent chemoradiation, especially in advanced nodal disease (Figure 6.3).

RT Techniques

Preparation and Simulation

The following preparations are important prior to RT for patients:
- Dental evaluation, and if required, extractions or restorative procedures, should be performed. Dental education regarding maintenance of oral hygiene should also be emphasized.
- The patient should be assessed by a dietician, especially if total-mucosal irradiation is planned.
- Psychosocial and speech therapy support should be offered when indicated.

Immobilization with a customized head, neck, and shoulder shell is implemented while the patients is in a supine position, with orthogonal laser beams for reference (see Chap., Figure 2.10). Computed tomography (CT) simulation should be performed from the vertex to the carina, with a slice thickness of 5 mm or less. Consider 3 mm or thinner slices near the area of interest, e.g., frontal sinuses to the shoulders, for improved resolution. Intravenous contrast may be administered to improve soft tissue and vascular definition. Scars should be wired.

Target Volumes and Doses

The recommended clinical target volumes (CTVs) and doses for adjuvant RT are described in Table 6.11. (Delineation of the nodal groups is detailed in Chap. 2.) The planning target volumes (PTVs) are constructed with margins 3–5 mm, depending on the anticipated setup accuracy. Treatment to the postoperative or node-positive neck may require some changes in delineation, as compared with the node-negative neck, as described in Table 6.12.

For gross disease, typically 70 Gy in 2-Gy daily fractions is delivered 5 days a week. However, there may be a benefit from altered fractionation or the addition of chemotherapy – at the cost of increased toxicity. The dose to subclinical disease in the unresected neck should be 50 Gy in 2-Gy fractions or its biologic equivalent if altered fractionation is utilized.

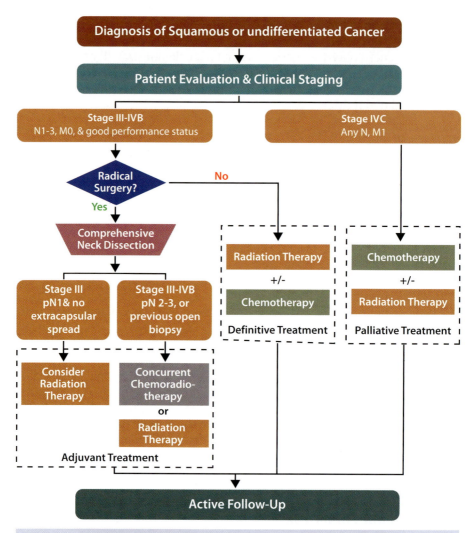

Figure 6.3 Proposed treatment algorithm for SCC of unknown head and neck primary

Table 6.11 Recommended CTVs and doses for adjuvant RT

RT	Phase 1	Dose (Gy)	Phase 2	Dose (Gy)	Total dose (Gy)
Unilateral neck	Unilateral neck levels Ib–V	50–60	Volume reduction optional after 50 Gy to involved levels only	10–16	60–66
Comprehensive	Bilateral levels Ib–V, RLN, pharyngolaryngeal mucosa[a]	50[b]	Levels Ib–V or only involved ipsilateral levels	10–16	60–66

CTVs: clinical target volumes; **RLN:** retropharyngeal lymph nodes

[a]*Some centers spare the hypopharynx and larynx to reduce treatment morbidity, because occult tumors in these sites are rare*
[b]*60–66 Gy may be recommended if there are areas particularly suspicious for disease*

Table 6.12 Considerations for the node-positive or postoperative neck

Situation	Proposed action
Level I node positive	Consider inclusion of oral cavity if comprehensive RT offered
Level II node positive	Include retrostyloid space cranially
Level IV or Vb node positive	Include supraclavicular fossa caudally
Postoperative setting	Include entire surgical bed
Extracapsular spread	Include adjacent muscles

[a]*Source: Grégoire V, Eisbruch A, Hamoir M, Levendag P (2006) Proposal for the delineation of the nodal CTV in the node-positive and the postoperative neck. Radiother Oncol 79:15–20*

Field Arrangements for Conventional RT or Three-Dimensional Conformal RT

Limited Unilateral RT

The radiation portal may be directed to the ipsilateral neck by direct photons, electrons, or a wedge pair.

Comprehensive RT

Upper Neck Fields
The superior border of the lateral opposing fields should encompass the nasopharynx with a margin of 1.5–2 cm, with the inferior border at the thyroid notch. Anteriorly, the oropharynx should be covered with a 2-cm margin. Posteriorly, the field should be placed at the C2 spinous process, with the cord shielded after 40–44 Gy, with posterior electron field matching to the required target dose (Figure 6.4a).

Lower Neck Fields
The field should match the upper fields with an isocentric or half-beam block technique superiorly, with the inferior border including the clavicular heads. Laterally, the field should cover the medial or entire supraclavicular region, depending on the extent of nodal involvement. A laryngeal block may be placed to spare the larynx and hypopharynx (Figure 6.4b).

Intensity-Modulated RT

Volumes for intensity-modulated RT (IMRT) is as described above, with dose constraints for normal tissue (as indicated in Table 6.11). Inverse planning is undertaken, with the plans generally normalized such that 95% the PTVs are covered by the intended dose.

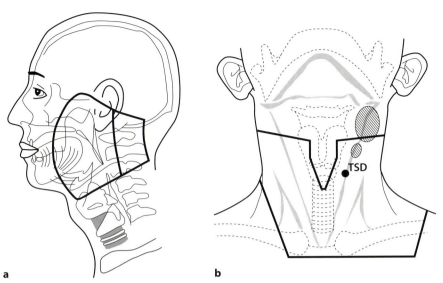

a   b

Figure 6.4 a, b   a Radiation treatment technique for CUP. Superiorly, the portal treats the nasopharynx and the jugular, and the spinal accessory lymph nodes at the base of the skull. The posterior border is behind the spinous process of C2. The inferior border is at the thyroid notch. Anteroinferiorly, the skin and subcutaneous tissues of the submentum are shielded, except in the case of advanced neck disease. The anterior tongue margin is set to obtain a 2-cm margin on the base of the tongue and tonsillar fossa, as well as the nasopharynx. One portal reduction is shown. **b** Fields for bilateral lower-neck radiotherapy. The larynx shield should be carefully designed. Because the internal jugular vein lymph nodes lie adjacent to the posterolateral margin of the thyroid cartilage, the shields cannot cover the entire thyroid cartilage without producing a low-dose area in these nodes. A common error in the treatment of the lower neck is to extend the low-neck portal laterally out to the shoulders, encompassing lateral supraclavicular lymph nodes, which are at negligible risk, while partially shielding the high-risk mid-jugular lymph node with a large, rectangular laryngeal block. The inferior extent of the shield is at the cricoid cartilage or first or second tracheal ring; the shield must be tapered because the nodes tend to lie closer to the midline as the lower neck is approached. Lateral borders of the low-neck portals are set to cover only the lymph nodes in the root of the neck when the risk of low-neck disease on that side is small (i.e., stage N0 or N1 disease). If there are clinically positive lymph nodes in the lower neck, or if major disease is present in the upper neck, the lateral border of the low-neck field is widened on that side to cover the entire supraclavicular region out to the junction of the trapezius muscle and the clavicle

Source: Mendenhall WM, Mancuso AA, Amdur RJ, Stringer SP, Villaret DB, Cassisi NJ. Squamous cell carcinoma metastatic to the neck from an unknown head and neck primary site. Am J Otolaryngol 2001; 22:261–267. Used with permission

Normal Tissue Tolerance

The normal tissue tolerance to radiation in the head and neck region is detailed in Table 6.13

Table 6.13 Recommended dose constraints

Organ-at-risk	Dose	Endpoint
Brainstem	$D_{max} < 54$ Gy	Permanent neuropathy
Spinal cord	$D_{max} < 50$ Gy	Myelopathy
Optic nerves, chiasm	$D_{max} < 55$ Gy	Optic neuropathy
Brachial plexus	$D_{max} < 66$ Gy	Neuropathy
Retina	Mean dose < 45 Gy	Blindness
Cochlea	Mean dose < 45 Gy	Sensorineural hearing loss
Mandible, TM joint	$D_{max} < 70$ Gy	Joint dysfunction
Parotid glands	Combined mean parotid dose < 25 Gy, or at least 1 gland <20 Gy	Permanent xerostomia
Thyroid gland	Mean dose < 45 Gy	Clinical thyroiditis
Larynx[a]	Mean dose < 50 Gy	Aspiration
	$D_{max} < 66$ Gy	Vocal dysfunction
Pharyngeal constrictors[a]	Mean dose < 50 Gy	Dysphagia and aspiration

D_{max}: maximum dose; **TM:** temporomandibular

[a]Constraints apply only if not target structure

Sources: Marks LB, Yorke ED, Jackson A et al (2010) Use of normal tissue complication probability models in the clinic. Int J Radiat Oncol Biol Phys 76:S10–S19; Emami B, Lyman J, Brown A et al (1991) Tolerance of normal tissue to therapeutic irradiation. Int J Radiat Oncol Biol Phys 21:109–122

Toxicity

Expected acute toxicities include mucositis, dermatitis, xerostomia, and loss of taste. Severity of toxicity may depend on the RT volume and dose parameters, as well as the use of chemotherapy. Late toxicity may include hypothyroidism, neck fibrosis, xerostomia, dysphagia, strictures, aspiration pneumonia, impaired lymphatic drainage, second cancers, and psychosocial problems.

Follow-Up

After completion of definitive treatment, a patient should be offered long-term follow-up to detect second primary tumors, recurrences, or late side effects, according to the recommendations of Table 6.14.

Table 6.14 Recommendations for follow-up

Schedule	Frequency
Year 1	■ Every 1–3 months
Year 2	■ Every 2–4 months
Years 3–5	■ Every 4–6 months
5+ years	■ Every 6–12 months
Examinations	
History and physical	■ Complete history and physical examination
Imaging studies	■ Consider posttreatment baseline imaging of head and neck for N2–3 disease ■ Further imaging only when indicated
Laboratory tests	■ Thyroid function tests every 6–12 months if neck was irradiated
Speech, hearing, and swallowing evaluation	■ As clinically indicated
Dental evaluation	■ Every 6 months
Smoking cessation and alcohol counseling	■ As clinically indicated

Adapted from: National Comprehensive Cancer Network (NCCN) (2009) Clinical practice guidelines in oncology: head and neck cancers, version 1

7

Thyroid Cancer

Roger Ove[1] and Almond Drake III[2]

Key Points

- Thyroid cancer occurs in less than 1% of the population. Benign nodules are far more common, found in 19–67% of randomly selected individuals, with a higher frequency in women and the elderly.

- Thyroid cancer is more common in women, but mortality is higher in men.

- Differentiated, medullary, and anaplastic are the three main types of thyroid cancer. The differentiated histologies are classified as papillary, follicular, and Hürthle cell.

- Papillary thyroid carcinoma is the most favorable differentiated histology, followed by follicular and then Hürthle cell carcinoma.

- Differentiated histologies are the most common (90%). Of these, papillary carcinomas comprise 85%; follicular, 10%; and Hürthle cell carcinoma, 3%.

- Anaplastic carcinomas represent only 2% of cases.

- Surgery and adjuvant ^{131}I are the mainstays of treatment for papillary and follicular variants. Iodine imaging should be performed for all differentiated variants, although Hürthle cell carcinoma is avid only 25% of the time.

- ^{131}I typically delivers a dose of 80 Gy to the thyroid remnant or residual disease, for iodine avid tumors, when given therapeutically. When given for remnant ablation, the delivered dose is roughly 30 Gy.

- Fine-needle aspiration (FNA) is accurate for papillary and medullary carcinoma, but more tissue is required to diagnose follicular and anaplastic histologies.

- Medullary carcinoma is associated with multiple endocrine neoplasia and other familial syndromes (multiple endocrine neoplasia [MEN] 2A and 2B and familial medullary thyroid cancer [FMTC]), although 80% of cases are sporadic.

- Medullary thyroid cancer tends to progress indolently, but it is difficult to control.

- Anaplastic thyroid carcinoma is usually fatal and takes a rapid course. However, aggressive locoregional management is indicated to avoid airway compromise.

- No prospective randomized trials have been performed to evaluate the role of external-beam radiotherapy.

[1] Roger Ove, MD, PhD
Email: rove@usouthal.edu

[2] Almond Drake III, MD
Email: drakea@ecu.edu

J. J. Lu, L. W. Brady (Eds.), *Decision Making in Radiation Oncology*
DOI: 10.1007/978-3-642-13832-4_8, © Springer-Verlag Berlin Heidelberg 2011

Epidemiology and Etiology

Thyroid cancer is a relatively uncommon malignancy, occurring in about 1% of the population, and accounting for 2% of malignancies. Although palpable thyroid nodules are found in up to 7% of the population, only 4–6.5% of these nodules are malignant. However, thyroid cancer is by far the most common endocrine malignancy, accounting for 95% of cases. Risk factors for thyroid cancer are listed in Table 7.1.

Table 7.1 Risk factors for thyroid cancer

Factor	Description
Patient related	**Age and gender:** differentiated thyroid cancers are more common in females, which led to speculation that estrogen levels may increase the risk
	Familial syndromes: ~20% of medullary thyroid cancer are associated with familial syndromes such as multiple endocrine neoplasia (MEN) 2A and 2B, and familial medullary thyroid cancer (FMTC). MEN 2A and 2B are associated with medullary carcinoma and pheochromocytoma, and the MEN 2A variant is also associated with parathyroid tumors. Familial tumors often present at earlier ages, are often bilateral, and have a more favorable prognosis than does sporadic medullary thyroid cancer
	Genetic predisposition: specific mutations of the RET proto-oncogene on chromosome 10 are associated with MEN 2 and FMTC (codes for a membrane-associated tyrosine kinase receptor that expressed in neuroendocrine cells). Thus, the diagnosis of medullary carcinoma warrants genetic testing
Environmental	**Radiation exposure:** exposure to radiation during childhood increases the risk. Such exposures are no longer common since use of radiotherapy for benign disease in childhood is no longer practiced. An increased incidence of thyroid cancer has been seen after exposure to radiation after nuclear bomb tests and detonations, and also nuclear reactor accidents. This is particularly so when exposure occurs prior to 12 years of age
	Dietary iodine: has been linked to thyroid cancer, and affects the distribution of prevalent histologies

Anatomy

Figure 7.1 details thyroid anatomy.

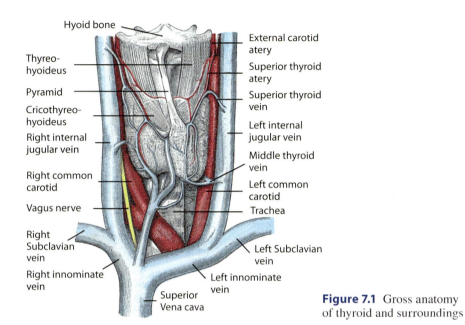

Hyoid bone

Thyreo-
hyoideus

Pyramid

Cricothyreo-
hyoideus

Right internal
jugular vein

Right common
carotid

Vagus nerve

Right
Subclavian
vein

Right innominate
vein

External carotid
atery

Superior thyroid
atery

Superior thyroid
vein

Left internal
jugular vein

Middle thyroid
vein

Left common
carotid

Trachea

Left Subclavian
vein

Left innominate
vein

Superior
Vena cava

Figure 7.1 Gross anatomy
of thyroid and surroundings

Pathology

Well-differentiated thyroid cancers include papillary and follicular carcinoma, accounting for ~80% and 10–15% of thyroid cancer cases, respectively.
Approximately 4% of thyroid cancers are medullary carcinomas, and less
than 2% are anaplastic thyroid carcinoma.

The majority of thyroid cancers including anaplastic thyroid cancer are derived from follicular cells. Pathological features of the commonly diagnosed
thyroid cancers are detailed in Table 7.2.

Table 7.2 Pathological features of commonly diagnosed thyroid cancer

Tumor type	Features
Papillary carcinoma	■ Most common type of thyroid cancer
	■ Arise from the endodermally derived follicular cell that synthesizes thyroxine and thyroglobulin
	■ Frequently multifocal, and histologically featured with nuclear crowding, ground glass nuclei, and psammoma bodies
	■ May have a pure papillary histopathology, but >50% contain an admixture of follicular elements (mixed papillary–follicular), which is classified under papillary and not follicular carcinoma
	■ Follicular variant papillary carcinoma has a purely follicular architectural pattern but may be recognized by the typical cellular features of papillary carcinoma
	■ Diffuse sclerosing variant occurs at a younger age and may cause a diffuse goiter without palpable nodules that can be mistaken for goitrous autoimmune thyroiditis. Diffuse involvement of one or both lobes occurs with dense sclerosis, patchy lymphocytic infiltration, and abundant psammoma bodies. Prognosis is less favorable than it is for typical papillary thyroid carcinoma
	■ Tall cell carcinoma is more aggressive and differs from the usual form by showing tall columnar cells
	■ Columnar cell carcinoma is a distinctly more aggressive form of papillary thyroid carcinoma that occurs more often in older males and is associated with a poor prognosis
Follicular carcinoma	■ Arises from the endodermally derived follicular cell that synthesizes thyroxine and thyroglobulin
	■ Often aneuploid and higher grade, as compared with papillary tumors, which more commonly are diploid
	■ Similar to a benign adenoma pathologically
	■ It is encapsulated, but is distinguished from a benign adenoma by the presence of extracapsular penetration or vascular invasion
	■ Fine-needle aspiration (FNA) is inadequate for diagnosis, histological sections being required to assess morphology and distinguish from adenoma

Table 7.2 *(continued)*

Tumor type	Features
Hürthle cell carcinoma	■ An uncommon variant of differentiated thyroid cancer, also called oncocytic carcinoma ■ Oncocytes are cells that are swollen due to accumulation of mitochondria, and an abundance of these cells defines Hürthle cell carcinoma ■ Oncocytes can also appear in benign tumors or can be associated with other malignancies ■ Similar to mixed-papillary follicular variants of more common histologies, Hürthle cell tumors exhibit follicular morphology and papillary cytology ■ Histological sections are required to make a diagnosis (FNA inadequate)
Medullary thyroid cancer	■ Derived from the neuroendocrine C cells of the thyroid, cells that produce calcitonin ■ While the majority of medullary thyroid cancer cases (75–80%) are sporadic, the remaining are associated with familial syndromes (Table 7.1)
Anaplastic carcinoma	■ An undifferentiated carcinoma, which can arise from transformation of better-differentiated histologies, or occur in isolation ■ Often found in association with papillary carcinoma or other favorable types ■ Subtypes of anaplastic carcinoma have been described (spindle cell, giant cell, squamoid), but all have a similar and dismal prognosis ■ Anaplastic thyroid cancers are unencapsulated, grow rapidly, and infiltrate adjacent tissue
Other thyroid cancer types	■ Nonepithelial malignancies may also occur in the thyroid, such as lymphoma, sarcoma, and malignant hemangio-endothelioma

Routes of Spread

Local extension is observed in all subtypes of thyroid cancer. Lymphatic (nodal) metastasis is a common route of spread in papillary and medullary thyroid cancer, but less commonly observed in follicular cancer. Distant metastasis is rare in papillary but more common in follicular thyroid cancer. Anaplastic thyroid cancer is extremely locally aggressive, as well as prone to early distant metastasis, and there is a substantial risk of death from locoregional progression and airway compromise. Routes of disease spread in commonly diagnosed thyroid cancers are detailed in Table 7.3.

Diagnosis, Staging, and Prognosis

Clinical Presentation

Benign thyroid nodules occur in up to two thirds of the population, depending on the age group studied. The majority of lesions found incidentally are asymptomatic, usually detected during routine physical exam or neck imaging performed for other reasons. For these incidentally found nodules (incidentalomas), biopsy is not recommended if the lesions are smaller than 1 cm, without other risk factors. Clinical presentations and routes of spread are briefed in Table 7.3.

Table 7.3 Clinical presentation and behavior of thyroid cancers including routes of spread based on pathologic diagnoses

Cancer	Description
Papillary carcinoma	■ Usually presents with early stage disease ■ Up to a third (depending on the nature of preoperative imaging) will have clinically apparent cervical adenopathy at presentation, and 50% will have positive nodes microscopically at neck dissection ■ 15% have disease directly extending beyond the thyroid capsule ■ In patients under the age of 20, nodal involvement is as high as 90% ■ Rarely presents with disease beyond the neck, but extensive neck disease is associated with an increased risk of mediastinal involvement ■ Roughly 2–5% of patients present with hematogenous metastases, typically in the lung
Follicular thyroid cancer	■ Has a lower incidence of clinical adenopathy (5%) than papillary thyroid cancer ■ Presentation with hematogenous metastases is more common (roughly 10%) than for papillary cancers ■ The most common sites of metastases are lung and bone
Anaplastic carcinoma	■ Anaplastic thyroid cancer has a tendency for rapid growth ■ Local and regional extension is the common mode of progression and often compromising the airway ■ Rapid hematogenous spread to multiple distant organs
Medullary thyroid cancer	■ Commonly can be found early if genetic screening is done after a diagnosis of MEN syndrome ■ Can be surgically cured if detected early, while still confined to the thyroid gland ■ Prophylactic surgery (total thyroidectomy) is indicated in family members of individuals with MEN 2, at an early age, when that family member also tests positive on genetic testing for the RET mutation ■ Hyperplasia of the C-cells is often present prior to the development of medullary thyroid cancer, and can be an indication for prophylactic surgery given a family history of medullary thyroid cancer ■ Calcitonin will be elevated for both C cell hyperplasiaand medullary thyroid carcinoma, though detection of elevation in early hyperplasia may require stimulation testing ■ Frequently associated with cervical lymph node spread ■ The most common sites for distant metastasis include liver, lung, and bone

Diagnosis and Staging

Figure 7.2 and Table 7.4 illustrate the suggested diagnostic work-up of a thyroid nodule and possible resulting malignancy, including suggested examinations and tests.

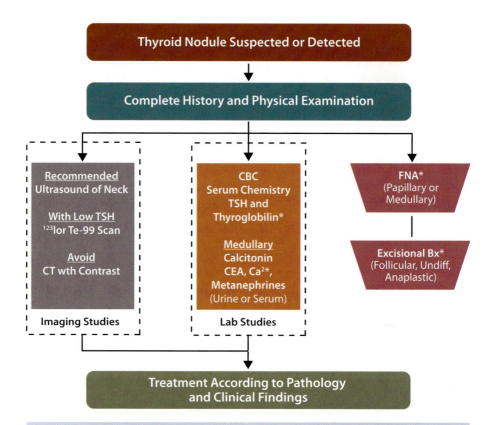

* Indications for a biopsy of a thyroid nodule:
- Nodule > 5mm, with high risk features such at childhood or adolescent exposure to radiation, positive family history for thyroid cancer, prior hemithyroidectomy with discovery of thyroid cancer, incidental PET scan avidity, MEN or other familial medullary thyroid cancer history, RET protooncogene mutation, calcitonin > 100pg/ml
- Nodule > 1cm, with microcalcifications
- Nodule > 1cm, solid and hypoechoic. If iso or hyperechoic by ultrasound, the threshold is 1.0-1.5cm
- Nodule > 2cm, mixed cystic and solid. Suspicious US characteristics would reduce the threshold to 1.5cm
- Purely cystic nodules need not be biopsied, although FNA may be therapeutic
- Suspicious US characteristics include internal hypervascularity, irregular borders, hypoechoic, microcalcifications, taller than wide on transverse view
- Nodules that are fixed to adjacent structures or associated with regional adenopathy
- Symptomatic nodules (pain, hoarseness, and/or dysphagia)
- Nodules found incidentally on positron emission tomography (PET) scans carry a high probability of being malignant (33%)

Table 7.4 Procedures, tests, and examinations used for thyroid cancers

Technique	Description
Fine-needle aspiration (FNA)	■ Accurate for papillary and medullary carcinoma, but not for follicular cancer ■ Distinguishing follicular carcinoma from benign follicular adenomas is not possible by FNA, as the cytology is similar, the distinction resting on histologic demonstration of vascular invasion or penetration of the capsule of the nodule ■ A surgical biopsy may also be necessary to distinguish anaplastic carcinoma from undifferentiated variants of more a favorable histology ■ Recommendations for FNA are detailed in the diagnostic algorithm (Figure 7.2) ■ In the case of a nondiagnostic or inadequate FNA or biopsy, repeating it with ultrasound guidance can yield a diagnosis for 75% of solid nodules, less reliably for cystic nodules ■ Indeterminate cytology, such as suspicion for neoplasm, follicular or Hürthle cell features, or atypia, should be followed by a surgical biopsy (typically a hemithyroidectomy) to make a definitive diagnosis
Excisional biopsy or surgical procedure	■ Indicated for potential follicular carcinoma, as distinguishing follicular carcinoma from benign adenomas by vascular invasion or penetration of the capsule is not possible by FNA due to similar cytology ■ A more substantial biopsy than FNA is required to establish the diagnosis for Hürthle cell carcinoma ■ Surgical resection is often necessary to distinguish anaplastic carcinoma from undifferentiated variants of more a favorable histology
Lab tests	■ Thyrotropin (thyroid stimulating hormone, or TSH), should be measured as one of the first tests in evaluation of a thyroid nodule. ■ Thyroglobulin (Tg), useful for following treated thyroid cancer, is not necessary at initial diagnosis ■ Calcitonin should be measured if medullary carcinoma is being considered ■ Carcinoembryonic antigen (CEA), calcium, and urine or serum metanephrines should also be measured if medullary carcinoma is confirmed ▶

Figure 7.2 Proposed algorithm for diagnosis of a thyroid mass

Revised American Thyroid Association Management Guidelines for Patients with Thyroid Nodules and Differentiated Thyroid Cancer, The American Thyroid Association (ATA) Guidelines Taskforce on Thyroid Nodules and Differentiated Thyroid Cancer, THYROID Volume 19, Number 11, 2009

Table 7.4 *(continued)*

Technique	Description
Radiology studies	■ Ultrasound is the imaging modality of choice to evaluate the primary site and neck ■ Ultrasound is also useful after therapy to monitor for recurrent disease ■ CT with contrast should be avoided, as it would interfere with potential treatment with radioactive iodine, iodine scanning, and remnant ablation ■ Magnetic resonance imaging (MRI) can be useful in evaluating the neck
^{131}I or ^{123}I scans	■ In the setting of a low TSH, it is recommended to perform a thyroid ^{123}I or technetium-99m scan, which can identify a patient with a hot nodule, almost invariably a benign follicular adenoma ■ A cold nodule is an indication for FNA ■ A cold nodule with a suspicious or indeterminate fine needle aspiration biopsy is an indication for an excisional biopsy (usually in the form of a hemi-thyroidectomy) ■ After surgical resection, ^{131}I or ^{123}I scans are useful in assessing for residual disease or a residual thyroid remnant ■ ^{123}I is more expensive, but has the potential advantage of decreased interference with subsequent radioactive iodine therapy
Genetic testing	■ Indicated in medullary thyroid cancer, to identify possible familial cancer syndromes including FMTC and MEN 2 ■ FMTC and MEN-2 can be associated with mutations in the RET proto-oncogene on chromosome 10, which are an indication for prophylactic surgery in family members who are found to also carry the mutation

Tumor, Node, and Metastasis Staging

Multiple staging systems or risk stratification systems for thyroid carcinoma have been developed. The most widely used is the American Joint Committee on Cancer (AJCC) system (currently, the 7th edn., Tables 7.5 and 7.6), which includes age as an important factor for the well-differentiated malignancies.

Table 7.5 American Joint Committee on Cancer (*AJCC*) TNM staging for thyroid cancer

Stage	Description
Primary tumor (T)	
TX	Primary tumor cannot be assessed
T0	No evidence of primary tumor
T1a	1 cm or less, limited to the thyroid
T1b	More than 1 cm, limited to the thyroid
T2	More than 2 cm, less than or equal to 4 cm, limited to thyroid
T3	More than 4 cm or minimal extrathyroid extension
T4a	Moderately advanced disease: Invasion of larynx, trachea, esophagus, recurrent laryngeal nerve, or subcutaneous soft tissues Anaplastic carcinoma contained by thyroid capsule
T4b	Very advanced disease: Invasion of prevertebral fascia, encasement of carotid or mediastinal vessels Anaplastic carcinoma with extrathyroidal extension
Regional lymph nodes (N)[a]	
NX	Regional nodes cannot be assessed
N0	No regional node metastases
N1a	Regional node metastases to level VI
N1b	Regional node metastases to cervical outside of level VI or superior mediastinal
Distant metastases (M)	
MX	Distant metastases cannot be assessed
M0	No distant metastases
M1	Distant metastases

[a]Regional nodes: central compartment, lateral cervical, upper mediastinal

Source: Edge SB, Byrd DR, Compton CC et al (2009) American Joint Committee on Cancer, American Cancer Society. AJCC cancer staging manual, 7th edn. Springer, Berlin Heidelberg New York

Table 7.6 AJCC stage grouping

Stage	Group		
Papillary or follicular, under 45 years of age			
I	Any T	Any N	M0
II	Any T	Any N	M1
Papillary or follicular, 45 years and older			
I	T1	N0	M0
II	T2	N0	M0
III	T3	N0	M0
	T1--3	N1a	M0
IVA	T4a	Any N	M0
	T1–3	N1b	M0
IVB	T4b	Any N	M0
IVC	Any T	Any N	M1
Medullary carcinoma			
I	T1	N0	M0
II	T2–3	N0	M0
III	T1–3	N1a	M0
IVA	T4a	Any N	M0
	T1–3	N1b	M0
IVB	T4b	Any N	M0
IVC	Any T	Any N	M1
Anaplastic carcinoma			
IVA	T4a	Any N	M0
IVB	T4b	Any N	M0
IVC	Any T	Any N	M1

Hürthle cell carcinoma is equivalent to follicular carcinoma with regard to staging. All anaplastic carcinomas are by definition stage IV

Source: Edge SB, Byrd DR, Compton CC et al (2009) American Joint Committee on Cancer, American Cancer Society. AJCC cancer staging manual, 7th edn. Springer, Berlin Heidelberg New York

Prognosis

The prognosis varies widely depending upon histology (Table 7.7).

Table 7.7 Prognostic factors of thyroid cancers

Factor	Description
Histology	■ Papillary differentiation is favorable. Mixed papillary follicular subtypes have a similar prognosis, and are characterized by being follicular in morphology with papillary cellular features ■ Survival for low-risk follicular or papillary carcinoma approaches 100%, with long term follow-up. ■ Although treated similarly to papillary thyroid cancer, invasive follicular carcinoma is more aggressive and carries a worse prognosis ■ Columnar and tall cell variants of papillary histology have a higher risk of recurrence ■ Hürthle cell carcinoma has worse prognosis than follicular histology, with twice the incidence of distant metastases. It is staged as follicular thyroid carcinoma in the AJCC staging system ■ Anaplastic thyroid cancer patients usually survive <1 year despite aggressive therapy with a median survival of 6 months ■ If a mixed population exists including anaplastic elements, the anaplastic feature dictates a poor outcome
Age	■ An important prognostic factor for differentiated thyroid cancer ■ Patients younger than 45 years of age with papillary or follicular carcinoma can have a surprisingly good outcome despite having systemic metastases
Treatment	■ Completeness of surgical resection is prognostically important ■ Iodine avidity is an important prognostic factor predicting the outcome of patients with metastatic disease ■ Medullary or anaplastic thyroid cancer does not concentrate iodine, which limits therapeutic options
Other	■ Include tumor size, nodal metastases, extent, invasion, and completion of dissection ■ For medullary carcinomas < 1cm, disease-free survival (DFS) is 90%, but is only 50% for primary tumors >1 cm ■ In addition to stage, alternative risk classification systems include MACIS (metastases, age, completeness of resection, invasion, size), AMES (age, metastases, extent, size), and AGES (age, grade, extent, size), each generating a numerical score correlated with outcome

Survival rates at 5 years by histology and group stage is detailed in Table 7.8.

Table 7.8 Survival at 5 years by histology and group stage

Histology	Group stage (%)			
	I	II	III	IV
Papillary	97%	93%	82%	41%
Follicular	97%	89%	58%	41%
Medullary	100%	88%	74%	25%
Anaplastic	–	–	–	6%

Source: Harrison LB, Mendenhall W, Hong WK, Medina J, Sessions RB (eds) (2003) Head and neck cancer: a multidisciplinary approach. Lippincott Williams & Wilkins, Philadelphia

Treatment

Principle and Practice

Surgery is the mainstay treatment of most thyroid cancer. Adjuvant treatment of thyroid cancer depends on the histology of disease. Systemic chemotherapy has limited use in thyroid cancer treatment.

Treatment of Papillary and Follicular Thyroid Cancer

The treatment of papillary and follicular thyroid cancer is outlined in Table 7.9.

Table 7.9 Treatment modalities used in papillary and follicular thyroid cancer

Aspect	Description
Surgery	
Indications	■ Mainstay treatment for most thyroid cancer. Total thyroidectomy is usually recommended
	■ Lobectomy is used for low-risk cases only, and can be considered for a solitary differentiated lesion <1 cm, with no evidence of vascular invasion, capsule involvement, or suspicious nodes
	■ If higher-risk features materialize, complete thyroidectomy should be undertaken (followed by remnant ablation). Remnant ablation with ^{131}I should not be performed after lobectomy
Techniques and facts	■ Neck dissection typically involves a central neck dissection (level VI), and functional lateral neck dissection including levels II through V
	■ Subtotal thyroidectomy reduces the risk of recurrent laryngeal nerve injury and hypoparathyroidism
	■ Surgical experience reduces complications. In the hands of surgeons performing greater than 100 cases per year, there is a 2–5% complication rate
External-beam radiation therapy	
Indications	■ Poor iodine uptake and incomplete resection, invasion of adjacent neck structures, extracapsular extension of nodal disease, salvage surgery
	■ There is compelling evidence to offer radiotherapy to papillary patients older than 40 years of age, with T4 disease or positive nodes. Also consider radiotherapy for cases with positive margins, N1b disease (lateral cervical nodes), or nodes > 2cm
	■ The benefit of adjuvant radiotherapy is less well established for follicular histologies, but is supported for patients older than 40 with T4 disease. It is also indicated for cases with positive margins
	■ Gross residual disease
Technique	■ EBRT using 3D-CRT or IMRT
Medical treatment	
Indications	■ Cytotoxic chemotherapy is usually not indicated for follicular
	■ Thyroid hormone replacement with levothyroxine is indicated after total thyroidectomy
	■ For differentiated or follicular cell derived thyroid cancer, thyroid replacement should be sufficient to suppress TSH below the lower limit of normal
Medication	■ Levothyroxine for hormone replacement

Adjuvant Radioactive Therapy

Adjuvant radioactive iodine is typically delivered to papillary and follicular thyroid cancer patients, with a positive iodine imaging after completion of resection. To facilitate follow-up, patients with a risk for recurrence should undergo ^{131}I to ablate any remnant of normal thyroid (Table 7.10).

Table 7.10 Radioactive therapy (^{131}I)

Aspect	Description
Characteristics	■ ^{131}I is a beta emitter (electron emitter) with a half-life of 8 days ■ There is little tissue penetration or systemic dose
Indications	■ As adjuvant therapy for residual microscopic disease, as well as residual thyroid remnant after incomplete resection ■ To facilitate follow-up, patients with a risk for recurrence should undergo ^{131}I treatment to ablate a possible remnant of normal thyroid ■ Typically delivered to patients with a positive iodine imaging after completion of resection ■ May not be indicated for patients with low risk Stage I tumors confined to the thyroid that are <2 cm and is not recommended for low risk Stage 1 tumors with primary <1 cm
Doses	■ The typical dose of ^{131}I is 100–200 mCi, which delivers roughly 80 Gy to the surgical bed or residual disease. For remnant ablation, 30–100 mCi is used, which delivers approximately 20–60 Gy to the remnant ■ The lifetime limit of ^{131}I is 1,000 mCi. The bone marrow dose per therapeutic course is only 2 Gy, and there is complete recovery ■ The limit is based on estimates of radiation induced malignancies, and possible pulmonary injury for patients with lung metastases
Treatment process	■ Withhold Synthroid (T4) for 6 weeks prior to treatment, along with a low-iodine diet. CYTOMEL (T3) is typically given for the first 3–4 weeks of this period ■ A diagnostic iodine scan is often done prior to the therapeutic dose, and treatment is given within 5 days of the scan ■ Some clinicians do not perform the pretreatment diagnostic iodine scan due to concern over inhibiting uptake of iodine during therapy, i.e., "stunning." The alternative isotope ^{123}I reduces this potential problem

^{131}I is used as adjuvant therapy to treat residual microscopic disease, as well as to ablate the residual thyroid remnant after resection. ^{131}I is ineffective in treating medullary, Hürthle cell (a variant of follicular thyroid cancer), or anaplastic carcinoma, as these thyroid cancer types are not iodine avid. A ^{131}I or ^{123}I body scan is typically done 4–6 weeks after thyroidectomy. To improve sensitivity, prior to the iodine body scan, the thyroid stimulating hormone (TSH) is raised with recombinant TSH (Thyrogen) or by withholding thyroid replacement therapy, and the patient is generally placed on a low-iodine diet for at least 2 weeks prior to the scan. Hürthle cell thyroid cancer (a variant of follicular thyroid cancer) is usually not iodine avid, but is avid often enough that iodine imaging should be performed.

After delivery of ^{131}I, a posttreatment scan is done at 1 week, which may show additional findings, due to the higher dose used (Figure 7.3).

Treatment of Medullary Thyroid Cancer

The treatment of medullary thyroid cancer is illustrated in Table 7.11. Neither radiation therapy nor chemotherapy can eradicate gross disease. However, even for locally advanced disease, long-term local control can be excellent after maximal surgery, followed by radiotherapy.

A proposed treatment algorithm for medullary thyroid carcinoma is illustrated in Figure 7.4.

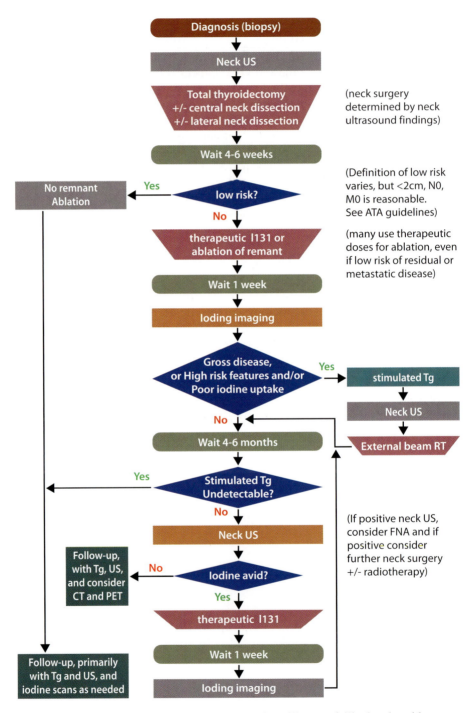

Figure 7.3 Proposed algorithm for treatment of papillary or follicular thyroid cancer. This diagram gives a general outline, and in practice clinical factors often dictate a more complex approach. More definitive guidance can be obtained from the American Thyroid Associaton (ATA)

Table 7.11 Treatment modalities used in medullary thyroid cancer

Aspect	Description
Surgery	
Indications	■ Surgery is the primary treatment, and resection of all gross disease is desirable ■ Total thyroidectomy is recommended, with at least a level VI neck dissection ■ Dissection of the lateral cervical neck (levels II–V) is indicated for primaries greater than 1 cm or positive nodes at level VI ■ More extensive neck dissections are performed for patients with MEN 2B, as these patients tend to have a higher incidence of positive nodes ■ Radical dissection is not recommended unless there is evidence invasion of adjacent structures
Techniques and facts	■ Calcitonin should be measured a few months postoperatively ■ Elevated calcitonin is an indicated for additional imaging (resection if gross disease present then adjuvant radiation therapy) ■ The serum half-life of calcitonin is 12 min
External-beam radiation therapy	
Indications	■ No universally accepted guidelines for exist for postoperative radiotherapy ■ Definite indications for adjuvant radiation therapy include gross residual disease or positive margins, cervical or mediastinal nodes, T3 or T4 disease; extracapsular extension of nodal disease, and after salvage surgery ■ Royal Marsden Hospital has studied adjuvant radiation therapy for an elevated calcitonin, which improved local control from 40 to 70% (Figure 7.4) ■ Due to the indolent nature of the disease, radiation therapy to improve locoregional control should be considered even with distant metastases
Techniques	■ EBRT using 3D-CRT or IMRT
Medical treatment	
Indication	■ Thyroid hormone replacement with levothyroxine is indicated after total thyroidectomy, but suppression of TSH for medullary carcinomas is not indicated
Medication	■ Synthroid for hormone replacement

Source: Revised American Thyroid Association Management Guidelines for Patients with Thyroid Nodules and Differentiated Thyroid Cancer, The American Thyroid Association (ATA) Guidelines Taskforce on Thyroid Nodules and Differentiated Thyroid Cancer THYROID Volume 19, Number 11, 2009

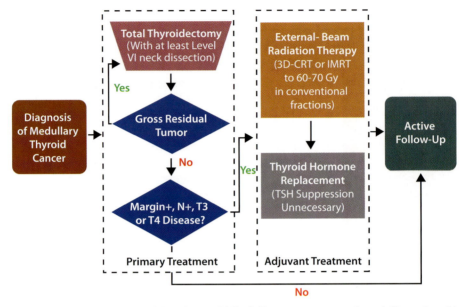

Figure 7.4 Proposed algorithm for multidisciplinary treatment of medullary thyroid carcinoma

Source: Fersht N, Vini L, A'Hern R et al (2001) The role of radiotherapy in the management of elevated calcitonin after surgery for medullary thyroid cancer. Thyroid 11:1161–1168

Treatment of Anaplastic Thyroid Cancer

Treatment of anaplastic thyroid carcinoma using surgery, radiation therapy, and chemotherapy is illustrated in Table 7.12 and Figure 7.5.

Table 7.12 Treatment for anaplastic thyroid carcinoma

Aspect	Description
Surgery	
Indications	■ Indicated for resectable small primary tumor ■ If resectable, total thyroidectomy and selective neck dissection of involved levels is recommended ■ Important for diagnosis of other pathology with similar morphology (e.g., lymphoma) using surgical specimen ■ Palliative surgery with the intent of protecting the airway is appropriate for unresectable cases
Facts	■ Surgery does not improve survival in most cases ■ However, completely resected small primaries are the only cases where prolonged survival has been observed ■ Aggressive locoregional management is appropriate, despite the dismal prognosis, to prevent death from airway compromise
External-beam radiation therapy	
Indications	■ An important treatment modality for anaplastic thyroid cancer ■ Radiation therapy should be initiated swiftly, due to the rapid rate of tumor proliferation that is observed, as this can rapidly compromise the airway ■ The best results have been obtained with hyperfractionated radiotherapy and concurrent doxorubicin (10 mg/m^2), improving median survival to 1 year at the price of considerable morbidity
Techniques	■ Hyperfractionated radiation with 3D-CRT ■ Dose is typically given at 1.6 Gy, twice a day, to a total of 57.6 Gy ■ IMRT should not be used if planning will delay onset of treatment
Chemotherapy	
Indications	■ Has not been shown to improve survival ■ Used concurrently with radiation therapy as radiosensitizer
Medication	■ Optimal cytotoxic agent(s) or regimens unknown. ■ Low dose doxorubicin (10 mg/m^2) is often used as a radiosensitizer, typically with hyperfractionated radiotherapy ■ For good performance status patients, systemic chemotherapy or biologic agents could be considered on clinical trial ■ Clinical trials are not readily available, due to the rarity of this malignancy

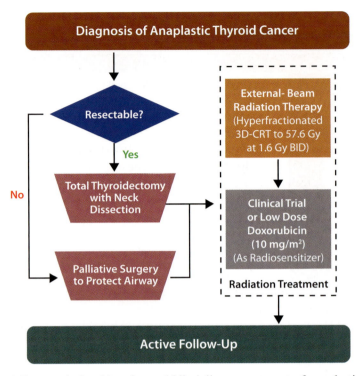

Figure 7.5 Proposed algorithm for multidisciplinary treatment of anaplastic thyroid carcinoma

Sources: Heron DE, Karimpour S, Grigsby PW (2002) Anaplastic thyroid carcinoma: comparison of conventional RT and hyperfractionation chemoradiotherapy in two groups. Am J Clin Oncol 25:442–446; Kim JH, Leeper RD (1987) Treatment of locally advanced thyroid carcinoma with combination doxorubicin and RT. Cancer 60:2372–2375; De Crevoisier R, Baudin E, Bachelot A et al (2004) Combined treatment of anaplastic thyroid carcinoma with surgery, chemotherapy, and hyperfractionated accelerated external RT. Int J Radiat Oncol Biol Phys 60:1137–1143

Radiation Therapy Techniques

Radiation Therapy for Adjuvant Treatment

Simulation and Target Volume Delineation

Computed tomography (CT) simulation for adjuvant radiation therapy, particularly three-dimensional (3D) conformal technique, in thyroid cancer is similar to those used for other head and neck malignancies such as hypopharyngeal cancer.

Definitions of gross target volume (GTV), clinical target volume (CTV), and planning target volume (PTV) in 3D-CRT and intensity-modulated radiation therapy (IMRT) for papillary, follicular, and medullary thyroid cancer (if indicated) are as follow:

■ GTV: gross tumor on imaging studies
■ CTV (for residual primary after surgery and RAI): GTV plus 1.5–2 cm and regional neck nodes of the same level of disease
■ CTV (for residual or recurrent cervical adenopathy after surgery and radioactive iodine imaging [RAI] or anaplastic carcinoma): bilateral cervical nodal regions and superior mediastinum
■ PTV: CTV plus 0.5–1cm

Dose and Treatment Delivery

For postoperative gross residual disease after surgery and RAI for papillary and follicular carcinoma, a total dose of 60–70 Gy in conventional fractions (1.8–2.0 Gy per fraction) covering the gross disease is recommended for external-beam radiation therapy (EBRT).

For persistent or recurrent cervical lymphadenopathy after surgery and RAI, a total dose of 50 Gy in 25 daily fractions to bilateral and superior mediastinal nodal regions, followed by 10- to 16-Gy boost to the gross adenopathy is recommended.

A similar regimen as described above can be used for medullary carcinoma after surgery. For anaplastic carcinoma, hyperfractionated radiation therapy (1.6 Gy twice a day) to a total dose of 57.6 Gy can be considered, to with concurrent chemotherapy (Table 7.12).

IMRT

IMRT for thyroid cancer treatment is feasible and effective in selected cases (Figure 7.6). However, it is not recommended for anaplastic carcinoma if planning will delay the initiation of treatment.

Normal Tissue Tolerance

Organs at risk (OARs) in EBRT for head and neck cancer is detailed in Chap. 6, "Squamous Cell Carcinoma of Unknown Head and Neck Primary," Table 6.13.

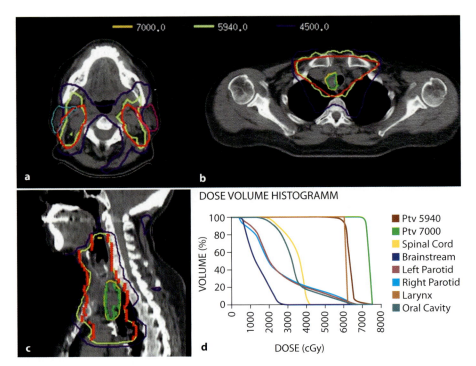

Figure 7.6 a–d A case of multiple recurrent tall cell variant papillary thyroid carcinoma presented with gross disease recurrence in the right tracheoesophageal groove. Intraoperatively, the disease was adherent to the trachea and esophagus and was deemed unresectable. She received 59.4 Gy to the upper neck and mediastinum, and 70 Gy to the area of gross disease, in 33 fractions, using a "dose-painting" technique. **a** A high-neck axial slice, demonstrating the planning target volume (*PTV*) 59.4 (*red*) and parotid (*cyan and pink*) contours, and representative isodose curves. **b** Upper mediastinal axial slice, demonstrating the PTV59.4 (*red*) and PTV70 (*green*) contours, plus isodose curves. **c** Sagittal slice, demonstrating the PTV59.4 (*red*) and PTV70 (*green*) contours, plus isodose curves. **d** Dose–volume histogram for the patient's treatment plan. *Adapted from Rosenbluth BD, Serrano V, Happersett L et al (2005) IMRT for the treatment of nonanaplastic thyroid cancer. Int J Radiat Oncol Biol Phys 63:1419–1426. Used with permission*

Follow-Up

Schedule and suggested examination during follow-up is presented in Table 7.13. Examination during follow-up depends on the pathology of the disease. Clinical responses after EBRT for papillary, follicular, or medullary thyroid carcinoma can take up to 12 months to appear.

Common radiation-induced adverse effects after EBRT include those observed after treatment of other types of malignancies in the lower neck, such as hypopharyngeal or laryngeal cancer.

Table 7.13 Follow-up schedule and examinations

Schedule	Frequency
First follow-up	■ 4–6 Weeks after radiation therapy
Years 0–1	■ Every 3–4 months
Years 2–5	■ Every 6 months
Years 5+	■ Annually
Examinations	
History and physical	■ Complete history and physical examination
Laboratory tests	■ TSH and free T4 ■ Thyroglobulin for differentiated thyroid cancer ■ Calcitonin for medullary thyroid cancer
Imaging studies	■ Neck ultrasound. May be omitted if stimulated thyroglobulin is undetectable (differentiated cases) ■ I-131 imaging used selectively ■ PET/CT if suspected disease (elevated thyroglobulin) with negative US and I131 scans

Source: Ove R, Allison RR (2008) Thyroid cancer. In: Lu JJ, Brady LW (eds) Radiation oncology: an evidence-based approach. Springer, Berlin Heidelberg New York

Section III
Breast Cancer

8

Breast Cancer

Manjeet Chadha[1]

Key Points

- Breast cancer is the most commonly diagnosed malignancy in women in the Western countries, and accounts for more than 25% of cancers diagnosed in women worldwide.

- Early-stage breast cancer and ductal carcinoma in situ (DCIS) are usually asymptomatic, and diagnosed via screening programs. Common clinical signs and symptoms include breast lumps, axillary mass, nipple discharge, or bleeding. Inflammatory breast cancer may present with erythema, pain, and peau d'orange in the affected breast.

- Work up for diagnosis of breast includes complete history and physical examination, imaging studies, and laboratory tests. Tissue diagnosis is mandatory prior to initiating treatment. Results from pathology are also critical for determining prognosis and tailoning systemic therapy (chemotherpay, hormonal therapy, and targeted therapy).

- Stage at diagnosis is the most important prognostic factor. Overall survival (OS) rates at 5 years range from >95% in stage I to <15% in stage IV diseases. Other important prognostic factors include molecular markers, oncogenes, as well as estrogen-receptor (ER), progesterone-receptor (PR), and HER2 status.

- The probabilities of regional lymph node (including axillary, supraclaviclar, and internal mammary nodes) metastases depend on the size and location of the primary disease. The commonly observed distant metastatic sites include liver, brain, lung, and bone.

- For early stage disease, breast-conserving therapy (BCT) using lympectomy and radiation therapy is the preferred approach. Adjuvant hormonal and/or chemotherapy further improves overall survival (OS) in selected stages I–IIA cases.

- Mastectomy followed by chemotherapy with/without radiation therapy is the treatment of choice for locally advanced breast cancer. Neoadjuvant chemotherapy followed by BCT (if feasible) or mastectomy. Postmastectomy radiation improves disease free survival and overall survival (OS) according to published metanalysis. Inflammatory breast cancers are usually treated with neoadjuvant chemotherapy followed by mastectomy and radition therapy.

[1] Manjeet Chadha, MD
Email: mchadha@chpnet.org

J. J. Lu, L. W. Brady (Eds.), *Decision Making in Radiation Oncology*
DOI: 10.1007/978-3-642-13832-4_9, © Springer-Verlag Berlin Heidelberg 2011

Key Points *(continued)*

- Hypofractionated radiation therapy or standard dose-fractionation can be considered for BCT in early-stage invasive breast cancer. 3D-conformal radiation therapy or intensity-modulated radiation therapy (forward plan or inverse planning) is recommended for whole-breast irradiation.
- Accelerated partial-breast irradiation can be used in select patients with early-stage disease after lumpectomy
- In locally advanced disease standard RT dose fractionation is recommended after mastectomy.
- Systemic hormonal therapy and chemotherapy, with or without targeted therapy, are the mainstay treatments for non-metastatic high risk node negative disease, node positive disease, and all metastatic breast cancer.

Epidemiology and Etiology

Worldwide, breast cancer accounts for approximately 25% of all cancers diagnosed in women, and almost 15% of all cancer deaths. It is one of the most common malignancies in the Western world with the highest incidence in North America. In the USA, approximately 62,030 in situ cancers and 178,400 new invasive cases are diagnosed, and an estimated 41,000 deaths per year are reported.

The lifetime risk of an American female developing breast cancer is 13.1 %. In 7–10% of cases, breast cancers present bilaterally as synchronous or metachronous primaries. A number of risk factors have been identified for breast cancer (Table 8.1).

A detailed discussion on risk for developing breast cancer is beyond the scope of this chapter. Recommendation for breast cancer screening is detailed in Table 8.2. In addition to mammography, there are identified clinical scenario in which the use of breast MRI has been considered useful as an additional imaging modality for screening or diagnosis (Table 8.3).

Table 8.1 Risk factors for breast cancer

Factor	Risk factors of breast cancer
Patient related	**Age and gender:** Incidence of breast cancer increases with advancing age. Female:male ratio of breast cancer is 100:1
	Race: Fivefold difference is observed in the incidence between the Western countries and Japan, Thailand, and India
	Past medical history: Prior history of ipsilateral or contralateral breast cancer significantly increases the incidence. History of atypical hyperplasia
	Hormonal milieu: Early age of menarche, late menopause, nulliparity, late primi (pregnancy >30 years of age), obesity, and hormone replacement therapy are adverse factors that increase incidence
	Lifestyle: Moderate exercise reduces risk; obesity and diet rich in animal fat increase risk
	Family medical history: two- to threefold increased incidence with known first-degree relatives
	Genetic predisposition: BRCA1 (chromosome 17q21) and BRCA2 (chromosome 13q12.3) mutation carriers have a high risk at a younger age
	Familial syndromes: Ataxia telangiectasia gene (*ATM*), chromosome 11 (11q22.3) Li Framini syndrome gene *TP53* (or p53), chromosome 17 (17p13.1) PTEN hamartoma tumor syndrome (*PHTS*): gene *PTEN*, chromosome 10 (10q23.3) includes Cowden syndrome (*CS*), Bannayan–Riley–Ruvalcaba syndrome (BRRS), Proteus syndrome (PS), and Proteus-like syndrome
Environmental	**Environmental exposure:** Prior radiation exposure has increased risk, with a latency period of 15–20 years

Table 8.2 Screening schedules and examinations for routine- and high-risk patients

Age (years)	Schedule and frequency
Routine-risk patients	
20–40	Clinical breast exam and directed imaging for palpable abnormality
>40	Annual mammogram and clinical breast exam
High-risk patients	
20–35[a]	Clinical breast exam and directed imaging, i.e., MRI or sonography for palpable abnormality
≥35	Annual mammogram/MRI and annual physical exam

[a]At an age 10 years younger than the age of the youngest relative diagnosed with breast cancer

Table 8.3 Breast MRI imaging in addition to mammography

Description
BRCA mutation or a first-degree relative of a BRCA carrier
When the personal lifetime risk is >20%, the clinical scenarios may include a known mutation carrier, a strong family history of breast cancer among first-degree relatives and those with family history of breast cancer diagnosed at a young age
History of mantle radiation therapy for hodgkins disease
Mammographer's recommendation based on dense breast tissue and mammography images inadequate for interpretation

Anatomy

Mammary glands lie over pectoralis major muscle and extend from the second to the sixth rib vertically, and laterally from the sternum to anterior or mid-axillary line. The anatomy composition of human breast and adjacent structures are presented in Figure 8.1.

The breast can be divided into quadrants for describing the primary site of breast cancer into upper inner quadrant (UIQ), lower inner quadrant (LIQ), upper outer quadrant (UOQ), lower outer quadrant (LOQ), and the central region.

The gross probabilities of breast incidence in different quadrants/regions are presented in Figure 8.2.

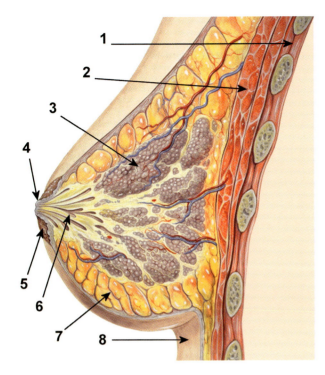

Figure 8.1 Composites of human breast and its adjacent structures. *1* Chest wall, *2* pectoralis muscles, *3* lobules, *4* nipple surface, *5* areola, *6* lactiferous duct, *7* fatty tissue, *8* skin

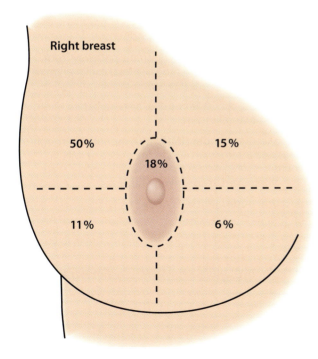

Figure 8.2 Breast quadrants and breast cancer rates per quadrant

Pathology

More than 95% of breast malignancies arise from the breast epithelial elements and are therefore carcinomas. Breast carcinomas can be divided into two major groups, *in situ carcinoma* and *invasive (infiltrating) carcinoma*.

The in situ subtypes are *primarily ductal* carcinoma in situ (DCIS) and *lobular* carcinoma in situ. The distribution of the invasive subtypes includes 70–80% infiltrating duct cell cancers, approximately 10% infiltrating lobular, and the remaining infiltrating subtypes are mucinous, tubular, papillary, and medullary. Further, estrogen-receptor (ER), progesterone-receptor (PR), and human epidermal growth factor receptor (HER)2 status are identified as important molecular features, and now considered mandatory in the complete pathologic evaluation of breast cancer.

Routes of Spread

Local extension, regional (lymphatic), and distant (hematogenous) metastases are the three major routes of spread.

Table 8.4 Routes of spread in breast cancer

Route	Description
Local extension	■ Direct involvement of overlying skin and underlying chest wall may occur in advanced primary diseases (T4 lesions)
Regional lymph node metastasis	■ **Axillary nodes:** The principal lymphatic pathway from the breast parenchyma is to the ipsilateral axillary lymph node ■ **Supra- and infra-clavicular nodes:** by lymphatics through the pectoralis muscle ■ **Internal mammary nodes (IMN):** by lymphatics through pectoralis and intercostal muscle. Incidence of IMN involvement is ≤10% and ≥30% when axillary node(s) are negative or involved, respectively (Table 8.4) ■ **Interpectoral nodes (Rotter's node):** by lymphatics through the pectoralis muscle
Distant metastasis	■ Common sites of metastasis include bone , brain, liver, and lung ■ Metastasis to other organs and tissues is relatively uncommon

Lymph Node Metastasis

Pattern of lymphatic spread depends on the location of the primary tumor in the breast. Commonly involved lymph nodes in breast cancer are illustrated in Figure 8.3a, b and Tables 8.4 and 8.5. The overall incidence of lymph node metastases is summarized in Table 8.6.

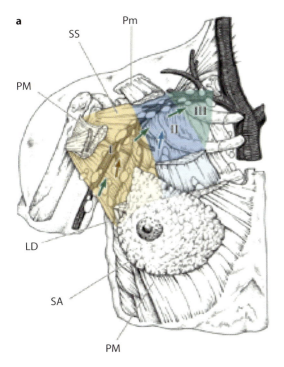

Figure 8.3 a, b **a** Lymphatic drainage of the breast. Axillary lymph nodes alone the axillary vein and may be divided into three regions (Table 8.3). **b** Lymph node groups commonly involved in breast cancer seen on CT scan

Source: Dijkema IM, Hofman P, Raaijmakers CP et al (2004) Loco-regional conformal therapy of the breast: delineation of the regional lymph nodes clinical target volumes in treatment position. Radiother Oncol 71:287–295. Used with permission from Elsevier

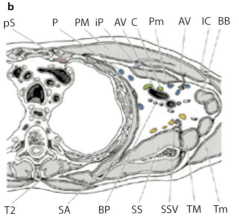

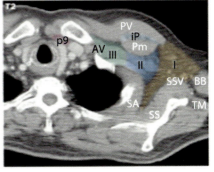

Table 8.5 Regions of lymphatic drainage in breast cancer and their boundaries (used for delineation in radiation therapy)

Nodal groups (levels)	Boundaries
Low axilla (I)	Lymph nodes lateral to the lateral border of the pectoralis minor muscle
Mid axilla (II)	Lymph nodes between the medial and lateral borders of the pectoralis minor muscle
Apical axilla (III)	Lymph nodes medial to the medial margin of the pectoralis minor muscle
Supraclavicular	Lymph nodes in the supraclavicular fossa (triangle), which is defined by the omohyoid muscle and tendon, the internal jugular vein, and the clavicle and subclavian vein
Internal mammary	Lymph nodes in the intercostal spaces along the edge of the sternum in the endothoracic fascia

Table 8.6 Incidence of lymph node metastasis in invasive breast carcinoma

Incidence of lymph node metastasis in breast cancer by size of the primary disease					
Tumor size (cm)	<0.5	0.6–1	1.1–2	2.1–3	3.1–5
Incidence (%)	3–7%	12–17%	20–30%	35–45%	40–60%
Incidence of IMN metastasis by origin of primary breast cancer and axillary nodal status (%)					
Axillary nodes	UIQ	LIQ	Central	UOQ	LOQ
Negative	14%	6%	7%	4%	5%
Positive	45%	72%	46%	22%	19%

UIQ: upper inner quadrant; **LIQ:** lower inner quadrant; **UOQ:** upper outer quadrant; **LOQ:** lower outer quadrant

Source: Handley RS (1975) Carcinoma of the breast. Ann R Coll Surg Engl 57:59–66

Diagnosis, Staging, and Prognosis

Clinical Presentation

With widespread use of screening mammography, a significant number of patients are asymptomatic at presentation, and the diagnosis is made from an abnormal finding on screening mammogram. The findings on mammogram are most commonly reported using the American College of Radiology, Breast Imaging Reporting and Data System (BI-RADs) Table 8.7.

Table 8.7 American College of Radiology, Breast Imaging Reporting, and Data System (BI-RADs)

Category	Assessment	Recommendation
0	Incomplete study	Need additional imaging or prior studies
1	Negative	Routine screening
2	Benign	Routine screening
3	Probably benign	Short-term follow-up to establish stability
4	Suspicious abnormality	Biopsy should be considered
5	Highly suggestive of malignancy	Appropriate action should be taken
6	Known, suggestive of malignancy	Appropriate action should be taken

Source: American College of Radiology (2003) Breast imaging reporting and data system atlas (BI-RADS Atlas). American College of Radiology, Reston, VA

Clinical Presentation

The common clinical presentations are detailed in Table 8.8. The distribution of breast cancer by its location in the breast is UOQ, ~50%; UIQ, ~15%; LOQ, ~11%; LIQ, ~6%; and central; ~18% (Figure 8.2). Approximately 3% of breast cancers are multicentric.

Table 8.8 Common presentation in breast cancer

Findings	Description
Abnormal mammography	■ Architectural distortion ■ Nodule ■ Density ■ Calcification (spiculated) ■ Other (abnormal axillary nodes)
Clinical	■ Palpable mass ■ Nipple discharge ■ Skin changes ■ Nipple areola changes (Paget's disease) ■ Erythema with classical inflammatory changes with or without palpable mass (Inflammatory breast cancer)

Diagnosis and Staging

Patient history and physical should be followed by bilateral mammogram. Additional imaging by ultrasound or magnetic resonance imaging (MRI) should be directed based on clinical findings, i.e., dense breast tissue, high-risk patients, and those in whom there is a clinical mass but the mammogram is negative.

Figure 8.4a, b illustrates the algorithm for workup when patient presents with a nonpalpable or palpable mass.

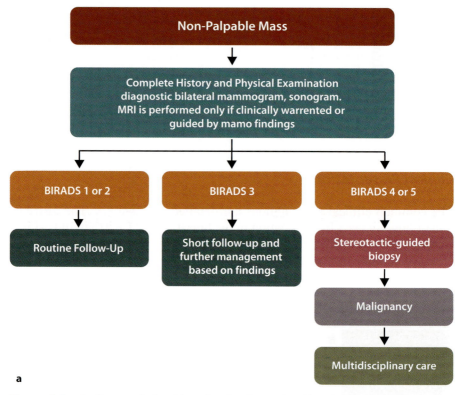

a

Figure 8.4 a, b Proposed algorithms for the diagnosis of breast cancer for non-palpable **a** and palpable **b** masses

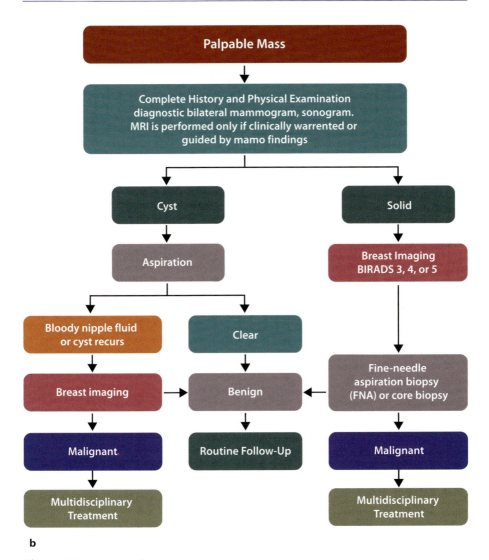

Figure 8.4 (*continued*)

Patients identified as carriers of the breast cancer *BRCA1* and *BRCA2* gene mutations have higher risk as compared with the general breast cancer risk population. The risk of genetic mutations as well as its impact on the treatment recommendations has evolved to identifying a high-risk population for whom genetic counseling and testing is advised as part of their initial workup (Table 8.9).

Table 8.9 Genetic counseling and testing in breast cancer

Description
Personal history of breast cancer diagnosed $\leq$40 years of age
Strong familial history of breast cancer at early age (<50 years) or ovarian cancer
Women <50 years of age, with Ashkenazi Jewish or Polish ancestry with known breast cancer
Relatives of known *BRCA1/BRCA2* mutation carriers
Personal history of male breast cancer
Patient with two primary cancers, i.e., breast and ovarian
Patient with cancer of the fallopian tube

Tumor, Node, and Metastasis Staging

Diagnosis and clinical staging depends on findings from history and physical examination, imaging, and laboratory tests. Pathological staging depends on findings during surgical resection and patholigcal examination, in addition to those required in clinical staging.

The 7th edn. of the tumor, node, and metastasis (TNM) staging system of American Joint committee on cancer (AJCC) is presented in Table 8.10.

Table 8.10 AJCC TNM classification of adenocarcinoma of the breast

Stage	Description
Primary tumor (T)	
TX	Primary tumor cannot be assessed
T0	No evidence of primary tumor
Tis (DCIS)	Ductal carcinoma in situ
Tis (LCIS)	Lobular carcinoma in situ

Table 8.10 *(continued)*

Stage	Description
Primary tumor (T)	
Tis (Paget's)	Paget's disease of the nipple *not* associated with invasive carcinoma and/or carcinoma in situ (DCIS and/or LCIS) in the underlying breast parenchyma. Carcinomas in the breast parenchyma associated with Paget's disease are categorized based on the size and characteristics of the parenchymal disease, although the presence of Paget's disease should still be noted
T1mic	Tumor ≤1 mm in greatest dimension
T1a	Tumor >1 mm but ≤5 mm in greatest dimension
T1b	Tumor >5 mm but ≤10 mm in greatest dimension
T1c	Tumor >10 mm but ≤20 mm in greatest dimension
T2	Tumor >20 mm but ≤50 mm in greatest dimension
T3	Tumor >50 mm in greatest dimension
T4a	Extension to the chest wall, not including only pectoralis muscle adherence/invasion
T4b	Ulceration and/or ipsilateral satellite nodules and/or edema (including *peau d'orange*) of the skin, which do not meet the criteria for inflammatory carcinoma. Invasion of the dermis alone does not qualify
T4c	Both T4a and T4b
T4d	Inflammatory carcinoma
Regional lymph nodes (N)	
NX	Regional lymph nodes cannot be assessed
N0	No regional lymph node metastasis
N1	Metastases to movable ipsilateral level I, II axillary lymph node(s)
N2a	Metastases in ipsilateral level I, II axillary lymph nodes fixed to one another (matted) or to other structures
N2b	Metastases only in clinically detected ipsilateral internal mammary nodes and in the absence of clinically evident axillary lymph node metastases
N3a	Metastases in ipsilateral infraclavicular (Level III axillary) lymph node(s)
N3b	Metastases in ipsilateral internal mammary lymph nodes(s) and axillary lymph node(s)
N3c	Metastases in ipsilateral supraclavicular lymph node(s) ▶

Table 8.10 *(continued)*

Stage	Description
Distant metastasis (M)	
M0	No distant metastasis
cM0(i plus)	No clinical or radiographic evidence of distant metastases, but deposits of molecularly or microscopically detected tumor cells in circulating blood, bone marrow, or other non-regional nodal tissue that are no larger than 0.2 mm in a patient without symptoms or signs of metastases
M1	Distant detectable metastases as determined by classic clinical and radiographic means and/or histologically proven larger than 0.2 mm

Table 8.11 Stage grouping of breast carcinoma

Stage Grouping				
	T1	T2	T3	T4
N0	IA	IB	IIA	III
N1	IIB	IIB	IIB	III
M1	IV	IV	IV	IV

Source: Edge SB, Byrd DR, Compton CC et al (2009) American Joint Committee on Cancer, American Cancer Society. AJCC cancer staging manual, 7th edn. Springer, Berlin Heidelberg New York

The overall survival of breast cancer patients according to presenting stage is presented in Table 8.12.

Table 8.12 Survival by presenting stage of breast cancer

Stage	5-year survival (%)
0	100%
I	98%
IIA	88%
IIB	76%
IIIA	56%
IIIB, IIIC	49%
IV	16%

Source: Bach PB et al (2002) American Joint Committee on Cancer (AJCC) cancer staging manual, 6th edn., Springer, Berlin Heidelberg New York

Prognosis

Prognosis of breast cancer depends on a number of factors. The most significant prognostic factor is the axillary lymph node status, followed by tumor size, histologic grade, and age of the patient. Other prognostic factors include biologic subtypes as defined by molecular markers, and oncogenes. Based on these molecular markers, four prognostic subtypes of breast have been identified (Table 8.13). ER and PR are growth-regulating nuclear transcription factors that are usually measured by immunohistochemistry (IHC), and the amount of protein expressed is directly related to responsiveness to endocrine therapy. Over-expressed and/or amplified HER2 is a strong predictor of response to targeted therapies such as trastuzumab.

Table 8.13 Biologic subtypes based on ER PR and HER2 status that are predictive factors for therapy and outcomes

Subtype	Predictive factors
Luminal A	ER positive, PR positive, HER2 negative
Luminal B	ER positive, PR positive, HER2 positive
HER2	ER negative, PR negative, HER2 positive
Triple negative (basal)	ER negative, PR negative, HER2 negative

Source: Sorlie T, Tibshirani R, Parker J et al (2003) Repeated observation of breast tumor subtypes in independent gene expression data sets. Proc Natl Acad Sci USA 100:8418–8423

The association between the Oncotype DX recurrence score assay (RS) and patient risk for distant disease has been identified by studying the outcomes in a population of node-negative ER-positive patients and has been validated with the data from the NSABP B-14 trial (Figure 8.5).

Genetic profile of the tumors as well as the host provides important prognostic information previously not identified.

Currently in the USA, the clinical relevance of the intermediate score is being studied in a randomized trial (Tailor-Rx).

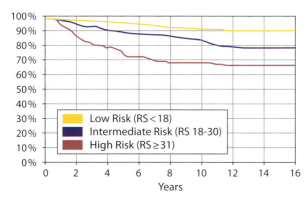

Figure 8.5 The prognostic significancee of Onco-type DX

Source: Paik S, Shak S, Tang G et al (2004) A multigene assay to predict recurrence of tamoxi-fen-treated, node-negative breast cancer. N Engl J Med 351:2817–2826

Treatment

Principles and Practice

Table 8.14 presents the commonly used treatment modality in breast cancer. For early stages, breast conservative treatment includes a combination of the three treatment modalities surgery, radiation therapy, and chemotherapy. For advanced stages, the primary treatment includes a combination of surgery and chemotherapy, with selective use of postmastectomy radiation therapy in high-risk populations.

Table 8.14 Treatment modalities used in breast cancer and their indications

Modality	Description
Surgery	
Indications	■ Lumpectomy is appropriate for DCIS, and stages T1, T2 invasive ductal or lobular breast cancer ■ Mastectomy is indicated in all patients who are not suitable for breast conservation ■ For invasive cancers, sentinel axillary lymph node sampling with our without subsequent axillary dissection for positive sentinel node is routinely completed
Facts/issues	■ Locoregional recurrence after lumpectomy alone without adjuvant therapy approaches 40% for invasive disease ■ When the sentinel lymph node has metastases an adequate axillary dissection requires 10 or more lymph node examined pathologically ■ For the sentinel lymph node that is positive only by immunohistochemistry without evidence of metastases on H&E, the role of additional axillary dissection is controversial

Table 8.14 *(continued)*

Modality	Description
Radiation therapy	
Indications	■ Adjuvant treatment after lumpectomy for DCIS and early stage invasive breast cancer ■ Adjuvant treatment after mastectomy for high risk locally advanced disease (including inflammatory breast cancer) ■ Palliative treatment for metastatic disease
Techniques	■ Whole-breast EBRT is delivered using 3D-CRT or IMRT for DCIS and early-stage invasive breast cancer. ■ Selected nodal irradiation to the supraclavicular, axilla, and internal mammary nodes is indicated only when there is pathologically documented metastatic disease in the lymph nodes ■ Partial breast irradiation using brachytherapy or EBRT can be considered in selected cases ■ In locally advanced disease, irradiation of breast (or chest wall), supraclavicular, axilla, with or without internal mammary lymph nodes is planned
Chemo-/hormonal/targeted therapy	
Indications	■ Adjuvant hormonal therapy as chemoprevention in DCIS ■ Adjuvant hormonal therapy for low- and intermediate-risk early-stage disease ■ Adjuvant chemotherapy[a] for intermediate- and high-risk early-stage breast cancer and advanced-stage disease ■ Neoadjuvant breast cancer is indicated for locally advanced disease (down staging to allow breast conservation) and inflammatory breast cancer
First-line active agents	■ Hormonal therapy: tamoxifen, arimidex, raloxifine ■ Chemotherapy first line: anthracycline-based and taxane-based multi-agent chemotherapy ■ Biologic therapy: Herceptin for HER2-positive tumor combined with multi-agent chemotherapy

[a]Adjuvant chemotherapy is usually give prior to radiation therapy; however, the benefit of such schedule for survival is controversial

3D-CRT: 3D conformal radiation therapy; **EBRT:** external-beam radiation therapy; **IMRT:** intensity-modulated radiation therapy; **DCIS:** ductal carcinoma in situ

In Situ Carcinoma

Approximately 20–22% of all breast cancers diagnosed are in situ. The diagnosis of in situ cancer is generally made on mammography.

Lobular carcinoma in situ (LCIS) is managed by active surveillance. The option of bilateral mastectomy may be considered by individualized risk assessment under special circumstances like *BRCA1* and *BRCA2* mutations or strong family history. Local therapy for LCIS at diagnosis is not indicated. Risk reduction may be achieved by use of chemoprevention strategy using tamoxifen or raloxifene (Table 8.15).

Table 8.15 Randomized data on chemoprevention

Randomized trial	Description
NSABP P1[a]	■ Randomized study delivered placebo versus tamoxifen in 13,388 females for 5 years ■ The relative risk of invasive and non-invasive breast cancer was reduced by 49 and 50%, respectively, with the use of tamoxifen ■ After 7 years of follow-up, tamoxifen led to a 32% reduction in osteoporotic fractures. However, it also led to a number of side effects such as endometrial cancer, deep-vein thrombosis, etc. ■ The study concluded that tamoxifen use as a breast cancer preventive agent is appropriate in many women at increased risk for the disease
NSABP P2[b]	■ A prospective, double-blind, randomized trial involved 19,747 postmenopausal females and studied tamoxifen versus raloxifene in preventing breast cancer ■ The final analysis initiated after at least 327 incident invasive breast cancers were diagnosed: 163 and 168 cases of invasive breast cancer in tamoxifen and raloxifene treated groups ■ There were fewer cases of noninvasive breast cancer in the tamoxifen than in the raloxifene group (nonsignificant) ■ No differences were found for other invasive cancer sites, ischemic heart disease events, or stroke. Thromboembolic events occurred less often in the raloxifene group, and the number of osteoporotic fractures in the groups was similar ■ Generally, tamoxifen is more often recommended in the premenopausal patients, and raloxifene for the postmenopausal patients

[a] *Source: Fisher B, Costantino JP, Wickerham DL et al (2005) Tamoxifen for the prevention of breast cancer: current status of the National Surgical Adjuvant Breast and Bowel Project P-1 study. J Natl Cancer Inst 97:1652–1962*
[b] *Source: Vogel VG, Costantino JP, Wickerham DL et al (2006) Effects of tamoxifen vs raloxifene on the risk of developing invasive breast cancer and other disease outcomes: the NSABP Study of Tamoxifen and Raloxifene (STAR) P-2 trial. JAMA 295:2727–2741*

Adjuvant Radiation Therapy

Adjuvant radiation therapy is indicated for all subgroups of DCIS patients after lumpectomy, according to the results of phase III randomized clinical trials (Table 8.16).

Table 8.16 Clinical evidence for the use of adjuvant radiation therapy for DCIS after breast conservation surgery

Randomized trial	Description
NSABP 17[a]	■ Randomized 813 patients; median follow-up of 128 months ■ Local recurrence without RT 32% and with RT 16% ($p < 0.000005$)
EORTC 10853[b]	■ Randomized 1,010 patients; median follow-up of 126 months ■ Local recurrence without RT 26% and with RT 15% ($p < 0.0001$)
SweDCIS[c]	■ Randomized 1,046 patients; mean follow-up of 96 months ■ Local recurrence without RT 27% and with RT 12% ($p < 0.0001$)
UK trial[d]	■ Randomized 1,030 patients; median follow-up of 53 months ■ Local recurrence without RT 14% and with RT 6% ($p < 0.0001$)

[a] *Source: Fisher B et al (2001) Prevention of invasive breast cancer in women with ductal carcinoma in situ: Update of the NSABP experience. Semin Oncol 28:400–418*
[b] *Source: Bijker N et al (2006) Breast conserving treatment with or without radiation therapy in DCIS: 10 year results of the EORTC randomized phase III trial. J Cancer Oncol 234:3381–3387*
[c] *Source: Holmberg L et al (2008) Absolute reductions for local recurrence after post operative radiotherapy after sector resection for DCIS of the breast. J Cancer Oncol 26:1247–1252*
[d] *Source: Houghton J et al (2003) Radiotherapy and tamoxifen in women with completely excised DCIS of the breast in UK, Australia and New Zealand: randomized control trial. Lancet 36295–102*

There is single-institution experience that has tried to classify DCIS into categories by a given score, categories of score range, with the goal of individualizing therapy recommendations (Table 8.17). Furthermore, results of a recent single-arm observation trial indicate that observation after lumpectomy may be appropriate only for a very small, select group of elderly patients with DCIS (Table 8.18).

Table 8.17 Modified Van Nuys Prognostic Index

Score	I	II	III
Size (mm)	≤1.5 mm	1.6–4.0 mm	≥4.1 mm
Group	No necrosis	Necrosis	Grade 3
Margins	>10	1–9	<1
Age	>60	40–60	<40
Overall Score		**Treatment**	
Total score 4–6 in the postmenopausal		May consider lumpectomy alone, followed by active surveillance	
Total score 7 or higher any age group		Appropriate treatment is lumpectomy followed by RT or mastectomy	
Comment: Limitations of the Van Nuys criteria that preclude wide acceptance in clinical practice is that it is not validated on external datasets			

Source: Silverstein MJ, Buchanan C (2003) Ductal carcinoma in situ: USC/Van Nuys Prognostic Index and the impact of margin status. Breast 12:457–471

Table 8.18 Nonrandomized DCIS trial: ECOG 5194 observational study

Grade	Grades 1–2	Grade 3
Patients (n)	580	102
Median tumor size (mm)	6 mm	7 mm
Median margin (mm)	5–10 mm	5–10 mm
Tamoxifen use (%)	31%	30%
5-Year LC rate (%)	6.8%	13.7%

LC: local control
Source: Hughes, SABSCS 2006

Adjuvant Hormonal Therapy

A number of studies have also evaluated the additional role of tamoxifen in reducing recurrence (Table 8.19).

Table 8.19 Clinical evidence for the use of tamoxifen in DCIS

Randomized trial	Description
NSABP 24[a]	■ 1,804 patients treated with lumpectomy and radiation therapy were randomized to observation ($n = 902$) and tamoxifen for 5 years ($n = 902$) ■ With tamoxifen the ipsilateral breast recurrence rate decreased from 11 to 8%, and in the contralateral breast cancer events decreased from 4.9 to 2.3% ■ The protective effect from tamoxifen was more profound in ER-positive patients as compared with ER-negative patients
UKCCCR[b]	■ Randomized controlled trial with 2 ×2 factorial design recruited 1,701 patients into 4 arms after lumpectomy with negative margins ■ Local relapse rates were 22%, 18%, 8% and 6% for patients enrolled to observation, tamoxifen alone, RT alone, and both RT and tamoxifen, respectively ■ Ipsilateral invasive disease was not reduced by tamoxifen but recurrence of overall ductal carcinoma in situ was decreased (HR of 0.68 [0.49–0.96]; $p = 0.03$) ■ Radiotherapy reduced the incidence of ipsilateral invasive disease (HR of 0.45 [0.24–0.85]; $p = 0.01$) and ipsilateral ductal carcinoma in situ (HR [0.19–0.66]; $p = 0.0004$), but there was no effect on the occurrence of contralateral disease ■ There was no evidence of interaction between radiotherapy and tamoxifen

UKCCCR: UK Coordinating Committee on Cancer Research; **NSABP**: National Surgical Adjuvant Breast and Bowel Project

[a] *Source: Fisher B, Dignam J, Wolmark N et al (1999) Tamoxifen in treatment of intraductal breast cancer: NSABP B-24 randomised controlled trial. Lancet 353:1993–2000; Allred et al (2002)*
[b] *Source: Houghton J, George WD, Cuzick J et al (2003) Radiotherapy and tamoxifen in women with completely excised DCIS of the breast in the UK, Australia, and New Zealand: randomised controlled trial. Lancet 362:95–110*

It must be noted that tamoxifen cannot replace radiation therapy for risk reduction in local recurrence. Patients' recurrence rate in the UKCCR study was 6% after radiation, as compared with 14% for those who received no radiation.

A treatment algorithm for LCIS and DCIS, based on the best available clinical evidence, is illustrated in Figure 8.6.

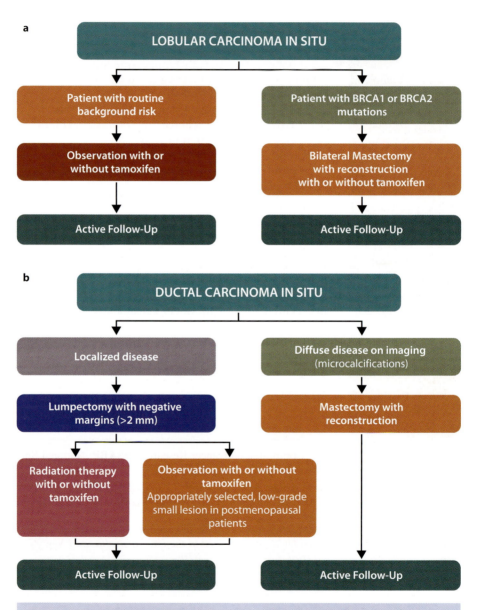

Treatment of Early-Stage Breast Cancer (Stage I and IIA)

Lumpectomy with Radiation Therapy

Breast conservation surgery (BCS) followed by adjuvant radiation therapy is the preferred treatment for early-stage invasive breast cancer. The relative contraindications include gross multicentric disease, pregnancy, prior irradiation, and scleroderma.

The standard regimen in BCS includes irradiation of the whole breast, with or without including regional nodes, as defined by extent of disease. Table 8.20 summarizes the level I clinical evidence from randomized trials. The results support the use of breast-conserving surgery and radiation therapy for early-stage disease.

Mastectomy radiation therapy (PMRT) is not indicated for early stage disease treated with mastectomy.

Table 8.20 Clinical evidence for the use of radiation therapy after lumpectomy for early-stage invasive breast cancer

Trial	Description
NSABP-B06 (1976–1980)[a]	■ 25-Year follow-up of a randomized trial of 590, 632, and 629 patients treated with mastectomy, lumpectomy alone, or lumpectomy followed by adjuvant RT ■ Cumulative incidence of recurrence in the ipsilateral breast was 14.3 versus 39.2% after lumpectomy with or without RT, respectively ($p < 0.001$) ■ No significant differences were observed with respect to DFS, DDFS, or OS ■ OS was ~ 60% for all 3 groups (at 12 years follow-up)
Milan (1973–1980)[b]	■ 20-Year follow-up of a randomized trial of 349 patients and 352 patients treated with mastectomy or quadrantectomy followed by adjuvant RT, respectively ■ Cumulative incidence of same-breast recurrence was 8.8 versus 2.3%, respectively ■ Overall survival 65 and 65% ($p = $ NS) ■ Rates of death from all causes was 41.7 versus 41.2% ($p = 1.0$) and rates of death from breast cancer were 26.1 versus 24.3% ($p = 0.8$) for the two groups ■ No significant difference between the two groups in the rates of contralateral-breast carcinomas, distant metastases, or second primary cancers ▶

Figure 8.6 a, b Proposed treatment algorithm for carcinoma in situ. **a** Lobular carcinoma in situ. **b** Ductal carcinoma in situ

Table 8.20 *(continued)*

Trial	Description
DBCG (1983–1987)[c]	■ Randomized 429 patients to mastectomy and 430 to lumpectomy, followed by radiation therapy ■ At 6 years of life-table analysis, the probability of recurrence-free survival favored lumpectomy and RT (70%) against mastectomy (66%) ■ Overall survival rates were 82 versus 79% at 6 years
IGR Breast Cancer Group (1972–1979)[d]	■ 15-Year follow-up of a randomized trial of 91 and 88 patients with breast cancer (<2 cm) treated with mastectomy or lumpectomy followed by adjuvant RT, respectively ■ pN$^+$ patients were further randomized to nodal irradiation versus no regional treatment ■ Cumulative incidence of same-breast recurrence was 8.8 versus 2.3%, respectively ■ OS were 65 and 73% (p = NS) at 15 years, respectively ■ OS, distant metastasis, contralateral breast cancer, new primary malignancy, and locoregional recurrence rates were not significantly different between any study groups ■ Most recurrences appeared during the first 10 years
NCI (1980–1986)[e]	■ Randomized trial for stages I-II breast cancer patients treated with mastectomy (n=247) or lumpectomy, followed by adjuvant RT (n=237) ■ Node-positive patients on axillary dissection received adjuvant chemotherapy ■ Overall survival was 75% versus 77% at 10 years ■ No difference between OS (75 versus 77%) or DFS observed ■ The probabilities of failure in the irradiated breast were 12 and 20% by 5 and 8 years, respectively
EORTC 10801[e]	■ Randomized trial for stages II breast cancer (<5cm) patients treated with mastectomy (n=426) or lumpectomy followed by adjuvant RT (n=456) ■ At 10 years, OS (66 versus 65%) and DDFS (66 versus 61%) were not different statistically ■ Locoregional recurrence after mastectomy was 12 versus 20% after lumpectomy and RT (p = 0.01)

RT: radiation therapy; **OS:** overall survival; **DFS:** disease-free survival; **DDFS:** distant-disease–free survival; **NSABP:** National Surgical Adjuvant Breast and Bowel Project; **IGR:** Institute Gustave-Roussy; **NCI:** National Cancer Institute; **EORTC:** European Organization for Research and Treatment of Cancer; **DBCG:** Danish Breast Cancer Co-operative Group

[a] *Source: Fisher B, Anderson S, Bryant J et al (2002)Twenty-year follow-up of a randomized trial comparing total mastectomy, lumpectomy, and lumpectomy plus irradiation for the treatment of invasive breast cancer. N Engl J Med 347:1233–1241*

Based on the long-term results of the Early Breast Cancer Trialists' Collaborative Group (EBCTCG) and overview of 78 randomized trials (42,000 patients), reduction in 5-year local recurrence is associated with reduction in mortality at 15 years:

- For Node– patients: 19% reduction in risk of local recurrence at 10 years translated to a 5% decrease in risk of death at 15 years (4:1 ratio)
- For Node+ patients: 33% reduction in risk of local recurrence at 10 years translated to a 7% decrease in risk of death at 15 years

(Clarke M, Collins R, Darby S et al (2005) Effects of radiotherapy and of differences in the extent of surgery for early breast cancer on local recurrence and 15-year survival: an overview of the randomised trials. Lancet 366:2087–2106; Punglia RS, Morrow M, Winer EP et al (2007) Local therapy and survival in breast cancer. N Engl J Med 356:2399–2405)

---

[b] *Source: Veronesi U, Cascinelli N, Mariani L et al (2002) Twenty-year follow-up of a randomized study comparing breast-conserving surgery with radical mastectomy for early breast cancer. N Engl J Med 47:1227–1232*

[c] *Blichert-Toft M, Rose C, Andersen JA et al(1992) Danish randomized trial comparing breast conservation therapy with mastectomy: six years of life-table analysis. J Natl Cancer Inst Monogr 11:19–25*

[d] *Source: Arriagada R, Lê MG, Rochard F et al (1996) Conservative treatment versus mastectomy in early breast cancer: patterns of failure with 15 years of follow-up data. Institut Gustave-Roussy Breast Cancer Group. J Clin Oncol 14:1558–1564*

[e] *Source: Lichter AS, Lippman ME, Danforth DN Jr et al (1992) Mastectomy versus breast-conserving therapy in the treatment of stage I and II carcinoma of the breast: a randomized trial at the NCI. J Clin Oncol 10:976–983*

[e] *Source: van Dongen JA, Voogd AC, Fentiman IS et al (2002) Long-term results of a randomized trial comparing breast-conserving therapy with mastectomy: EORTC 10801 trial. J Natl Cancer Inst 92:1143–1150*

Partial-Breast Irradiation

Single institution experience suggests that whole-breast irradiation (WBI) and partial-breast irradiation (PBI) result in equivalent local control and survival among appropriately selected patients (Table 8.21).

Table 8.21 Single-institutional randomized experience of PBI versus WBI

Endpoint	258 Patients with low-risk (T1N0–1, grades 1–2) invasive breast cancer	
Patients	PBI (n = 130)	WBI (n = 128)
5-Year LR rates (actuarial) (%)	4.7%	3.4% ($p = 0.50$)
5-Year CSS rates (%)	98.3%	96%
5-Year DFS rates (%)	88.3%	70.3%

PBI: partial-breast irradiation; **WBI:** whole-breast irradiation; **LR:** local recurrence; **CSS:** cancer specific survival; **DFS:** disease-free survival

Source: Polgár C, Fodor J, Major T et al (2007) Breast-conserving treatment with partial or whole breast irradiation for low-risk invasive breast carcinoma – 5-year results of a randomized trial. Int J Radiat Oncol Biol Phys 69:694–702

Longer follow-up and results from the ongoing randomized trial NSABP B39/RTOG0413 are required in order to establish the definitive role of PBI in early stage disease (Figure 8.7).

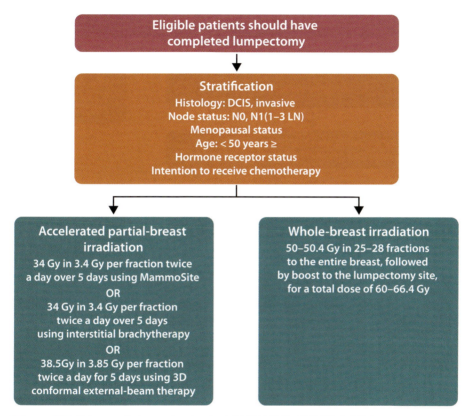

Figure 8.7 Schema of the randomized trial NSABP B-39/RTOG 0413.

Source: A randomized phase III study of conventional whole breast irradiation (WBI) versus partial breast irradiation (PBI) for women with stage 0, I, or II breast cancer. Radiation Therapy Oncology Group. Available at: http://www.rtog.org/members/protocols/0413/0413.pdf. Cited 1 May 2010

Lumpectomy Alone (Without Radiation Therapy)

A few recently published randomized trials have studied the value of lumpectomy alone (i.e., omitting adjuvant radiation) and concluded uniformly that the use of radiation therapy significantly reduces recurrence rates. However, selected elderly, early-stage breast cancer patients with severe comorbidities and limited life spans who have an overall low risk of failure may be candidates for lumpectomy alone (Table 8.22).

A proposed treatment algorithm, based on the best available clinical evidence, is presented in Figure 8.8.

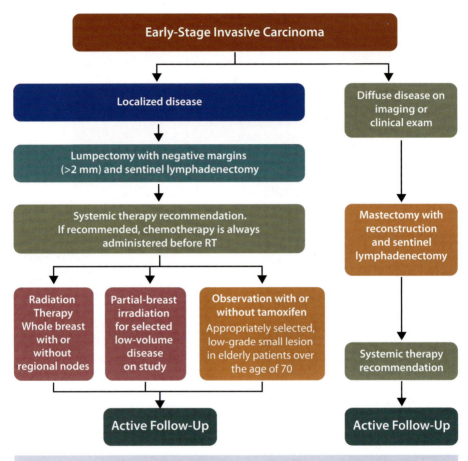

With lumpectomy and mastectomy, sentinel node (SLN) is always performed. The current standard is to perform a formal axillary dissection when the SLN are positive for metastases. Alternatively, patients not undergoing nodal dissection with positive SLN can receive nodal irradiation

Figure 8.8 Proposed treatment algorithm for stages I and II invasive breast cancer.

Table 8.22 Randomized studies for stage I breast cancer comparing surgery and hormone therapy to surgery, radiation therapy, and hormones

Randomized trial	Description
CALGB/ECOG trial[a]	■ 636 Stage T1N0 and ER$^+$ breast cancer patients over 70 years of age were randomized to tamoxifen (TAM) alone ($n = 319$) or RT plus TAM ($n = 317$) ■ The 5-year LR rates were 1 and 7% (p <0.001), and favored the RT plus TAM group ■ No significant differences in mastectomy for LR, distant metastasis, or 5-year OS (86 versus 87%) were observed
PMH[b]	■ 769 Early-stage breast cancer (tumor ≤ 5 cm) patients were randomized to TAM alone ($n = 383$) or RT plus TAM ($n = 386$) ■ The 5-year LR rates were 7.7 versus 0.6% ($p < 0.001$), with a corresponding 5-year DFS rates of 84 versus 91% ($p = 0.004$), favoring the irradiation group ■ The 5-year axillary recurrence rates (0.5 versus 2.5%) also favored combined RT plus TAM ($p = 0.049$) ■ Patients with stage T1 and ER positive disease also benefited from RT (5-year LR rates of 0.4 versus 5.9%, $p < 0.001$) ■ No significant differences in distant metastasis or OS rates were observed
NSABP B21[c]	■ Randomized 1,099 patients with N negative invasive breast cancer (tumor ≤1 cm) to TAM alone ($n = 336$), RT plus placebo ($n = 336$), or RT plus TAM ($n = 337$) ■ Cumulative incidence of IBTR through 8 years was 16.5, 9.8, and 2.8% for TAM, RT alone, and RT plus TAM, respectively ■ RT reduced IBTR below the level achieved with TAM alone, regardless of estrogen receptor (ER) status ■ TAM provided a significant reduction in contralateral breast cancer ($p = 0.039$) ■ OS rates were 93, 94, and 93% in the 3 groups ($p = 0.93$)

LR: local recurrence; **OS:** overall survival; **IBTR:** ipsilateral breast tumor recurrence

[a]*Source: Hughes KS, Schnaper LA, Berry D et al (2004) Lumpectomy plus tamoxifen with or without irradiation in women 70 years of age or older with early breast cancer. N Engl J Med 351:971–977*
[b]*Source: Fyles AW, McCready DR, Manchul LA et al (2004) Tamoxifen with or without breast irradiation in women 50 years of age or older with early breast cancer. N Engl J Med 351:963–970*
[c]*Source: Fisher B, Bryant J, Dignam JJ et al (2002) Tamoxifen, radiation therapy, or both for prevention of ipsilateral breast tumor recurrence after lumpectomy in women with invasive breast cancers ≤1 cm. J Clin Oncol 20(:4141–4149*

Adjuvant Chemotherapy

Adjuvant chemotherapy is indicated in early-stage disease for high-risk patients. If chemotherapy is used, current practice is to current practice is to deliver chemotherapy followed by radiation therapy followed by hormonal therapy. A detailed discussion on clinical evidences of chemotherapy or hormonal therapy regimen is beyond the scope of this chapter.

Treatment of Locally Advanced Breast Cancer (Stages IIB–III)

Locally advanced breast cancer represents a heterogeneous cohort of diseases, from large primary tumor with or without extensive regional lymph node metastases and also include distinguishable aggressive subtypes clash inflammatory breast cancer. A multimodality treatment approach is usually required for achieving optimal control of local, regional, and distant disease (Figure 8.9).

The protocol of combined-modality therapy for any given patient is individualized over a wide range of clinical scenarios, ranging from surgery followed by adjuvant chemotherapy to neoadjuvant chemotherapy followed by surgery. In all cases, the application of radiation therapy is tailored to the extent of disease at initial presentation.

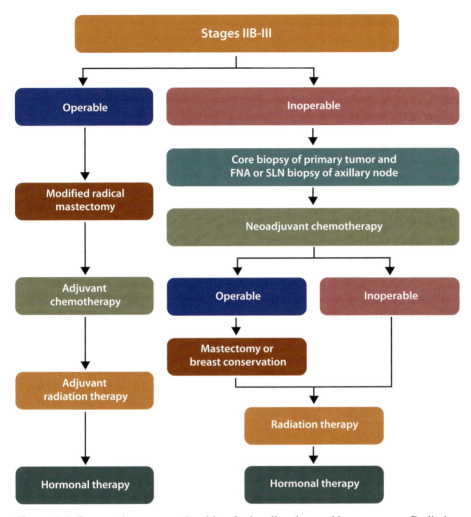

Figure 8.9 Proposed treatment algorithm for locally advanced breast cancer. Radiation therapy generally begins after 3–4 weeks of the last adjuvant chemotherapy cycle. In addition, for patients receiving Herceptin, the RT course is administered concomitantly

The most significant factor in achieving the best outcome for any individual patient is the collaborative role of the surgeon, radiation oncologist, and medical oncologist at the initial presentation.

Adjuvant Systemic Treatment

A detailed discussion on systemic treatment in locoregionally advanced breast cancer is beyond the scope of this chapter. The current practice routinely recommends adjuvant chemotherapy before radiation therapy (Table 8.23). Recent studies have also documented a significant benefit from incorporating trastuzumab in HER2-positive disease.

Table 8.23 Selected clinical evidence for the use of adjuvant chemotherapy, hormonal therapy, or targeted therapy, or their combination

Randomized trial	Description
NSABP B31[a]	■ Randomized 3,351 patients to receive either adriamycin, cyclophosphamide, and paclitaxel or the same chemotherapy plus trastuzumab ■ 3-Year DFS and OS rates were 87 and 94%, respectively with trastuzumab versus 75 and 92% after chemotherapy alone ■ Trastuzumab was associated with a higher cardiac toxicity
EBCTCG trial[b]	■ This meta-analysis included 194 randomized trials. The results reported a benefit to using anthracycline-based chemotherapy and hormone therapy in the ER-positive patients ■ With anthracycline-containing chemotherapy regimen, a reduction by 38 and 20% in the breast cancer mortality was observed among the premenopausal and postmenopausal women, respectively ■ 5-Year duration of tamoxifen is more effective than the 1–2 year course. The absolute benefits at 5 years without chemotherapy were 12%, and with chemotherapy 11%

DFS: disease-free survival; **OS:** overall survival; **EBCTCG:** Early Breast Cancer Trialists' Collaborative Group

[a]*Source: Romond EH, Perez EA, Bryant J et al (2005) Trastuzumab plus adjuvant chemotherapy for operable HER2-positive breast cancer. N Engl J Med 353):1673–1684*
[b]*Source: EBCTCG (2005) Effects of chemotherapy and hormonal therapy for early breast cancer on recurrence and 15-year survival: an overview of the randomized trials. Lancet 365:1687–1717*

Post Mastectomy Radiation Therapy

Locally advanced breast cancers are commonly treated with modified radical mastectomy, followed by adjuvant chemotherapy and post mastectomy radiation therapy. In this scenario, radiation therapy is administered within 6 months postoperatively.

For patients with positive or close surgical margins, post mastectomy radiation should be incorporated in the early postoperative period, either prior to starting chemotherapy or concomitant with a modified chemotherapy schedule.

Clinical evidence for post mastectomy radiation therapy after mastectomy is detailed in Table 8.24.

Table 8.24 Clinical evidence support the use of post-mastectomy radiation therapy

Randomized trial	Description and results
British Columbia trial[a]	■ Randomized 318 premenopausal breast cancer patients (N) to PMRT versus observation ■ RT fields included chest wall, supraclavicular, and internal mammary lymph node regions versus no PMRT ■ The 20-year LR rates were 13 versus 39%, and favored adjuvant RT ($p = 0.0005$) ■ The 20-year OS rates were 47 versus 37%, and favored PMRT ($p = 0.03$)
DBCG 82b trial[b]	■ Randomized 1,708 premenopausal patients with stage II and III breast cancer to PMRT versus observation ■ RT fields included chest wall, supraclavicular, and internal mammary lymph node regions ■ All patients received adjuvant chemotherapy ■ The 10-year LR rates were 9 versus 32%, and favored adjuvant RT ($p < 0.0001$) ■ The 10-year OS rates were 45 versus 54%, favored adjuvant RT ($p < 0.0001$)
DBCG 82c trial[c]	■ Randomized 1,375 postmenopausal patients with stage II and III breast cancer to PMRT versus observation ■ RT fields included chest wall, supraclavicular, and internal mammary lymph node regions ■ All patients received hormonal therapy with tamoxifen ■ The 10-year LR rates were 8 versus 35%, and favored PMRT ($p < 0.0001$) ■ The 10-year OS were 45 versus 36%, and favored adjuvant RT ($p = 0.03$)

[a]*Source: Ragaz J, Olivotto IA, Spinelli JJ et al (2005) Locoregional radiation therapy in patients with high-risk breast cancer receiving adjuvant chemotherapy: 20-year results of the British Columbia randomized trial. J Natl Cancer Inst 97:116–126*
[b]*Source: Overgaard M, Hansen PS, Overgaard J et al (1997) Postoperative radiotherapy in high-risk premenopausal women with breast cancer who receive adjuvant chemotherapy. N Engl J Med 337:949–955*
[c]*Source: Overgaard M, Jensen MB, Overgaard J et al (1999) Postoperative radiotherapy in high-risk postmenopausal breast-cancer patients given adjuvant tamoxifen. Lancet 353:1641–1648*

Neoadjuvant Chemotherapy

There is accumulating evidence on the role of neoadjuvant chemotherapy (Table 8.25). Neoadjuvant therapy followed by mastectomy is still commonly used for this group of patients. However, with adequate down-staging of disease breast conserving surgery followed by radiation therapy can be an alternative to mastectomy (Table 8.26).

Table 8.25 Clinical evidences for the use of neoadjuvant therapy in locally advanced breast cancer (excluding inflammatory breast cancer)

Randomized trial	Description
NSABP B-27[a]	■ Randomized 2411 operable cancers to AC versus AC → D versus AC → S → D ■ Breast conservation rate was same between arms. ■ The pCR rate favored AC over D over AC ($p < 0.001$)
MDACC trial[b]	■ Randomized 258 patients with stages I–IIIa ■ Weekly P–FAC versus every 3 week P –> FAC ■ Breast conservation 47 versus 38% favor weekly P–FAC ($p = 0.05$) ■ The pCR rate favored weekly P –> FAC ($p = 0.02$)
ECTO trial[c]	■ Randomized 1,355 patients with stages T2–T3, N0–N1 ■ AP → CMF → S versus S → AP→CMF versus S → A → CMF ■ Breast conservation 65 versus 34% in favor of AP → CMF → S ($p < 0.001$)
Gerpar–DUO trial[d]	■ Randomized 913 patients with stages T2–T3, N0–N2 ■ Dose dense AD → S versus AC → D → S ■ Breast conservation 63 vs 58% in favor of AC → D → S ($p = 0.05$) ■ The pCR rate favored AC → D → S ($p < 0.001$)

A: adriamycin; **C:** cyclophosphamide; **D:** docetaxel; **V:** vincristine; **P:** paclitaxel; **F:** 5-fluorouracil; **M:** methotrexate; **pCR** pathologic complete response; **S:** surgery

[a] *Source: Bear HD et al (2006) Sequential preoperative or postoperative docetaxel added to preoperative doxorubicin plus cyclophosphamide for operable breast cancer: National Surgical Adjuvant Breast and Bowel Project protocol B-27. NSABP B-27. J Clin Oncol 24:2019–2027*
[b] *Source: Greene MC et al (2005) Weekly paclitaxel improves pathologic complete remission in operable breast cancer when compared with paclitaxel once every 3 weeks. J Clin Oncol 23:5983–5992*
[c] *Source: Gianni L et al (2005) Feasibility and tolerability of sequential doxorubicin/paclitaxel followed by cyclophosphamide, methotrexate, and fluorouracil and its effects on tumor response as preoperative therapy. Clin Cancer Res 11:8715–8721*

Table 8.26 Selected clinical evidence on local control rates for breast conservation treatment following neoadjuvant chemotherapy

Trials	Description
Institut Curie (Paris, France)[a]	■ 257 Patients with T1–3 invasive breast carcinoma treated with neoadjuvant chemotherapy, lumpectomy, and radiation therapy ■ The IBTR rates were 16% at 5 years and 21.5% at 10 years
MDACC[b]	■ 340 Cases of breast cancer were treated with neoadjuvant chemotherapy followed by conservative surgery and radiation therapy ■ 5-Year actuarial rates of IBTR-free and LRR-free survival were 95 and 91%, respectively.
Milan Cancer Institute[c]	■ 536 Breast cancer patients enrolled in 2 nonrandomized trials (tumor >2.5 cm) were analyzed ■ Patients were treated with primary chemotherapy followed by breast-sparing surgery (if feasible), then additional postoperative chemotherapy for patients with high risk of disease recurrence ■ The 5-year IBTR rate was 7% after breast-conserving therapy and neoadjuvant chemotherapy
University of North Carolina[d]	■ 62 Patients with locally advanced breast cancer (LABC) treated with neoadjuvant chemotherapy (doxorubicin) followed by breast-conserving therapy (if feasible), followed by adjuvant chemotherapy and radiation therapy ■ IBTR rate of 10% was observed, and OS was 76% at 5 years

IBTR: ipsilateral breast tumor recurrence; **LRR:** locoregional recurrence; **OS:** overall survival; **MDACC:** MD Anderson Comprehensive Cancer Center

[a]*Source: Rouzier R, Extra JM, Carton M et al (2001) Primary chemotherapy for operable breast cancer: incidence and prognostic significance of ipsilateral breast tumor recurrence after breast-conserving surgery. J Clin Oncol 19:3828–3835*
[b]*Source: Chen AM, Meric-Bernstam F, Hunt KK et al (2004) Breast conservation after neoadjuvant chemotherapy: the MDACC experience. J Clin Oncol 22:2303–2312*
[c]*Source: Bonadonna G, Valagussa P, Brambilla C et al (1998) Primary chemotherapy in operable breast cancer: 8.year experience at the Milan Cancer Institute. J Clin Oncol 16:93–100*
[d]*Source: Cance WG, Carey LA, Calvo BF et al (2002) Long-term outcome of neoadjuvant therapy for locally advanced breast carcinoma: effective clinical downstaging allows breast preservation and predicts outstanding local control and survival. Ann Surg 236:295–303*

Treatment of Inflammatory Breast Cancer (T4d, N0–3, M0)

The most significant factor in achieving the best outcome for any individual patient is the collaborative role of the surgeon, radiation oncologist, and medical oncologist at the initial presentation. Treatment of inflammatory cancer requires combined modality therapy. The 5-year overall survivals range between 30 and 50% (Table 8.27).

Patients are usually treated with neoadjuvant chemotherapy followed by local regional treatment individualized by response, i.e., mastectomy followed by adjuvant radiation therapy or primary radiation therapy.

Table 8.27 Inflammatory breast cancer treated with combined modality therapy

Trial	Description
Attia-Sobol et al[a]	■ 109 Patients with inflammatory breast cancer (IBC) or "neglected" LABC treated with doxorubicin, vincristine, cyclophosphamide, and 5-FU chemotherapy, followed by local treatment ■ Local treatment included mastectomy and radiation (pre- or postsurgical) ■ With a median follow-up of 10 years, the median OS and DFS were 70 and 45 months, respectively; IBC and LABC do not behave differently ■ Multivariate analysis showed peau d'orange, menopausal status and clinical node involvement predicted DFS and OS
MDACC[b]	■ Study included 178 patients with IBC treated in 7 prospective trials at MDACC ■ All patients received local therapy after 3–4 cycles of chemotherapy ■ DFS was 30% beyond the 10-year follow-up

Table 8.27 *(continued)*

Trial	Description
Thomas et al[c]	■ Study of 125 patients with nonmetastatic IBC treated with alternating schedule of RT and chemotherapy ■ Treatment consisted of 3 cycles of induction chemotherapy followed by 3 series of RT to a total of 65–75 Gy to the breast tumor, followed by 5 cycles of chemotherapy administered in between the first two and after the third radiotherapy course ■ 82% of the patients achieved CR, and 5-year local and distant failure rates were 27 and 53%, respectively ■ The 5-year OS and DFS rates were 50 and 38%, respectively
Centre H. Becquerel[d]	■ 178 Patients with IBC treated with neoadjuvant chemotherapy followed by RT or mastectomy, followed by adjuvant chemotherapy ■ A number of combinations were used with regard to chemotherapy and radiation ■ The 5-year OS and DFS approximated 32 and 20%, respectively

OS: overall survival; **DFS:** disease–free survival; **LABC:** locally advanced breast cancer; **IBC:** inflammatory breast cancer

[a] *Source: Attia-Sobol J, Ferrière JP, Curé H et al (1993) Treatment results, survival and prognostic factors in 109 inflammatory breast cancers: univariate and multivariate analysis. Eur J Cancer 29:1081–1088*

[b] *Source: Buzdar AU, Singletary SE, Booser DJ et al (1995) Combined modality treatment of stage III and inflammatory breast cancer. MD Anderson Cancer Center experience. Surg Oncol Clin N Am 4:715–734*

[c] *Source: Thomas F, Arriagada R, Spielmann M et al (1995) Pattern of failure in patients with inflammatory breast cancer treated by alternating radiotherapy and chemotherapy. Cancer 76:2286–2290*

[d] *Source: Chevallier B, Bastit P, Graic Y et al (1993) The Centre H. Becquerel studies in inflammatory non metastatic breast cancer. Combined modality approach in 178 patients. Br J Cancer 67:594–601*

Clinical evidence for treatment of inflammatory breast cancer is detailed in Table 8.27. The treatment algorithm for inflammatory breast cancer, based on the best available clinical evidence, is presented in Figure 8.10.

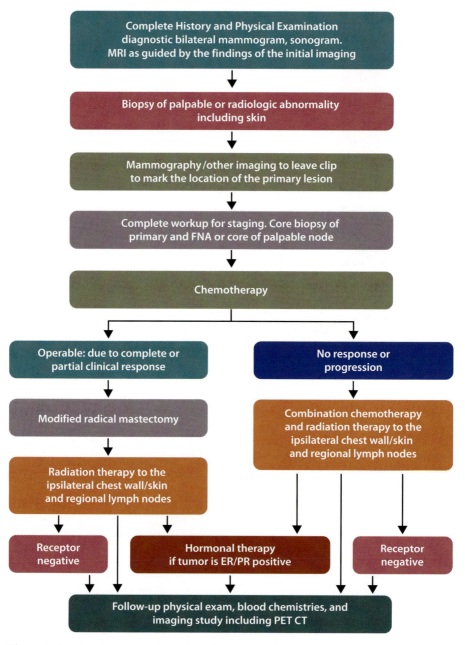

Figure 8.10 Treatment algorithm for inflammatory breast cancer

Treatment of Locally Recurrent Disease

With the prevailing use of breast conservation therapy and improved outcome, an increased number of patients in follow up have an intact irradiated breast. Up to 10–15% of patients will experience a subsequent in-breast local recurrence. Although mastectomy is the current standard of care, many patients desire repeat breast conservation.

Experience from various single-institution reports suggest that there may be a second chance at breast conservation for patients who have history of prior radiation therapy. A detailed discussion of the brachytherapy technology is beyond the scope of this chapter. Results of clinical evidences are summarized in Table 8.28.

Currently the RTOG is conducting a phase II trial to study this important question. http://www.rtog.org/members/protocols/1014/1014.pdf

Table 8.28 Brachytherapy alone after second lumpectomy for breast cancer

Author	Patients (n)	Brachytherapy technique	Median follow-up (months)	Mastectomy-free survival (%)
Maingnon et al	32	LDR	55	73%
Hannoun-Levi et al	69	LDR	50.2	77.4%
Resch et al	17	PDR ± ERT	59	76%
Chadha et al	38	LDR	45.5	94.4%

Sources: Hannoun-Levi JM, Houvenaeghel G, Ellis S et al (2004) Partial breast irradiation as second conservative treatment for local breast cancer recurrence. Int J Radiat Oncol Biol Phys 60:1385–1392; Resch A, Fellner C, Mock U et al (2002) Locally recurrent breast cancer: pulse dose rate brachytherapy for repeat irradiation following lumpectomy – a second chance to preserve the breast. Radiology 225:713–718; Chadha M, Trombetta M, Boolbol S et al (2009) Managing a small recurrence in the previously irradiated breast. Is there a second chance for breast conservation? Oncology 23:933–940

Treatment Planning of Delivery

Radiation Therapy

The indications for irradiation to various clinical target volumes are detailed in Table 8.29.

Table 8.29 Indications for RT to various CTVs

CTV	Indications
Breast only with or without boost	■ Pathologically negative nodes or SLN positive by IHC only
Axillary nodes	■ No pathologic sampling of axilla ■ Positive SLN and no axillary dissection ■ >2-mm extranodal extension
Supraclavicular nodes	■ All patients with >3 nodes positive ■ Selectively in high-risk patients with 1–3 nodes positive
IMN	■ High number of metastatic axillary lymph nodes and inner quadrant lesions ■ Internal mammary nodes (IMN) involvement on positron-emission photography (PET)

The commonly used target volume are summarized in Tables 8.30 and 8.31. The goal of field definition is to encompass target while sparing as much adjoining and underlying normal structures as is feasible without compromising coverage of target volume.

Table 8.30 Guidlines for defining target volume for breast

Anatomical site	Defining target volume
Whole breast	■ Medial: mid sternum ■ Lateral: mid axilla line ■ Superior: 1–2 cm superior to palpable breast ■ Inferior: 1–2 cm inferior to palpable breast
Boost volume[a]	■ Identified by clips or seroma with 1.5- to 2-cm margin

[a]En face electron beam or two- to three-field photon technique

Table 8.31 Guidelines for defining teraget volume for regional lymph nodes (with arm placed in overhead abduction treatment position)

	Cranial	Caudal	Ventral	Dorsal	Lateral	Medial
Axilla level I	Caudal CT-slice tendon latissimus dorsi m.	Caudal CT-sclice free edge pectoralis major m., caudal CT-slice subscapular m.	Skin[a]	Dorsal border axillary vessels, subscapular m., serratur anterior m.	Latissimus dorsi m., teres major m., subscpular m.[b]	Biceps brachii m., coracobrachialis m., lateral border pectorales mm.[c] and breast
Axilla level II	Cranial CT-slice axillara vessels	Caudal CT-slice free edge pectoralis minor m.	Dorsal surface pectoralis minor m.	Dorsal border axillary vessels, rub, serratus anterior m.	Lateral border pectoralis minor m.[c]	Medial border pectoralis minor m.[d]
Axilla level II (including subclavian trunk)	Caudal CT-slice coracoid process	Caudal CT-slice axillary v.	Dorsal surface pectoralis major m.	Ventral border subclavius m., dorsal border suvclavian v. and axillary vessels, rib	Medial border pectoralis minor m.	Clavicle, rib, lateral border jugulo-subclavian junction
Medial SC LNs	Caudal CT-slice cricoid cartilage	Cranial CT-slice jugulo-subclavian junction, caudal CT-slice external jugular v.	Dorsal surface sternocleidomastoid m.	Dorsal border internal carotid a., ventral border scalenus anterior m.	Lateral border sternocleidosmatoid m. and scalenus anterior m.	Medial edge internal jugular v.
Lateral SC LNs	Cranial CT-clice omohyoid m.	Caudal CT-slice external jugular v., transverse cervical vessels	Clavicle, skin	Ventral surface omohyoid m., levator scapulae m., scalenus medius m.	Clavicle, trapezius m.	Lateral border sternocleidomastoid m. and scalenus anterior m.

Table 8.31 (continued)

	Cranial	Caudal	Ventral	Dorsal	Lateral	Medial
IC LNs	CT-slice caudal to deltoid m.	Caudal CT-slice coracoid process	Pectoralis major m., skin	Clavicle, subclavisu m.	Medial border coracoid process, pectoralis minor m.	Skin, origin pectoralis minor m.
Interpectoral LNs	Cranial CT-slice thoracoacromial vessels	Caudal CT-slice pectoralis minor m.	Dorsal surface pectoralis major m.	Ventral surface pectoralis minor m.	Lateral border pectoralis minor m.	Medial border pectoralis minor m.
IMN	Cranial CT-slice jugulo-subclavian junction	Cranial CT-slice 4th rib	Dorsal surface pectoralis major m., dosal surface sternum	Pleura or 5 mm fat tissue dorsal of IMV	5 mm lateral of IMV, lateral border or brachiocephalic v.	5 mm medial of IMV, medial border brachiocephalic v.

LNs: lymph nodes; **SC:** supraclavicular; **IC:** infraclavicular; **m.:** muscle; **a.:** artery; **v.:** vein; **IMN:** internal mammary nodes; **IMV:** interna mammary vessels

[a] ≤ 5 mm ventral of axillary vessels:

Dosimetry and RT Dose Fraction Schedule

The improved dosimetric coverage with associated reduction in hot spots and significant reduction in the incidence of moist desquamation supports the routine use of intensity-modulated radiation technique (IMRT) for intact breast, either using inverse planning or 3D-CRT forward planning with field-in-field technique (Table 8.32) (*Pignol JP, Olivotto I, Rakovitch E et al (2008) A multicenter randomized trial of breast IMRT to reduce acute radiation dermatitis. J Clin Oncol 26:2085–2892*).

The appropriateness of the treatment plan can be evaluated by reviewing the dose–volume histogram from the plan as illustrated in Figures 8.11c (supine) and 8.12 (prone).

Radiation Dose Fractionation

Intact Breast

A number of dose fractionation can be used for adjuvant WBI:
- A total dose of 50 Gy in 25 daily fractions, followed by a boost of 10 Gy in 5 daily fractions, or
- A total dose of 46.8 Gy in 26 daily fractions, followed by a boost of 14 Gy 7 daily fraction, or
- Accelerated schedule of 40.5–42.5 Gy in 15–16 daily fractions (2.7 Gy per fraction) with concomitant boost to 4.5–4.8 Gy in 15 fractions, or sequential boost to 10 Gy in 4 daily fractions

With an improved understanding of the α/β ratio of breast cancer and late-reacting tissues, there has been an interest in evaluating shorter WBI therapy schedules (Table 8.32).

Post Mastectomy Radiation Therapy

Conventional dose fraction regimen to a total of 50–50.4 Gy at 1.8 Gy to 2.0 Gy per daily fraction is recommended for postmastectomy adjuvant radiation therapy.

Regional Lymph Nodes

The dose prescribed to the IMN chain, supraclav, and axilla is in the range of 50.4 Gy in 1.8 Gy per fraction. Depending on the dosimetric coverage of the axillary target volume from the anterior field a posterior axilla boost may be added as supplement the therapeutic dose delivered to the axilla.

Table 8.32 Accelerated whole-breast radiation therapy dose fraction schedule

Randomized trial	Description
Whelan et al (Canada)[a]	■ Randomized studied the efficacy of hypofractionated versus standard radiation dose regimen in whole breast irradiation for N negative breast cancer after lympectomy (margin negative) ■ Radiation regimens were 42.5 Gy in 16 fractions versus 50 Gy in 25 fractions ■ The risks of local recurrence at 10 years were 6.7 and 6.2% respectively, after standard or hypofractionated regimens ■ Good or excellent cosmetic outcome was seen in 71.3 and 69.8% of patients after standard or hypofractionated regimens, respectively ■ Thus, accelerated, hypofractionated whole-breast irradiation was not inferior to standard radiation treatment in women who had undergone breast-conserving surgery at 10 years
START A, (UK)[b]	■ Randomized trial studied standard versus hypofractionated adjuvant RT in 2,236 women with pT1–3a, pN0–1 breast cancer ■ After surgery, patients were randomized to 50 Gy in 25 fractions versus 41.6 Gy in 13 fractions versus 39 Gy in 13 fractions ■ The rate of 5-year local-regional tumor relapse at 5 years was 3.6 versus 3.5% versus 5.2%, after 50, 41.6, and 39 Gy of radiation; the estimated absolute differences in 5-year local-regional relapse rates compared with 50 Gy were 0.2% (95% CI, 1.3–6%) after 41.6 Gy and 0.9% (95% CI, 0.8–3.7%) after 39 Gy ■ Lower rates of late adverse effects were reported with 39 Gy and 50 Gy ■ Thus, a lower total dose in a smaller number of fractions offered similar rates of tumor control and side effects as the standard dose regimen for breast cancer
START B (UK)[c]	■ Similar study setting as in START A but tested 50 Gy in 25 fractions versus 40 Gy in 15 fractions in 2,215 patients with pT1–3a, pN0–1 breast cancer ■ The rate of locoregional tumor relapse at 6 years was 2.2 versus 3.3% in the 40- and 50-Gy groups, respectively. The estimated absolute differences in 6-year locoregional relapse rates compared with 50 Gy was −0.7% after 40 Gy ■ Lower rates of late adverse effects after 40 than with 50 Gy were reported

[a] *Source: Whelan TJ, Pignol JP, Levine MN et al (2010) Long-term results of hypofractionated radiation therapy for breast cancer. N Engl J Med 362:513–520*
[b] *Source: START Trialists' Group (2008) The UK Standardization of Breast Radiotherapy (START) trial A of radiotherapy hypofractionation for treatment of early breast cancer: a randomized trial. Lancet Oncol 9:331–341*
[c] *Source: START Trialists' Group (2008) The UK Standardization of Breast Radiotherapy (START) trial B of radiotherapy hypofractionation for treatment of early breast cancer: a randomized trial. Lancet 371:1098–1107*

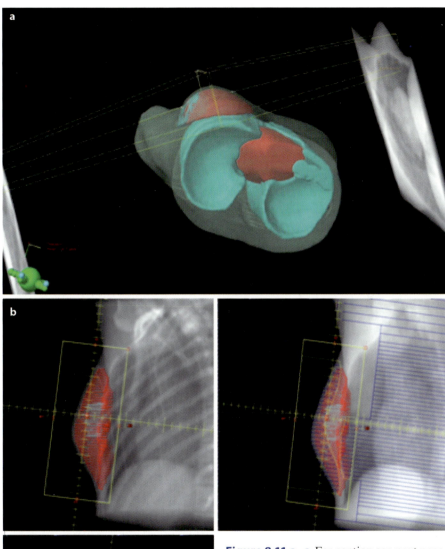

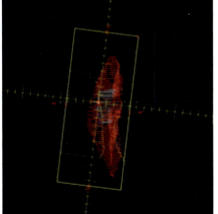

Figure 8.11 a–c For caption see next page

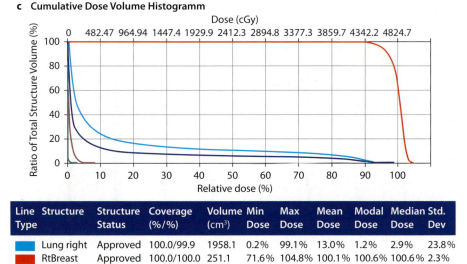

Line Type	Structure	Structure Status	Coverage (%/%)	Volume (cm³)	Min Dose	Max Dose	Mean Dose	Modal Dose	Median Dose	Std. Dev
🟦	Lung right	Approved	100.0/99.9	1958.1	0.2%	99.1%	13.0%	1.2%	2.9%	23.8%
🟥	RtBreast	Approved	100.0/100.0	251.1	71.6%	104.8%	100.1%	100.6%	100.6%	2.3%
🟦	Total lungs	Approved	100.0/100.0	3692.7	0.0%	99.1%	7.0%	0.0%	1.0%	18.5%
🟫	Heart	Approved	100.0/100.0	618.9	0.0%	8.5%	0.7%	0.0%	0.4%	0.9%
🟩	Lung left	Approved	100.0/100.0	1734.6	0.0%	2.9%	0.1%	0.0%	0.1%	0.1%

Figure 8.11 a–c a Tangent beams set up in supine position, **b** Segments of the field in field beam arrangement used in forward plan dosimetry. **c** Dose–volume histogram evaluation reporting dose to target and normal structures.

Normal Tissue Tolerance

Organs at risk (OARs) in radiation therapy of breast cancer include brachial plexus, lung, heart, and skin. In the setting of adjuvant radiation therapy, the planned radiation dose and fractionation postlumpectomy and postmastectomy does not exceed the tolerance of the OARs.

The prescription dose of 50–54 Gy in 1.8–2.0 Gy per fraction to the brachial plexus falls within tolerance. The dose to the entire breast is generally limited to 50 Gy, and boost dose up to 66 Gy is known to be well tolerated, with good cosmetic results. More recent data suggest that a large fraction size of 2.7-Gy fractions to a dose of 40.5–42 Gy delivered to the whole breast is also well tolerated by the breast parenchyma and skin. The dose to lung and heart is kept well below the threshold for these OARs.

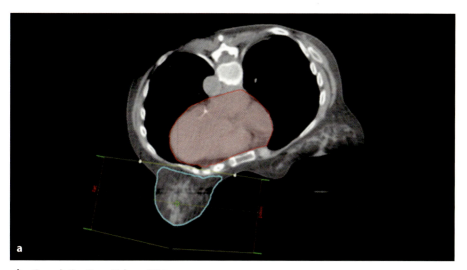

b   Cumulative Dose Volume Histogramm

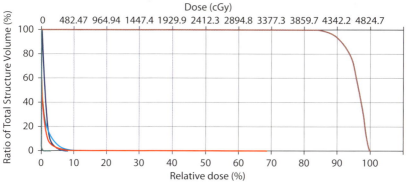

Line Type	Structure	Structure Status	Coverage (%/%)	Volume (cm³)	Min Dose	Max Dose	Mean Dose	Modal Dose	Median Dose	Std. Dev
	LtBreast	Approved	100.0/100.0	257.2	74.9%	100.4%	95.8%	97.9%	96.6%	3.1%
	Lung left	Approved	100.0/99.9	1332.8	0.0%	66.8%	1.4%	0.0%	0.7%	2.4%
	Total lungs	Approved	100.0/99.9	2612.3	0.0%	66.8%	0.7%	0.0%	0.2%	1.8%
	Heart	Approved	100.0/100.0	501.6	0.0%	13.4%	0.9%	0.0%	0.5%	1.1%
	Lung right	Approved	100.0/99.9	1279.5	0.0%	2.4%	0.0%	0.0%	0.0%	0.0%

Figure 8.12 a, b Tangent field irradation for whole-breast irradation in prone position. **a** Patient set up prone with lateral beams, and **b** dose–volume histogram of the same patient

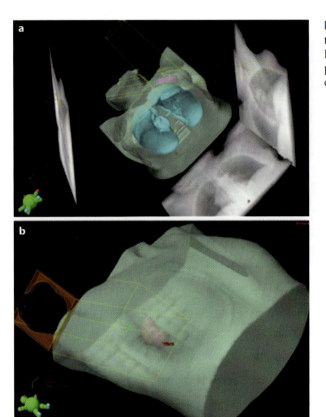

Figure 8.13 a, b Boost to tumor bed can be delivered using **a** oblique photon beams or **b** enface electron beam

The objective of the ideal plan is to keep the radiation therapy dose to these organs as low as reasonably achievable by using collimation, blocks, and IMRT to improve dose homogeneity.

The choice of the beam electrons or photons for the boost is individualized by the size and depth characteristics of the target (Figure 8.13).

When treating the lymph nodes in addition to the breast, a match line between the tangents and the supraclavicular anterior field is achieved by using the mono-isocenter technique. In the case example shown in Figure 8.14, the level I nodes are encompassed in part in the tangent beam and in part by the anterior field, whereas levels II–III and supraclavicular are encompassed in the anterior field only.

When the internal mammary chain is within the planned target, the options for the beam arrangement include deep tangents with block added to the lower half of the field (Figure 8.15a) or a combination of medial electron beam matching a shallow photon tangent beam (Figure 8.15b).

The RTOG breast atlas is a helpful guide in standardizing treatment plans (*http://www.rtog.org/Atlases/breastCancer/main.html*).

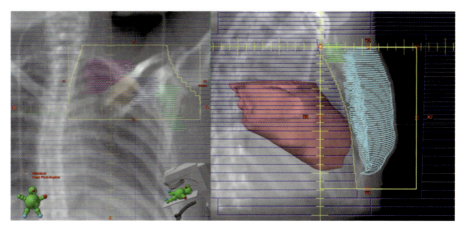

Figure 8.14 Three-field setup using mono-isocenter technique for regional nodes and tangent fields

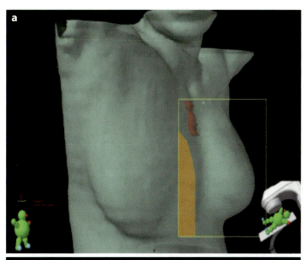

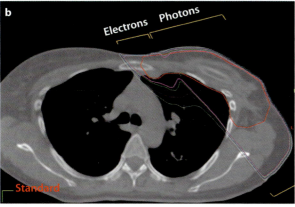

Figure 8.15 a, b Treatment of Internal Mammary Chain may be accomplished by **a** deep tangents using photon beam to encompass the internal mammary nodes (IMN) target with a heart and lung block below the IMN. **b** Combination photon and electron-beam arrangement to encompass the IMN target

Simulation and RT Beam Arrangement

Patients may be positioned in supine (Figure 8.11) or prone (Figure 8.12) position for treatment. Simulation technique in most cases involves a supine setup with immobilization that ensures the arm positioned in abduction with hand over the head. A computed tomography (CT) scan (3- to 5-mm cut) should be performed without contrast from the angle of the mandible to the level of the xyphoid bone.

Follow-Up

Long-term follow up after definitive or palliative treatment of breast cancer is recommended. Schedule and suggested examinations during follow-up is presented in Table 8.33.

Table 8.33 Follow-up schedule and examinations

Schedule	Frequency
First follow-up	■ 4–6 Weeks after radiation therapy
Years 0–1	■ Every 3–4 months
Years 2–5	■ Every 6 months
Years 5+	■ Annually
Examination	
History and physical	■ Complete history and physical examination
Laboratory tests	■ Complete blood counts (CBC) ■ Hepatic and metabolic panels ■ Tumor markers including CA 15-3
Imaging studies	■ Chest X-ray (if clinically indicated) ■ Bone scan (if clinically indicated) ■ CT of the abdomen and pelvis (if clinically indicated)

Source: Chadha M. Breast cancer. In: Lu JJ, Brady LW (eds) (2008) Radiation oncology: an evidence-based approach. Springer, Berlin Heidelberg New York

Male Breast Cancer

Male breast cancer often presents with a palpable mass and have a higher incidence of lymph node metastases at presentation. High incidence of male breast cancer is associated with positive family history, BRCA2 mutation, Klinefelter's syndrome, and testicular dysfunction.

Treatment

The majority of the patients are treated with mastectomy with either sentinel lymph node sampling or a levels I–II axillary dissection. Most of the treatment guidelines are drawn from relatively large retrospective series (Table 8.34). The treatment algorithm for male breast cancer is summarized in Table 8.35. The follow-up scheme are similar to those recommended for female patients as detailed in Table 8.33.

Table 8.34 Selected clinical evidence of the treatment of breast cancer

Published experience	PMH review[a]	French multi-institutional review[b]
Patients (*n*)	229	397 patients (382 IDC and 15 DCIS)
Median age (years)	63	64 (range of 25–93)
N[+] (%)	57%	56%
ER/PR status	90%	79%
Outcome	DFS and OS were 47% and 53%, respectively	5- and 10-year DSS were 74 and 51%, respectively

PMH: Princess Margaret Hospital; **OS:** overall survival: **DSS:** disease specific survival

[a]*Source: Goss PE, Reid C, Pintilie M et al (1999) Male breast carcinoma: a review of 229 patients who presented to the PMH during 40 years 1955–1996. Cancer 85:629–639*
[b]*Source: Cutuli B, Lacroze M, Dilhuydy JM et al (1995) Male breast cancer: results of the treatments and prognostic factors in 397 cases. Eur J Cancer 31:1960–1964*

Table 8.35 Male breast cancer treatment algorithm

Treatment	Indications and regimens
Surgery	■ Modified radical mastectomy or total mast plus SLNDP
Radiation therapy	■ Margin$^+$ or T3–T4 disease ■ >4 Positive lymph nodes
Systemic therapy	■ Chemotherapy: N$^+$ or tumor >1 cm ■ Hormonal therapy: ER$^+$
Options for hormone therapy	■ Orchiectomy ■ LHRH agonist plus anti-androgen ■ Selective estrogen-receptor modulators (SERMs) (tamoxifen) ■ Aromatase Inhibitors ■ Anti-estrogens

IV

Section IV
Tumors of the Thorax

9

Lung Cancer

Steven H. Lin[1] and Joe Y. Chang[2]

Key Points

- Lung cancer is the most common cancer worldwide and accounts for the most cancer-related deaths.

- Over 222,000 cases of lung cancer were diagnosed (the second most diagnosed cancer) in the USA in 2010, causing an estimated 157,000 deaths (making it the number one killer of Americans in terms of cancer-related deaths). The 5-year overall survival of lung cancer is 15%.

- Smoking is the highest risk factor, along with second-hand smoking, radon gas, asbestos, air pollution, and environmental and occupational chemical exposure among nonsmokers.

- Non–small cell lung cancers (NSCLC) account for over 85% of all cases; the rates of small cell lung cancers (SCLC) fall with the reduction in smoking rates.

- The most common presenting symptoms include dyspnea, cough, and weight loss.

- Paraneoplastic syndromes are commonly seen in SCLC.

- Lobectomy is the standard treatment for early-stage NSCLC, although stereotactic body radiation therapy is a good option for medically inoperable patients.

- The optimal management of locally advanced NSCLC is controversial. Treatment includes either definitive chemoradiation therapy or surgical resection and lymph node dissection, with either induction or adjuvant chemotherapy.

- Postoperative radiotherapy is controversial. It is indicated for positive-margin disease and perhaps for patients with pathologic N2 disease.

- After surgical resection for stages IIA–IIIA NSCLC, adjuvant therapy with platinum-based chemotherapy is now the standard of care.

- SCLC is best managed with upfront definitive chemoradiation immediately, using induction chemotherapy; however, the optimal radiotherapy schedule is unknown and is being investigated in cooperative clinical trials.

- Prophylactic cranial irradiation (PCI) is indicated for all stages of SCLC after response to primary therapy. PCI is not routinely recommended for NSCLC.

[1] Steven H. Lin, M.D., Ph.D.
Email: shlin@mdanderson.org

[2] Joe Y. Chang, M.D., Ph.D.
Email: jychang@mdanderson.org

J. J. Lu, L. W. Brady (Eds.), *Decision Making in Radiation Oncology*
DOI: 10.1007/978-3-642-13832-4_10, © Springer-Verlag Berlin Heidelberg 2011

Epidemiology and Etiology

Worldwide, lung cancer is the most common cancer in both incidence and mortality (1.35 million new cases and 1.18 million deaths annually). In the USA, it is the second most commonly diagnosed cancer, with approximately 222,520 new diagnoses in 2010, accounting for 105,770 female and 116,750 male patients; lung cancer is responsible for 28% of all cancer-related death each year (~160,000), more than all of breast, colorectal, and prostate cancers combined. While the incidence in men has decreased in the past 20 years, the incidence in women has increased; however, it has recently stabilized.

A number of risk factors have been associated with lung cancers (Table 9.1). Screening using imaging tests (chest X-rays, computed tomography [CT] scans) in high-risk patients remains controversial, and further studies are needed.

Table 9.1 Risk factors of lung cancer

Factor	Particulars
Patient related	**Lifestyle:** Smoking accounts for nearly 90% of cases of lung cancers (98% for small cell). Lifetime risk for developing lung cancer in smokers is 17.2% in males and 11.6% in females. Lung cancers from second-hand smoke exposure increases the relative risk to 1.2–1.3, and accounts for 20,000 to 30,000 cases annually
	Past medical history: "Scar cancer" has been reported for adenocarcinoma as a radiological-evident tuberculosis (*TB*) sequela
	Therapeutic radiation: Risks of developing breast and lung cancers are increased in patients exposed to therapeutic radiation for lymphoma during youth
	Viral infection: Viral infection with human papilloma virus (HPV), JC, simian virus 40 (*SV40*), BK, and cytomegalovirus (*CMV*) have been attributed to lung cancer development in some cases
Environmental	**Radon gas exposure:** a breakdown product of radioactive radium derived from the decay of uranium found in the earth's crust. Radon gas is the second most important risk factor for lung cancer in the USA
	Asbestos exposure: highest risk factor for mesothelioma, but has synergistic effect to cause lung cancer with smoking. It accounts for 2–3% of lung cancer cancers (other than mesothelioma)
	Occupational exposure: Arsenic, bischloromethyl ether, hexavalent chromium, mustard gas, nickel, polycyclic aromatic hydrocarbons are some of the chemicals linked to lung cancers

Anatomy

There are five lobes in the lung, three on the right and two on the left. Each lobe is divided by five segments, each supplied by tertiary bronchi, except for the right upper and right middle lobes, which are divided into three and two segments, respectively (Figure 9.1). Lymph nodes draining the lung are divided into intrapulmonary, hilar, and mediastinal nodal groups along the secondary bronchi, main stem bronchi, and surrounding tracheal and vascular structures within the mediastinum, respectively (Figure 9.2).

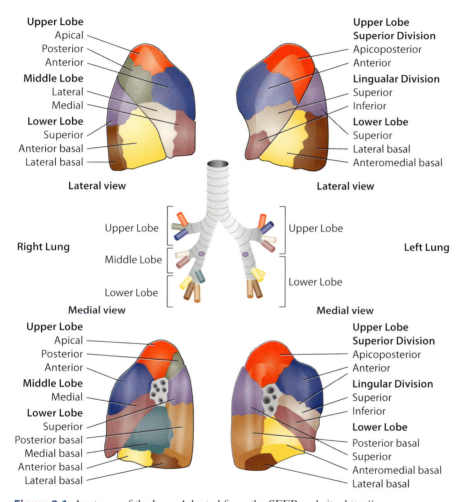

Figure 9.1 Anatomy of the lung. Adapted from the SEER website, http://seer.cancer.gov

Pathology

Lung cancers are broadly categorized as non–small cell (NSCLC) and small cell (SCLC) lung cancers, accounting for around 85 and 15% of all lung cancers, respectively. The most common histologic subtypes of NSCLC are

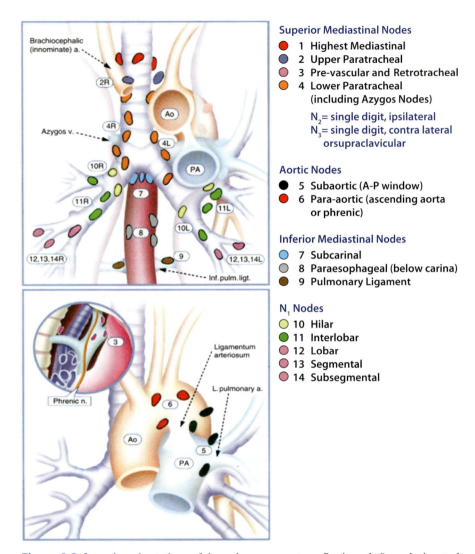

Superior Mediastinal Nodes

● 1 Highest Mediastinal
● 2 Upper Paratracheal
● 3 Pre-vascular and Retrotracheal
● 4 Lower Paratracheal
   (including Azygos Nodes)

   N_2= single digit, ipsilateral
   N_3= single digit, contra lateral
      orsupraclavicular

Aortic Nodes

● 5 Subaortic (A-P window)
● 6 Para-aortic (ascending aorta
   or phrenic)

Inferior Mediastinal Nodes

● 7 Subcarinal
● 8 Paraesophageal (below carina)
● 9 Pulmonary Ligament

N_1 Nodes

● 10 Hilar
● 11 Interlobar
● 12 Lobar
● 13 Segmental
● 14 Subsegmental

Figure 9.2 Lymph node stations of the pulmonary system. Stations *1–9* are designated N2 nodes; stations *10–14* are designated N1 nodes

adenocarcinoma (50%), squamous cell carcinoma (35%), and large cell lung cancer (15%). Subtypes of adenocarcinoma include broncho-alveolar, acinar, and papillary; subtypes of large cell lung cancer include giant cell and clear cell carcinomas, both of which carry poor prognosis. Adenocarcinomas are the histologic type least associated with smoking.

SCLC (a.k.a. *oat cell cancer*) contains dense neurosecretory granules containing neuroendocrine hormones such as adrenocorticotropic hormone (ACTH) and vasopressin.

Routes of Spread

Local extension, regional spread to the lymphatics (Figure 9.3), and distant metastasis are the three most common routes of spread in lung cancer (Table 9.2).

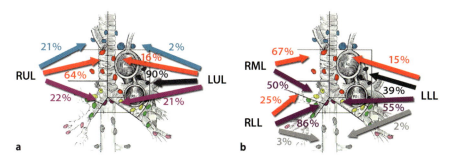

Figure 9.3 a,b a Lymph node stations with highest propensity of spread due to location of primary tumor, either in the upper lobes **b** or in the lower lobes. *Adapted from Asamura H, Nakayama H, Kondo H et al (1999) Lobe-specific extent of systematic lymph node dissection for non–small cell lung carcinomas according to a retrospective study of metastasis and prognosis. J Thorac Cardiovasc Surg 117:1102–1111 Used with permission from Elsevier*

Table 9.2 Route of spread in lung cancer

Route	Details
Local extension	▪ Direct involvement of pleural surfaces, chest wall, ribs, and mediastinal structures causing hemoptysis
	▪ Apical tumors can cause superior sulcus syndrome, with involvement of vertebral body, brachial plexus, stellate ganglion (causing Horner's syndrome), subclavian vasculature, and superior vena cava (causing SVC syndrome)
	▪ Direct extension to recurrent laryngeal nerve can cause vocal cord paralysis and hoarseness. Involvement of phrenic nerve causes diaphragmatic paralysis
Regional lymph node metastasis	▪ First echelon of lymph node drainage includes the hilar and interlobar nodes, followed by mediastinal lymph nodes
	▪ Mediastinal nodal routes of spread differ between upper and lower lobe tumors (Figure 9.3)
Distant metastasis	▪ The most common stage at presentation is with distant metastasis (~a third)
	▪ Most common sites of distant metastasis are contralateral lung, brain, bone, adrenals, and liver
	▪ Malignant pleural effusion, while strictly not defined as distant metastasis, has poor prognosis and behaves like stage IV disease

Diagnosis, Staging, and Prognosis

Clinical Presentation

Presenting signs and symptoms of lung cancer depend on the location and extent of disease. The symptoms can reflect locoregional spread of disease (either from primary mass or from location of distant metastasis) or systemic manifestation of disease (constitutional symptoms, paraneoplastic syndrome). The three most common presenting sign and symptoms of lung cancers are dyspnea, cough, and weight loss. Others include chest pain, hemoptysis, clubbing, and bone pain (Table 9.3).

Table 9.3 Common signs and symptoms of lung cancer

Disease manifestation	Particulars
Locoregional manifestation of disease	**Superior sulcus syndrome:** nvasion of apical structures to cause Horner's, brachial plexopathy, and bone pain
	Superior vena cava syndrome: venous distension of neck and chest wall, cyanosis, facial plethora, and upper extremity edema
	Nerve plexopathies: brachial plexopathy, recurrent laryngeal nerve, and phrenic nerve paralysis
	Local extension of disease: causes hemoptysis, chest wall pain, rib pain, post-obstructive pneumonia, headaches, nausea and vomiting, or focal neurologic signs/symptoms from brain metastasis
Systemic manifestation of disease	**Constitutional symptoms:** fever, weight loss, anorexia, weakness
	Paraneoplastic disorders (NSCLC): hypercalcemia of malignancy (HCM)
	Paraneoplastic disorders (SCLC): Lambert-Eaton myasthenic syndrome, hyponatremia due to syndrome of inappropriate antidiuretic hormone hypersecretion (SIADH), Cushing's syndrome (ACTH), several neurologic paraneoplastic disorders (encephalomyelitis, sensory neuropathies, cerebellar degeneration, limbic and brainstem encephalitis)

Workup and Staging

Complete history, physical examination, and diagnostic imaging and laboratory tests are necessary for the proper diagnosis and staging of lung cancers. Figure 9.4 summarizes the workup and Table 9.4 provides details on the various tests employed for the diagnosis and staging. The 7th edition of the American Joint Committee on Cancer (AJCC) staging and grouping of lung cancer (both NSCLC and SCLC) is presented in Tables 9.5 and 9.6. However, the clinical staging that is commonly used in SCLC is determined by whether the disease can be encompassed within a radiation portal (limited) or not (extensive).

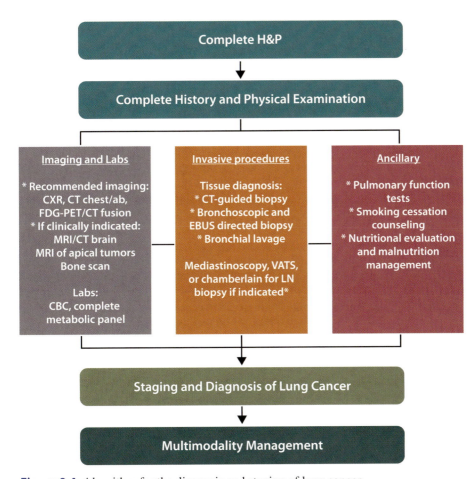

Figure 9.4 Algorithm for the diagnosis and staging of lung cancer

Table 9.4 Tests for workup of lung cancer

Modality	Test
Imaging	**Chest X-ray** is usually the first test ordered at first presentation. "Popcorn" calcification is commonly a radiologic sign of benign process
	CT scan of the thorax and abdomen to study the extent of the disease regionally and to rule out lesions in adrenals and liver. Sensitivity is 64% and specificity is 74%
	FDG-PET: approved by U.S. Food and Drug Administration (FDA) to workup pulmonary nodules. Limit of detection ~8-mm lesions. Rate of detection of occult metastasis range from 6 to 18%. Sensitivity and specificity for staging is 83 and 91%, respectively. Positive predictive value (PPV) is ~80% (false-positive rate ~10–20%) and negative predictive value (NPV) is ~95% (false-negative rate ~5–16%). Because FP rate is higher, a positive PET lesion needs to have pathologic confirmation if will impact management
	MRI is more sensitive than CT is to detect brain metastasis, should be done in patients with advanced disease. For superior sulcus tumors to rule out brachial plexus invasion. For symptomatic patients to rule out cord compression
	Bone scan can be done for symptomatic patients. More sensitive for blastic than lytic lesions. Bone scan is optional if FDG-PET is performed, as FDG-PET is more sensitive for detecting osseous metastasis
Invasive procedures	**Bronchoscopy:** Allows direct visualization and sampling of centrally located tumors. The use of fiberoptic techniques allows visualization and sampling of peripheral lesions.
	Endobronchial Ultrasound (EBUS): Visualize extent of invasion in centrally located tumors and mediastinal lymph nodes. Allows sampling of suspicious lymph nodes using fine needle aspiration. Generally stations 2, 3, 4, 7 and 10 could be interrogated.
	Mediastinoscopy: Done to evaluate status of enlarged mediastinal lymph nodes seen on CT and/or positive on PET. Can evaluate stations 2, 4, and 7.
	Chamberlain procedure (Anterior mediastinotomy): May be necessary to evaluate nodes in stations 5 and 6.
	Video Assisted Thorascopic Surgery (VATS): Reserved for tumors that remain undiagnosed after bronchoscopy or CT-guided biopsy. May also be important for management of malignant pleural effusions.
	CT guided biopsy: This procedure is generally necessary for peripherally-located lesions, or at sites of distant disease.

Table 9.5 AJCC tumor, node, and metastasis (*TNM*) classification of lung cancers (NSCLC and SCLC), 7th edition

Stage	Description
Primary tumor (T)	
Tx	Primary tumor cannot be assessed
T1	≤3-cm tumor, surrounded by lung parenchyma
T1a	≤-cm tumor
T1b	2.1- to 3-cm tumor
T2	>3- to 7-cm tumor, involvement of visceral pleura, invading main-stem bronchus >2 cm from carina, or causing atelectasis to a single lobe of the lung
T2a	3.1- to 5-cm tumor
T2b	5.1- to 7-cm tumor
T3	>7-cm tumor, tumor invading mainstem bronchus <2 cm from ca-rina, invasion of diaphragm, chest wall, pericardium, mediastinal pleura, or associated atelectasis or obstructive pneumonitis of en-tire lung, or satellite nodule in the same lobe
T4	Invasion of great vessels or adjacent organs, or nodules in separate lobe in the ipsilateral lung
Regional lymph nodes (N)	
Nx	Regional lymph nodes cannot be assessed
N0	No regional lymph nodes metastasis
N1	Ipsilateral hilar or peribronchial nodes
N2	Ipsilateral mediastinal or subcarinal nodes
N3	Any supraclavicular/scalene node or contralateral mediastinal/hilar nodes
Distant metastasis (M)	
M1a	Malignant pleural effusion, pericardial nodules/effusions, or lung nodules in contralateral lung
M1b	Metastasis to distant organs

Source: Edge SB, Byrd DR, Compton CC et al (2009) American Joint Committee on Cancer, American Cancer Society. AJCC cancer staging manual, 7th edn. Springer, Berlin Heidelberg New York

Table 9.6 AJCC stage grouping of lung cancers (NSCLC and SCLC), 7th edition

Stage Grouping						
	T1a	T1b	T2a	T2b	T3	T4
N0	IA	IA	IB	IIA	IIB	IIIB
N1	IIA	IIA	IIA	IIB	IIIA	IIIB
N2	IIIA	IIIA	IIIA	IIIA	IIIA	IIIB
N3	IIIB	IIIB	IIIB	IIIB	IIIB	IIIB
M1	IV	IV	IV	IV	IV	IV

Source: Edge SB, Byrd DR, Compton CC et al (2009) American Joint Committee on Cancer, American Cancer Society. AJCC cancer staging manual, 7th edn. Springer, Berlin Heidelberg New York

Prognosis

Overall survival is determined by treatment factors and patient factors. The four strongest adverse prognostic factors for survival in lung cancers are (1) advanced stage of disease, (2) poor performance status (Karnofsky Performance Status [KPS] <80%), (3) weight loss >5% in preceding 3 months, and (4) age >60 years. The survival of patients based on stage is summarized in Table 9.7.

Table 9.7 Overall survival (*OS*) based on the stage of presentation

Survival (years)	Extent of cancer				
	Early-stage (I-II) NSCLC	Locally advanced (III) NSCLC	Advanced (IV) NSCLC	Limited-stage SCLC	Extensive-stage SCLC
1	–	–	30–40%	50%	27–40%
3	–	15–22%	–	30–40%	0%
5	50–77%	9–16%	–	20–30%	0%
Median survival	36 Months (20–60 Months)	13–17 Months	8–10 Months	18 Months	7–10 Months

Survival based on the best treatment arms in various randomized trials and meta-analyses

Treatment

Principles and Practice

Management for lung cancers is largely dependent on whether the diagnosis is NSCLC or SCLC (Table 9.8). Surgery is the treatment of choice for early-stage NSCLC, and it is often incorporated for early locally advanced patients as well. In the past, conventional radiation therapy yielded poor outcomes for unresectable early-stage patients; however, technologic advances with the advent of stereotactic ablative radiation therapy have contributed to improvements in local control and survival. Locally advanced NSCLC is often managed with concurrent chemotherapy and radiation therapy. Postoperative radiotherapy is given for patients with positive-margin or pathologic N2 disease. Systemic agents (chemotherapy, targeted agents) are given in the adjuvant setting after surgical resection for stage Ib (tumors >4 cm) to IIIA patients, or palliatively for stage IV patients. For SCLC, definitive chemoradiation is usually employed for limited-stage SCLC or extensive-stage SCLC with good response to chemotherapy, although surgical resection for early-stage SCLC is being explored based on promising

Table 9.8 Treatment modalities used in lung cancer

Modality	Details
Surgical resection	
Indications	■ Treatment of choice for early stage NSCLC (stage I-II) ■ Maybe indicated for early stage IIIA after induction therapies (chemoradiation or chemotherapy) if lobectomy can be performed ■ Lobectomy preferred over wedge resection, with mediastinal lymph node dissection ■ Minimum FEV1 necessary for lobectomy >1.5 L and for pneumonectomy > 2.0 L. The marginal %FEV1 is 40% of predicted ■ Generally not indicated for SCLC, although can be considered for small lesions on clinical trial
Facts	■ For a T1N0 NSCLC, local control after lobectomy is 94%, and 82% after wedge resection[a] (Ginsberg RJ et al, NEJM 1995) ■ Around 5-25% of clinical stage I patients are upstaged after surgery ■ Factors that predict for postoperative complications include: 1) active smoking, 2) poor nutritional status, 3) advanced age, 4) poor lung function ■ Mortality rates range 1-4% after lobectomy, and 10-20% after pneumonectomy ▶

Table 9.8 *(continued)*

Modality	Details
Radiation Therapy	
Indications	■ Definitive treatment for medical inoperable stage I NSCLC using hypofractionated stereotactic body radiation therapy ■ Definitive treatment for NSCLC patients unable to tolerate chemotherapy ■ Definitive treatment for locally advanced (stage III) NSCLC and limited stage SCLC with concurrent chemotherapy ■ Prophylactic cranial irradiation in all stages of SCLC after response to primary treatment ■ Postoperative radiation after surgical resection with pathologic N2 disease, T4 disease except for separate nodules in the same lobe, close/positive surgical margins, gross residual disease ■ Palliation for pain, bleeding, SVC syndrome, brain metastasis, cord compression
Technique	■ External beam radiation with 3D-CRT, IMRT or Stereotactic body radiation therapy ■ Proton beam therapy is a promising modality for the management of thoracic malignancies ■ Intraoperative HDR used after wedge resection may improve local control rates
Endobronchial Brachytherapy	
Indications	■ Palliation of endobronchial disease recurrent after EBRT ■ Palliation of endobronchial disease from metastatic disease ■ Boost treatment after initial course of definitive EBRT for primary cancer with endobronchial component
Side Effects and Complications	■ Bronchial stenosis and radiation bronchitis (around 25%) ■ Fatal hemoptysis (~10-20%), but increases with prior RT, multiple brachy courses, longer segments of treatment
Chemotherapy/Targeted agents	
Indications	■ Adjuvant treatment after surgery for stage Ib (>4cm) to IIIA NSCLC patients ■ Added to radiation therapy for definitive management of NSCLC and SCLC patients ■ Mainstay of treatment for advanced stage lung cancers
Agents	■ Platinum-doublet is preferred over single agents ■ No additional benefits seen for > 4 cycles ■ Carboplatin-Paclitaxel is the most common regimen used in the US, while Cisplatin-Vinorelbine is the most common regimen in Europe for the management of NSCLC

Table 9.8 *(continued)*

Modality	Details
Chemotherapy/Targeted agents	
Agents	■ Cisplatin-Etoposide is the regimen of choice for SCLC ■ Erlotinib can be used in the first line setting for patients with documented EGFR mutation ■ Bevacizumab (Avastin) is used with carboplatin/paclitaxel in the first line metastatic setting ■ Erlotinib or Premetrexed (Alimta) is used in the second line setting ■ Biomarkers predict for response to systemic agents (ERCC1, EGFR mutation, KRas)

[a]*Source: Ginsberg RJ et al (1995) N Eng J Med*

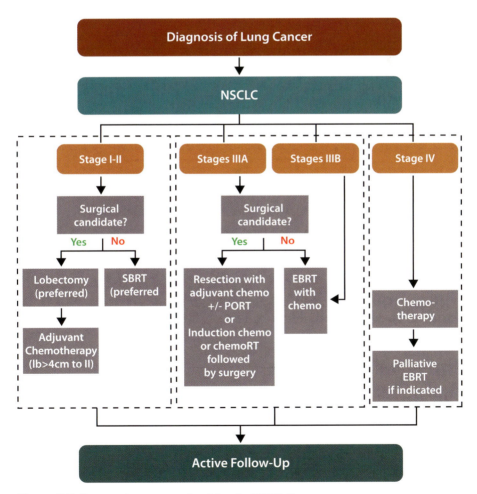

Figure 9.5 Proposed treatment algorithm for NSCLC

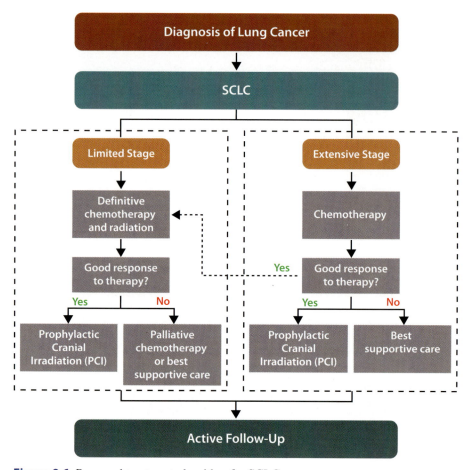

Figure 9.6 Proposed treatment algorithm for SCLC

single-institutional experiences. Figures 9.5 and 9.6 are proposed treatment approaches based on the best clinical evidence for NSCLC and SCLC, respectively.

Treatment of NSCLC (Stages I–III)

Surgical resection with lobectomy is preferred, based on a randomized trial (Table 9.9). Medical inoperable candidates with T1–T2a (<5 cm) N0M0 could be amendable for definitive management with stereotactic body radiation (SBRT). Randomized trials comparing surgery with SBRT for resectable patients are underway (Table 9.10). Adjuvant chemotherapy is indicated based on multiple randomized trials in Ib (>4 cm) to IIIa patients (Table 9.11).

Table 9.9 Treatment of early-stage NSCLC surgical resection

Trial	Description
LCSG 921	<ul><li>Randomized prospective trial</li><li>276 Patients randomized</li><li>Lobectomy versus wedge resection</li><li>Local recurrence: lobectomy, 6%; wedge resection, 18%</li><li>No difference in overall survival</li></ul>

Source: Ginsberg RJ, Rubinstein LV (1995) Randomized trial of lobectomy versus limited resection for T1N0 non-small-cell lung cancer. Lung Cancer Study Group. Ann Thorac Surg 60:615–622

Table 9.10 Treatment of early-stage NSCLC: SBRT

Trial	Description
RTOG 0236[a]	<ul><li>Phase II cooperative trial</li><li>T1–3N0 (up to 5 cm) patients, except patients with central lesions (T3 tumors invading mediastinum or those <2 cm from carina)</li><li>20 Gy × 3 fractions (actual treatment with heterogeneity correction is 18 Gy × 3 = 54 Gy)</li><li>Local failure defined as failures within 1 cm of treated area</li><li>55 Patients were evaluable (T1 = 44 patients), median age = 72 years old</li><li>Median follow-up of 34 months , 3-year LC = 98%</li><li>3-year DM = 20%</li><li>Median OS = 48 months , 2-year OS = 72%, and 2-year DFS = 67%</li></ul>
Onishi et al (Japan)[b]	<ul><li>Single-institutional, retrospective review</li><li>257 Patients with stage I NSCLC</li><li>18 to 75 Gy in 1 to 22 fractions, with median BED = 111 Gy (57–180 Gy), $\alpha/\beta = 10$</li><li>Median follow-up = 38 months</li><li>Local recurrence related to BED: LC for BED ≥ 100 = 92%; LC for BED <100 = 57%</li><li>5-year OS for BED ≥ 100 = 71%; BED < 100 = 30%</li></ul>
Nagata et al (Japan)[c]	<ul><li>Single institutional, phase I/II</li><li>45 Patients with stage I NSCLC</li><li>48 Gy in 4 fractions, 6–10 non-coplanar beams, prescribed to isocenter</li><li>Median follow-up = 30 months</li><li>Local control = 98%</li><li>3-Year OS for stage IA = 83%, IB = 72%</li><li>No grade 3 toxicities ▶</li></ul>

Table 9.10 *(continued)*

Trial	Description
RTOG 0618 (pending)	■ Phase II trial of SBRT in operable stage I/II NSCLC ■ Accrual goal: 33 patients ■ 18 Gy × 3 fractions
JCOG-0403 (pending)	■ Phase II trial of SBRT in T1N0M0 NSCLC ■ Accrual goal: 165 patients ■ 12 Gy × 4 fractions ■ Both operable (65) and Inoperable (100)
ROSEL (Dutch) (pending)	■ Phase III SBRT versus surgery for operable stage I ■ Radiation therapy (RT): 20 Gy × 3 for T1; 12 Gy × 5 for T2; 7.5 Gy × 8 for central tumors ■ Primary endpoint: 2 and 5 year LC, QOL, and cost
Accuray/MD Anderson (pending)	■ Phase III SBRT (CyberKnife) versus surgery in operable stage I patients ■ RT: 12.5 Gy × 4 for central lesion and 16.7 Gy × 3 fractions for peripheral lesion ■ Primary endpoint: OS, DFS and toxicity at 3 years
RTOG 0915 (pending)	■ Randomized phase II comparing two SBRT schedules ■ All inoperable stage I peripheral NSCLC ■ 34 Gy × 1 versus 12 Gy × 4 ■ Accrual goal: 88 patients

[a] *Source: Timmerman R, Paulus R, Galvin J et al (2009) Stereotactic body radiation therapy for medically inoperable early stage lung cancer patients: analysis of RTOG 0236. Presented at ASTRO, November 2009, Chicago*
[b] *Source: Onishi H, Shirato H, Nagata Y et al (2007) Hypofractionated stereotactic radiotherapy (HypoFXSRT) for stage I non–small cell lung cancer: updated results of 257 patients in a Japanese multi-institutional study. J Thorac Oncol 7:S94–S100*
[c] *Source: Nagata Y, Takayama K, Matsuo Y et al (2005) Clinical outcomes of a phase I/II study of 48 Gy of stereotactic body radiotherapy in 4 fractions for primary lung cancer using stereotactic body frame. Int J Radiation Oncol Biol Phys 63:1427–1431*
[d] *Source: Chang JY, Balter PA, Dong L et al (2008) Stereotactic body radiation therapy in centrally and superiorly located stage I or isolated recurrent non-small-cell lung cancer. Int J Radiation Oncol Biol Phys 72:967–971*

Table 9.11 Trials and meta-analyses of adjuvant chemotherapy after surgery

Trial	Description
IALT[a]	■ Prospective randomized phase III ■ 1,867 Patients randomized to cisplatin, vinorelbine, vinblastine, and etoposide versus observation after surgical resection in stages I–III patients ■ HR was 0.86 in favor of adjuvant chemotherapy
ANITA[b]	■ Prospective randomized phase III ■ 840 Patients with stages IB–IIIA randomized to cisplatin and vinorelbine versus observation after surgical resection ■ HR was 0.80 in favor of adjuvant chemotherapy
NCIC-CTG JBR.10[c]	■ Prospective randomized phase III ■ 482 Patients with IB–IIB NSCLC randomized to cisplatin and vinorelbine versus observation after surgical resection ■ HR was 0.69 in favor of adjuvant chemotherapy
CALGB 9633[d]	■ Prospective randomized phase III ■ 344 Patients with IB disease randomized to adjuvant carboplatin and Taxol versus observation ■ No difference in overall survival (HR of 0.83, $p = 0.12$) ■ Unplanned subset analysis of tumors ≥4 cm showed better outcomes (HR of 0.69, $p = 0.043$)
LACE meta-analysis	■ 4,584 Patients (stages I–IIIA) enrolled in 5 largest phase III adjuvant chemo trials ■ 5-Year OS benefit of 5.4% with the use of cisplatin-based chemotherapy ■ Overall HR was 0.89, $p = 0.004$

[a] *Source: Arriagada R, Bergman B, Dunant A et al (2004) Cisplatin-based adjuvant chemotherapy in patients with completely resected non–small cell lung cancer. N Engl J Med 350:351–360*
[b] *Source: Douillard JY, Rosell R, De Lena M et al (2006) Adjuvant vinorelbine plus cisplatin versus observation in patients with completely resected stage IB-IIIA Non–small cell lung cancer (Adjuvant Navelbine International Trialist Association (ANITA): a randomized controlled trial. Lancet Oncol 7:719–727*
[c] *Source: Winton T, Livingston R, Johnson D et al (2005) Vinorelbine plus cisplatin versus observation in resected non–small cell lung cancer. N Engl J Med 352:2589–2597*
[d] *Source: Strauss GM, Herndon JE, Maddaus MA et al (2008) Adjuvant paclitaxel plus carboplatin compared with observation in stage IB non–small cell lung cancer: CALGB 9633 with the Cancer and Leukemia Group B, Radiation Therapy Oncology Group, and North Central Cancer Treatment Group Study Groups. J Clin Oncol 26:5043–5051*

Management of Locally Advanced NSCLC Patients

Optimal management of locally advanced NSCLC patients is controversial. Primary surgery for resectable stage IIIA patients, followed by postoperative radiation therapy, is controversial, but may be indicated in patients with pathologic N2 disease, any T4 disease except separate nodules in the same lobe, close or positive margins, and gross residual disease. However, adding concurrent chemotherapy to postoperative radiation therapy (PORT) has no value (Table 9.12).

Table 9.12 Studies for postoperative radiotherapy in stage III patients

Trial	Description
LCSG 773[a]	■ Randomized phase III trial of 210 patients with resected stages II–IIIA (T3 or N2) SCC, randomized to PORT or observation ■ No adjuvant chemotherapy was given ■ Radiation therapy used Co-60 to mediastinum to 50 Gy POD 28 ■ Overall LR rate improved with PORT (3 versus 41%); no difference in OS observed between the 2 groups
PORT Meta-analysis Trialists Group[b]	■ Meta-analysis of 10 trials for PORT since 1965 ■ Suggested OS detriment for PORT overall, but subset analysis demonstrated detriment restricted to stages I–II disease, but no adverse effect in N2 disease ■ **Caveats:** 25% of patients were T1N0 (where PORT is generally not recommended); old RT techniques (large fields, high total doses, Co-60) were used; >30% of patients relied on a single study from Dautzenberg et al (1999) using poor techniques, causing 31% deaths to PORT due to cardiac and respiratory deaths.
SEER analysis[c]	■ Retrospective study based on SEER database ■ 7,465 Stage II-III NSCLC cased between 1988 and 2002 (more modern era than PORT meta-analysis group compared PORT versus observation after surgical resection ■ Overall PORT provided no effect on OS, but was associated with improved OS (HR = 0.85) for N2 disease; PORT was detrimental for N0–N1 patients

Table 9.12 *(continued)*

Trial	Description
PORT data from the ANITA trial[d]	■ Re-analysis of PORT data from phase III adjuvant chemo trial (i.e., the ANITA) ■ Stages IB–IIIA patients treated with adjuvant cisplatin and vinorelbine versus observation , with or without PORT (232 patients received PORT) ■ As a group, PORT was detrimental on survival (HR = 1.34) ■ Subset analysis based on pN stage showed PORT was detrimental for pN0, but improved survival in pN1 in observation arm but detrimental for adjuvant chemo-therapy arm ■ For pN2 patients, PORT improved survival for both observation and chemotherapy arms
INT0115/RTOG 9105[e]	■ Randomized trial of 488 patients with stages II–IIIA NSCLC to compare PORT versus postoperative chemoradiation therapy ■ Patients were randomized to either radiation alone or 4× cycles cisplatin/etoposide plus RT (same regimen) ■ Radiation regimen was 50.4 Gy in 30 daily fractions (con-ventional) ■ No differences in median survival (38–39 months) and in-field local recurrence (12–13%) were observed

[a] *Source: Weisenburger TH (1986) Effects of postoperative mediastinal radiation on completed resected stage II and stage III epidermoid cancer of the lung. LCSG 773. Chest 106:297S–301S*

[b] *Source: Burdett S, Stewart L (2005) PORT Meta-analysis Group. Postoperative radiotherapy in non-small-cell lung cancer: update of an individual patient data meta-analysis. Lung Cancer 47:81–83*

[c] *Source: Lally BE, Zelterman D, Colasanto JM et al (2006) Postoperative radiotherapy for stage II or III non-small-cell lung cancer using the surveillance, epidemiology, and end results database. J Clin Oncol 24:2998–3006*

[d] *Source: Douillard JY, Rosell R, De Lena M et al (2008) Impact of postoperative radiation therapy on survival in patients with complete resection and stage I, II, or IIIA non-small-cell lung cancer treated with adjuvant chemotherapy: the adjuvant Navelbine International Trialist Association (ANITA) Randomized Trial. Int J Radiat Oncol Biol Phys 72:695–701*

[e] *Source: Keller SM, Adak S, Wagner H et al (2000) A randomized trial of postoperative adjuvant therapy in patients with completely resected stage II or IIIA non–small cell lung cancer. N Engl J Med 343:1217–1222*

For treating patients in unresectable disease with radiation, at least 60 Gy should be administered (based on Radiation Therapy Oncology Group [RTOG] 73-01), although a number of subsequent studies have demonstrated that improvements can be made by altering the fractionation schedules and escalating the dose (Table 9.13). Adding chemotherapy to radiation does improve outcomes further, and several trials demonstrated that adding chemotherapy to radiation (in sequential fashion) is better than radiation alone is. Later studies demonstrated that concurrent chemoradiation is better than sequential is or with induction chemotherapy (Table 9.14). Adding surgery to induction therapy (chemotherapy or chemoradiation is an option for select patients with non-bulky, single-station N2 disease) (Table 9.15). Dose escalation and adding targeted agents such as cetuximab against epidermal growth factor receptor (EGFR) may improve concurrent chemoradiation therapy for stage III patients, and it is a subject of a current RTOG trial (0617) (Figure 9.7). There is currently no role for prophylactic cranial irradiation for patients with NSCLC, based on numerous clinical trials. Future developments include proton-beam therapy and incorporating novel targeted agents into a standard cytotoxic chemotherapy regimen.

Superior sulcus tumors are apical masses that involve the chest wall, ribs, vertebral body, brachial plexus, stellate ganglion, and subclavian vessels. They account for ~3% of all NSCLC. Management is controversial, with some advocating preoperative management using chemoradiation to 45 Gy, followed by surgical resection, based on promising results of Southwest Oncology Group (SWOG) 9416 (INT 0160) (Table 9.16), whereas others favor primary resection, followed with adjuvant therapy (chemotherapy and radiotherapy), based on a series from MD Anderson Cancer Center (MDACC) (Table 9.16). Hyperfractionation using 1.2 Gy twice daily to 69.6 Gy to minimize risk to the brachial plexus should be considered.

Table 9.13 Effect of radiation schedule and dose on tumor control in NSCLC

Trial	Description
RTOG 73-01[a]	■ Prospective randomized trial ■ 376 Patients with stages T1–3,N0-2 NSCLC were randomized to 4 arms: (1) 40 Gy/2 continuous, (2) 40 Gy/4 split course, (3) 50 Gy/2 continuous, and (4) 60 Gy/2 continuous ■ Increased survival found with 60 Gy (3-year OS = 15 versus <10% for other arms ■ Better response rate (24%) and local failure rate (33% [60Gy], 42% [50Gy], 44% ([40-Gy split, 52% [40Gy]) ■ Patients with response to therapy between 50 and 60 Gy had 3-year OS of 22 versus 10%

Table 9.13 *(continued)*

Trial	Description

RTOG 93-11[b]	■ Phase I–II dose escalation study
	■ 177 patients with inoperable NSCLC
	■ Patients stratified at escalating dose levels depending on %V20 irradiated
	  ■ Patients with V20 < 25% got successive dose escalation from 70.9, 77.4, 83.8, and 90.3 Gy
	  ■ Patients with V20 of 25–36% got 70.9 Gy and 77.4 Gy
	■ Doses of 83.8 and 77.4 Gy appeared safe for V20 < 25% and 25–36%, respectively

University of Michigan	■ Prospective phase I study ■ 106 Patients with stages I–III NSCLC treated 63–103 Gy in 2.1-Gy fractions with 3D-CRT ■ 81% did not get chemotherapy ■ Median survival 19 months ■ 5-Year OS was 4, 22, and 28% for patients receiving 63–69, 74–84, and 92–103 Gy, respectively
University of North Carolina[c]	■ Updated results of 4 dose-escalation phase I/II studies ■ Retrospective analysis of these studies in 112 patients with stage III NSCLC treated with high dose (60–90 Gy with chemotherapy) ■ Of 88 patients analyzed, 24% of patients developed some form of late complications (bronchial stenosis, fatal hemoptysis, esophageal stricture, cardiac related (MI, effusion, pericarditis), and second cancers ■ Median survival was 24.7 months , 5-year OS = 24%
RTOG 8311[d]	■ Randomized phase I/II trial ■ 850 Patients with unresectable N2 disease were treated at 1.2 Gy twice daily to 60, 64.8, 69.6, 74.4, and 79.2 Gy ■ Favorable patients that received 69.6 Gy had significantly better MS (13 months) and 2-year OS (29%) than lower total doses. No difference >69.6 Gy in survival. No increased normal tissue toxicities
CHART[e]	■ Prospective randomized trial ■ CHART trial (Continuous Hyperfractionated Accelerated Radiotherapy) ■ 563 Patients with unresectable NSCLC randomized to 54 Gy at 1.5 Gy TID × 12 Consecutive days (including weekends) versus 60 Gy/6 weeks ■ ~10% improvement in 2-year absolute survival for CHART (29 versus 20%, $p = 0.004$) ■ Severe esophagitis more common (19 versus 3%) ►

Table 9.13 *(continued)*

Trial	Description
ECOG 2597 (HART)[f]	■ Prospective randomized trial ■ HART trial (Hyperfractionated Accelerated Radiotherapy) ■ Trial closed early due to poor accrual, accruing 141 out of 388 planned ■ Stage IIIA/B unresectable patients randomized induction chemotherapy (carboplatin/Taxol) followed by: (1) 64 Gy/2 Gy per day, versus (2) 57.6 Gy (1.5 Gy three times daily × 2.5 weeks, Monday through Friday (aka HART). ■ Median survival better for HART (20 versus 15 months, $p = 0.28$). 3-Year OS was 24 versus 14% ■ Increased toxicity in HART mostly due to esophagitis, but not pneumonitis

[a] *Source: Perez CA, Bauer M, Edelstein S (1986) Impact of tumor control on survival in carcinoma of the lung treated with irradiation. Int J Radiat Oncol Biol Phys 12:539–547*

[b] *Source: Bradley J, Graham MV, Winter K et al (2005) Toxicity and outcome results of RTOG 9311: a phase I-II dose-escalation study using three-dimensional conformal radiotherapy in patients with inoperable non–small cell lung carcinoma. Int J Radiat Oncol Biol Phys 61:318–328*

[c] *Source: Lee CB, Stinchcombe TE, Moore DT et al (2009) Late Complications of high-dose (≥66 Gy) thoracic conformal radiation therapy in combined modality trials in unresectable stage III non–small cell lung cancer. J Thorac Oncol 4:74–79*

[d] *Source: Cox JD, Azarnia N, Byhardt RW et al (1990) A randomized phase I/II trial of hyperfractionated radiation therapy with total doses of 60 Gy to 79.2 Gy: possible survival benefit with greater than or equal to 69.6 Gy in favorable patients with Radiation Therapy Oncology Group stage III non-small-cell lung carcinoma: report of the Radiation Therapy Oncology Group 83-11. J Clin Oncol 8:1543–1555*

[e] *Source: Saunders MI, Dische S, Barrett A et al (1997) Continuous hyperfractionated accelerated radiotherapy (CHART) versus conventional radiotherapy in non–small cell lung cancer: a randomised multicentre trial. CHART Steering Committee. Lancet 350:161–165*

[f] *Source: Belani CP, Wang W, Johnson DH et al (2005) Phase III study of the Eastern Cooperative Oncology Group (ECOG 2597): induction chemotherapy followed by either standard thoracic radiotherapy or hyperfractionated accelerated radiotherapy for patients with unresectable stage IIIA and B non–small cell lung cancer. J Clin Oncol 23:3760–3767*

Table 9.14 Trials exploring sequential versus concurrent chemotherapy and radiation in stage III NSCLC patients

Trial	Description
CALGB 8433[a]	<ul><li>RT versus chemotherapy and RT</li><li>RT (60 Gy) versus chemo (cisplatin/vinblastine) plus RT (60 Gy)</li><li>155 Patients with stage IIIA (T3 or N2)</li><li>Sequential chemotherapy plus RT improved MS from 10 to 14 months, and 2/5 year OS from 13/7 to 26/19%</li></ul>
RTOG 88-08[b]	<ul><li>RT versus chemotherapy and RT</li><li>RT (60 Gy) versus altered fractionation RT (69.6 Gy at 1.2 Gy twice daily) versus chemotherapy (cisplatin/vinblastine) plus RT (60 Gy)</li><li>458 Patients with unresectable stages II–IIIB</li><li>MS better with sequential chemoradiation therapy (13.2 month) versus RT (11.4 month) or bid RT (12 month)</li></ul>
West Japan Lung Cancer Study Group[c]	<ul><li>Sequential chemoradiation therapy versus concurrent chemoradiation therapy</li><li>Sequential chemoradiation therapy (cisplatin/vindesine/mitomycin C) plus 56 Gy conventional RT versus concurrent chemoradiation therapy (cisplatin/vindesine/mitomycin C) plus split-course RT (28 Gy × 2)</li><li>320 Patients with stages II–III</li><li>Better OS and PFS in concurrent chemoradiation therapy (5-year OS = 15.8 versus 8.9%; MS was 16.5 versus 13.3 months)</li></ul>
RTOG 9410[d]	<ul><li>Sequential chemoradiation therapy versus Concurrent chemoradiation therapy</li><li>Three arms: (1) Dillman regimen with RT to 63 Gy, (2) concurrent chemoradiation therapy, (3) concurrent chemoradiation therapy with hypofractionated RT (1.2 Gy/69.6 Gy). Chemotherapy = cisplatin/vinblastine for arms 1, 2, and cisplatin/etoposide for arm 3</li><li>610 Patients with unresectable stage III</li><li>Better MS (17 months) in arm 2 (concurrent chemoradiation therapy) than in others (14.6 months in arm 1 and 15.2 months in arm 3)</li><li>4-Year OS was 21% in arm 2 versus 12% in other two arms. Increased toxicity in concurrent chemoradiation therapy ▶</li></ul>

Table 9.14 (*continued*)

Trial	Description
NPC95-01 (France)[e]	■ Sequential chemoradiation therapy versus concurrent chemoradiation therapy ■ Randomized phase III trial ■ 205 Patients with unresectable stage III NSCLC ■ Sequential chemotherapy (cisplatin/vinorelbine) × 4 plus RT (66 Gy) versus concurrent chemo × 2 plus RT, then chemotherapy × 2 ■ Median survival: sequential (14.5 months) versus concurrent (16.3 months) (p = 0.24) ■ 2-, 3-, and 4-year survival in sequential (26, 19, and 14%) versus concurrent (39, 25, and 21%) ■ Worse esophageal toxicity in concurrent (32%) than in sequential (3%)

LAMP trial[f]	■ Induction chemotherapy and chemoradiation therapy versus chemoradiation therapy alone
	■ Randomized phase II in 3 arms
	■ 276 Patients with stage IIIA/B
	  ■ Arm 1: Dillman regimen (chemo × 2 to 63-Gy RT)
	  ■ Arm 2: induction chemotherapy × 2 cycles then concurrent chemoradiation therapy (63 Gy)
	  ■ Arm 3: concurrent chemoradiation therapy and then consolidation chemotherapy for 2 cycles
	■ Chemotherapy included carboplatin and paclitaxel
	■ Arm 3 had better MS (16.3 months) versus 13 months (arm 1) or 12.7 months (arm 2)

CALGB 39801[g]	■ Induction chemotherapy plus chemoradiation therapy versus chemoradiation therapy alone
	■ Randomized phase III trial in 2 arms
	■ 366 Patients with unresectable stage IIIA/B
	  ■ Arm 1: chemoradiation therapy
	  ■ Arm 2: induction chemotherapy for 2 cycles then chemoradiation therapy
	■ Chemotherapy included carboplatin and paclitaxel
	■ No difference in MS or OS. Upfront chemotherapy increased G3/4 heme toxicity

Table 9.14 *(continued)*

Trial	Description
Cochrane review[h]	■ Concurrent chemoradiation therapy versus sequential chemoradiation therapy; concurrent chemoradiation therapy versus RT alone ■ Meta-analysis of 14 randomized trials (2,393 patients) using concurrent chemoradiation therapy versus RT alone ■ RR for death at 2 years = 0.93 (*p* = 0.005) (relative to RT alone), 2-year PFS = 0.90 ■ Greater benefit using daily fractionation and higher total chemotherapy dose ■ Meta-analysis of 3 trials comparing concurrent chemoradiation therapy versus sequential chemoradiation therapy ■ RR = 0.86, *p* = 0.003 ■ Conclusions: (1) chemoradiation therapy versus RT alone yielded 7% reduction in risk of death; (2) concurrent chemoradiation therapy versus sequential chemoradiation therapy yielded a 14% risk reduction

[a] *Source: Dillman RO, Seagren SL, Propert KJ et al (1990) A randomized trial of induction chemotherapy plus high-dose radiation versus radiation alone in stage III non-small-cell lung cancer. N Eng J Med 323:940–945*
[b] *Source: Sause W, Kolesar P, Taylor S et al (2000) Final results of phase III trial in regionally advanced unresectable non-small-cell lung cancer. Chest 117:358–364*
[c] *Source: Furuse K, Fukuoka M, Kawahara M et al (1999) Phase III study of concurrent versus sequential thoracic radiotherapy in combination with mitomycin, vindesine, and cisplatin in unresectable stage III non-small-cell lung cancer. J Clin Oncol 17:2692–2699*
[d] *Source: Curran W, Scott CB, Langer CJ et al (2003) Long-term benefit is observed in a phase III comparison of sequential versus concurrent chemo-radiation for patients with unresected stage III NSCLC: RTOG 9410. Proc Am Soc Clin Oncol 22:Abstract 2499*
[e] *Source: Fournel P, Robinet G, Thomas P et al. (2005) Randomized phase III trial of sequential chemoradiotherapy compared with concurrent chemoradiotherapy in locally advanced non-small-cell lung cancer: Groupe Lyon-Saint-Etienne d'Oncologie Thoracique-Groupe Francais de Pneumo-Cancerologie NPC 95-01 Study. J Clin Oncol 23:5910–5917*
[f] *Source: Belani CP, Choy H, Bonomi P et al. (2005) Combined chemoradiotherapy regimens of paclitaxel and carboplatin for locally advanced non-small-cell lung cancer: a randomized phase II locally advanced multi-modality protocol. J Clin Oncol 23:5853–5855*
[g] *Source: Vokes E, Herndon JE 2nd, Kelly MJ et al. (2007) Induction chemotherapy followed by chemoradiotherapy compared with chemoradiotherapy alone for regionally advanced unresectable stage III non-small-cell lung cancer: Cancer and Leukemia Group B. J Clin Oncol 25:1698–1704*
[h] *Source: Rowell NP, O'Rourke NP (2004) Concurrent chemoradiotherapy in non-small-cell lung cancer. Cochrane Database Syst Rev 18:CD002140*

Table 9.15 Trials adding induction therapy to surgery in stage III NSCLC patients

Trial	Description
Rosell (Madrid)[a]	■ Chemotherapy and surgery versus surgery alone ■ 60 Patients randomized to surgery alone versus 3 cycles cisplatin/ifosfamide/mitomycin C prior to surgery ■ All patients received thoracic RT after surgery ■ 32% had downstaging of N2 nodes after induction chemotherapy ■ At 7-year follow-up, the median overall survival was 22 months for chemotherapy versus 10 months for surgery alone. All surviving patients had squamous cell histology
Roth (MDACC)[b]	■ Chemotherapy and surgery versus surgery alone ■ 60 Patients randomized to surgery alone versus cisplatin/etoposide/cyclophosphamide × 1 prior to surgery ■ Median survival is 21 months for chemo group and 14 months for surgery alone ■ 5-year OS was 36% with chemotherapy versus 15% with surgery alone
JCOG 9209 (Japan)[c]	■ Chemotherapy and surgery versus surgery alone ■ 62 Patients with stage IIIA-N2 randomized to surgery alone versus 3× cisplatin/vindesine prior to surgery ■ Closed prematurely due to poor accrual ■ Median follow-up of 6.2 years ■ Median OS 17 months (chemotherapy) versus 16 months (surgery) ($p = $ NS) ■ 5-Year OS was 10% (chemotherapy) versus 22% (surgery) ($p = $ NS)
The Spanish Lung Cancer Group Trial 9901[d]	■ Chemotherapy and surgery improves outcome if complete resection can be obtained ■ 136 Patients with N2 IIIA or T4N0–1 IIIB enrolled in this phase II study ■ 3 Cycles cisplatin/gemcitabine/docetaxel prior to surgery ■ 13% pCR in induction chemo group ■ Median survival 48.5 months for R0 resection, versus 12.9 months for R1–2 resection ■ 5-Year OS was 41.4% for R0 resection, versus 11.5% for R1–2 resection, versus 0% for unresected

[a] *Source: Rosell R, Gomez-Codina J, Camps C et al. (1996) Preresectional chemotherapy in stage IIIA non-small-cell lung cancer: a 7-year assessment of a randomized controlled trial. Lung Cancer 26:7–14*
[b] *Source: Roth JA, Atkinson EN, Fossella F et al. (1998) Long-term follow-up of patients enrolled in a randomized trial comparing perioperative chemotherapy and surgery with surgery alone in resectable stage IIIA non-small-cell lung cancer. Lung Cancer 21:1–6*
[c] *Source: Nagai K, Tsuchiya R, Mori T (2003) A randomized trial comparing induction chemotherapy followed by surgery with surgery alone for patients with stage IIIA N2 non-small-cell lung cancer (JCOG 9209). J Thorac Cardiovasc Surg 125:254–260*

Table 9.15 *(continued)*

Trial	Description
INT-0139[e]	■ Chemoradiation therapy versus chemoradiation therapy before surgery ■ This trial follows phase II study RTOG 8805 demonstrating promising results for trimodality management of stage IIIA/B patients ■ 396 Resectable stage IIIA patients randomized to induction chemoradiation therapy to 45 Gy prior to surgery versus definitive chemoradiation therapy (61 Gy) ■ Chemotherapy: cisplatin/gemcitabine ■ LF rate reduced for surgery arm (10%) versus 22% ($p = 0.002$), but no difference in DM and OS ■ OS better in subset analysis of patients with lobectomy (5-year OS of 36% versus 18%; MS of 34 versus 22 months, $p = 0.002$), but not in patients with pneumonectomy
The German Lung Cancer Cooperative Group Trial[f]	■ Chemotherapy and Surgery versus chemoradiation therapy and surgery ■ 558 Patients, stage IIIA/B randomized to (1) induction chemotherapy PE × 3 cycles and surgery and RT versus (2) chemo –> chemoradiation therapy (bid RT with carboplatin/vindesine) and surgery ■ Higher pCR rate (60 versus 20%) and mediastinal downstaging (46 versus 29%) in chemoradiation therapy group, but no difference in PFS or OS ■ If patients required a pneumonectomy, postoperative mortality increased in chemoradiation therapy group
EORTC 08941[g]	■ Chemotherapy and surgery versus chemotherapy and RT ■ 579 Eligible patients, but only 321 patients who responded to induction chemotherapy (3 cycles of cisplatin or carboplatin doublet) were randomized (61% response rate) ■ All stage IIIA–N2 patients ■ In surgery arm, 5% pCR, 4% postoperative mortality, 50% radical resection ■ In RT group, only 55% compliant with RT ■ No difference in OS and PFS: median survival 16.4 versus 17.5 months; 5-year OS of 15.7 versus 14% (surgery versus RT)

[d] *Source: Garrido P, Gonzalez-Larriba JL, Insa A et al. (2007) Long-term survival associated with complete resection after induction chemotherapy in stage IIIA (N2) and IIIB (T4N0-1) non-small-cell-lung cancer patients: the Spanish Lung Cancer Group Trial 9901. J Clin Oncol 25:4736–4742*
[e] *Source: Albain KS, Swann RS, Rusch VW et al. (2009) Radiotherapy plus chemotherapy with or without surgical resection for stage III non-small-cell lung cancer: a phase III randomized controlled trial. Lancet 374:379–386*
[f] *Source: Thomas M, Rube C, Hoffknecht P et al. (2008) Effect of preoperative chemoradiation in addition to preoperative chemotherapy: a randomized trial in stage III non-small-cell lung cancer. Lancet Oncol 9:636–648*
[g] *Source: van Meerbeeck JP, Kramer GWPM, Van Schil PEY et al. (2007) Randomized controlled trial of resection versus radiotherapy after induction chemotherapy in stage IIIA–N2 non-small-cell lung cancer. J Natl Cancer Inst 99:442–450*

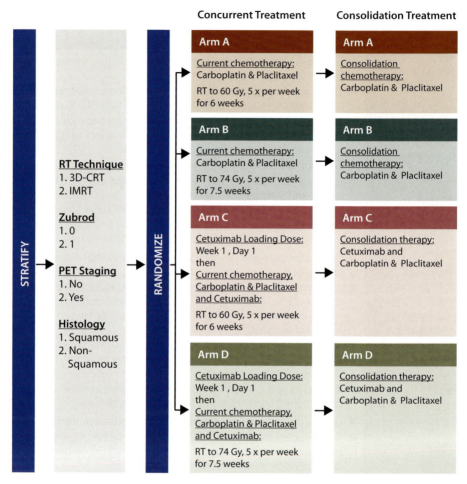

Figure 9.7 Dose escalation and adding targeted agents for NSCLC. Patient population: newly diagnosed unresectable stage IIIA or B non–small cell lung cancer. Ineligibility: supraclavicular or contralateral hilar adenopathy. Required sample size: 500. *Adapted from RTOG Study 0617: A randomized phase III comparison of standard-dose (60 Gy) versus high-dose (74 Gy) conformal radiotherapy with concurrent and consolidation carboplatin/paclitaxel +/− cetuximab (IND #103444) in patients with stage IIIA/ IIIB non–small cell lung cancer." http://www.grcop.org/Attachments/0617%20Fast-Facts.pdf*

Table 9.16 Neoadjuvant therapy for superior sulcus tumor

Trial	Description
SWOG 9416 (INT 0160)[a]	■ Single-arm phase II trial ■ 110 Patients with superior sulcus tumors (T3 [78] and T4 [32], N0-1) ■ Two cycles of cisplatin/gemcitabine plus RT to 45 Gy and then surgery (88 had resection) ■ 76% had complete resection, with pCR or minimal residual disease in 61% (pCR = 36%) ■ 5-Year OS = 44% for all patients, those with pCR had 5-year OS ~70% versus 40% without CR ($p = 0.02$)
MDACC[b]	■ Single-institutional retrospective review ■ 143 Patients with superior sulcus tumors treated with various methods ■ Primary resection, followed by adjuvant radiation was done in 20% of the patients, with definitive RT or chemo-radiation therapy for the remaining 53% who were unresectable ■ Patients treated with surgery, followed by adjuvant RT to 55–64 Gy had 5-year OS = 82%, versus 56% in patients who received 50–54 Gy ■ Of the 23 patients who survival longer than 3 years, 19 (83%) had primary surgery with RT or chemotherapy

[a]*Source: Rusch VW, Giroux DJ, Kraut MJ et al. (2007) Induction chemoradiation and surgical resection for non–small cell lung carcinomas of the superior sulcus: long term results of Southwest Oncology Group Trial 9416 (Intergroup Trial 0160). J Clin Oncol 25:313–318*
[b]*Source: Komaki R, Roth JA, Walsh GL et al. (2000) Outcome predictors for 143 patients with superior sulcus tumors treated by multidisciplinary approach at the University of Texas M.D. Anderson Cancer Center. Int J Radiat Oncol Biol Phys 48:347–354*

Management of SCLC

For patients present with T1–2N0M0 (stage I) SCLC (<5% in total incidences), complete surgical resection with a lobectomy, and mediastinal nodal dissection may be considered, based on promising outcomes from numerous surgical series. However, proper staging with mediastinoscopy or endobronchial ultrasound (EBUS) must rule out mediastinal nodal involvement. Postoperative chemotherapy must be considered even if surgical pathology demonstrates no mediastinal nodal involvement. Patients with pathologic mediastinal nodal involvement, adjuvant chemotherapy, and radiotherapy should be considered.

For patients with more advanced non-metastatic diseases (95% of limited-stage cases), definitive chemoradiation with cisplatin–etoposide is standard of care for the management. Thirteen randomized studies, included 2,140 patients, have investigated the role of thoracic radiotherapy in limited-stage SCLC. Two meta-analyses of these trials have demonstrated that adding radiation to chemotherapy is beneficial to local control and overall survival (Table 9.17).

The current standard of care is based on Intergroup 0096, using concurrent cisplatin–etoposide with radiotherapy to 45 Gy in 1.5-Gy, twice-daily fractionation (Table 9.17). Numerous other trials and meta-analyses have demonstrated that early utilization of radiation is better than delayed treatment is (Table 9.18).

Although the current standard of care is based on Intergroup 0096, the optimal schedule is unknown and possibilities are being tested in an ongoing randomized phase III trial (Cancer and Leukemia Group B [CALGB] 30610/ RTOG 0538) (Figure 9.8).

Table 9.17 Studies demonstrating importance of multimodality management of SCLC

Trial	Description
Pignon meta-analysis[a]	■ 2,103 Patients with limited-stage SCLC from 13 randomized trials compared chemotherapy alone to chemotherapy and RT ■ Chemotherapy regimen and RT timing/dose varied widely (most common drugs were cyclophosphamide, vincristine, adriamycin, and methotrexate) ■ Median follow-up was 43 months ■ RR of death with RT = 0.86 ■ Thoracic RT produced a 14% reduction in mortality rate ■ 3-Year OS benefit with RT = 5% (15 versus 10%) ■ Greatest benefit in patients between ages 55 and 70 years
Warde and Payne meta-analysis[b]	■ 1,911 Patients with limited-stage SCLC from 11 randomized trials comparing chemotherapy alone to chemotherapy and RT ■ RT doses 40–55 Gy, various chemotherapies ■ Overall increase in 2-year survival with RT = 5.4% ($p < 0.05$) (16% chemotherapy versus 23% chemotherapy and RT) ■ 2-year LR rate 77% (chemotherapy) versus 52% (chemotherapy and RT)
INT0096[c]	■ Prospective randomized trial ■ 381 Patients with limited-stage SCLC ■ Chemotherapy/QD RT to 45 Gy (1.8 Gy daily) versus chemotherapy and RT twice daily (1.5 Gy) to 45 Gy ■ Etoposide 120 mg/m^2 days 1–3 and cisplatin 60 mg/m^2 on day 1; every 3 weeks × 4 cycles ■ RT to begin with 1st chemotherapy cycle ■ PCI given for all patients with clinical CR after completion (25 Gy/10) ■ No difference in response rate ■ Median survival of 23 months twice daily versus 19 months every day ■ 5-Year OS = 26% twice daily versus 16% every day ■ Local failure rate = 36% twice daily versus 52% daily

[a] *Source: Pignon JP, Arriagada R, Ihde DC et al. (1992) A meta-analysis of thoracic radiotherapy for small-cell lung cancer. N Engl J Med 327:1618–1624*
[b] *Source: Warde P, Payne D (1992) Does thoracic irradiation improve survival and local control in limited-stage small-cell carcinoma of the lung? A meta-analysis. J Clin Oncol 10:890–895*
[c] *Source: Turrisi AT, Kim K, Blum R et al. (1999) Twice-daily compared with once-daily thoracic radiotherapy in limited small-cell lung cancer*

Table 9.18 Studies demonstrating early RT is better than late RT is for limited-stage SCLC

Trials	Description
NCIC[a]	<ul><li>Prospective randomized trial of 308 patients randomized to early RT (concurrent with 2nd cycle chemo) versus delayed RT (concurrent with 6th cycle chemo)</li><li>Chemotherapy: every 3 weeks × 6 cycles (cyclophosphamide, doxorubicin and vincristine [CAV] × 3 alternated with etoposide and cisplatin [EP] × 3)</li><li>Radiation therapy used: 40 Gy in 2.67 Gy for 15 fractions</li><li>PCI given to those without progressive disease after chemoradiation therapy</li><li>No difference in response rate</li><li>Median survival of 21 months of early versus 16 months of late RT</li><li>5-Year OS = 20% early versus 11% late</li></ul>
Yugoslavia[b]	<ul><li>Prospective randomized trial</li><li>103 Patients randomized to early chemoradiation therapy (weeks 1–4) versus late chemoradiation therapy (weeks 6–9)</li><li>Chemotherapy: carboplatin/etoposide with RT for 4 cycles PE</li><li>Radiation therapy used: 1.5 Gy twice daily to 54 Gy</li><li>PCI for all patients who had a response to treatment at weeks 16 to 17</li><li>Median survival of 34 months with early versus 26 months with late RT</li><li>5-Year OS = 30% early versus 15% late RT ($p = 0.027$)</li><li>Better LR in early RT but no difference in DM</li></ul>
Fried meta-analysis[c]	<ul><li>Meta-analysis of trials after 1985 testing early versus late thoracic RT in limited-stage SCLC</li><li>7 RCTs, with a total of 1,524 patients</li><li>Overall survival favored early versus late RT (RR = 1.17 at 2 years, $p = 0.03$, but trend at 3 years: RR = 1.13, $p = 0.2$)</li><li>Subset analysis of trials using hyperfractionated RT revealed better OS RR = 1.44, ($p = 0.001$) at 2 years and RR = 1.39 at 3 years. Once-daily RT had no difference in survival between groups</li><li>Platinum-based chemotherapy had better RR (1.35) at 3 years, favoring early RT. Studies using non-platinum–based chemotherapy had no difference in OS between groups</li><li>Conclusion: Early chemoradiation therapy is better than late chemoradiation therapy is, particularly if given with platinum-based agents</li></ul>

[a] *Source: Murray N, Coy P, Pater JL et al. (1993) Importance of timing for thoracic irradiation in the combined modality treatment of limited-stage small-cell lung cancer. The National Cancer Institute of Canada Clinical Trials Group. J Clin Oncol 11:336–44*
[b] *Source: Jeremic B, Shibamoto Y, Acimovic L et al. (1997) Initial versus delayed accelerated hyperfractionated radiation therapy and concurrent chemotherapy in limited small-cell lung cancer: a randomized study. J Clin Oncol 15:893–900*
[c] *Source: Fried DB, Morris DE, Poole C et al. (2004) Systemic review evaluating the timing of thoracic radiation therapy in combined modality therapy for limited-stage small-cell lung cancer. J Clin Oncol 22:4837–4845*

Schema (1 cycle = 21 days)
Patients will receive 4 cycles od chemotherapy on all arms

Part I:

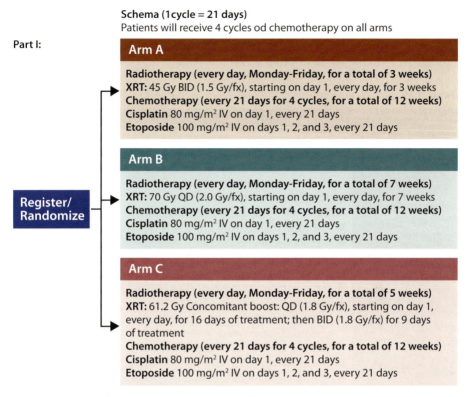

Arm A

Radiotherapy (every day, Monday-Friday, for a total of 3 weeks)
XRT: 45 Gy BID (1.5 Gy/fx), starting on day 1, every day, for 3 weeks
Chemotherapy (every 21 days for 4 cycles, for a total of 12 weeks)
Cisplatin 80 mg/m² IV on day 1, every 21 days
Etoposide 100 mg/m² IV on days 1, 2, and 3, every 21 days

Arm B

Radiotherapy (every day, Monday-Friday, for a total of 7 weeks)
XRT: 70 Gy QD (2.0 Gy/fx), starting on day 1, every day, for 7 weeks
Chemotherapy (every 21 days for 4 cycles, for a total of 12 weeks)
Cisplatin 80 mg/m² IV on day 1, every 21 days
Etoposide 100 mg/m² IV on days 1, 2, and 3, every 21 days

Arm C

Radiotherapy (every day, Monday-Friday, for a total of 5 weeks)
XRT: 61.2 Gy Concomitant boost: QD (1.8 Gy/fx), starting on day 1, every day, for 16 days of treatment; then BID (1.8 Gy/fx) for 9 days of treatment
Chemotherapy (every 21 days for 4 cycles, for a total of 12 weeks)
Cisplatin 80 mg/m² IV on day 1, every 21 days
Etoposide 100 mg/m² IV on days 1, 2, and 3, every 21 days

Register/ Randomize

Prophylactic cranial irradiation (PCI) should be offered to all patients with a complete or near complete response (see Section 8.2.9 for further details).

Part II: Based on the results of Part I, the experimental arm with the higher rate of toxic events will be discontinued and patients will be randomized as follows:

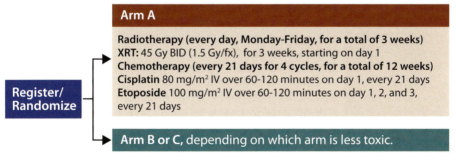

Arm A

Radiotherapy (every day, Monday-Friday, for a total of 3 weeks)
XRT: 45 Gy BID (1.5 Gy/fx), for 3 weeks, starting on day 1
Chemotherapy (every 21 days for 4 cycles, for a total of 12 weeks)
Cisplatin 80 mg/m² IV over 60-120 minutes on day 1, every 21 days
Etoposide 100 mg/m² IV over 60-120 minutes on day 1, 2, and 3, every 21 days

Register/ Randomize

Arm B or C, depending on which arm is less toxic.

Prophylactic cranial irradiation (PCI) should be offered to all patients with a complete or near complete response (see Section 8.2.9 for further details).

Figure 9.8 CALGB 30610/RTOG 0538 study: "Phase III comparison of thoracic radiotherapy regimens in patients with limited small cell lung cancer also receiving cisplatin and etoposide."

Prophylactic cranial irradiation (PCI) is given for both limited and extensive-stage SCLC after response to primary treatment, with 25 Gy in 10 fractions being the standard dosing, based on a randomized trial demonstrating no benefit to higher doses (Table 9.19).

Table 9.19 Studies demonstrating importance of adding PCI to SCLC of all stages

Trials	Description
Institute Gustave-Roussy (France)[a]	■ Prospective randomized trial ■ 300 Patients with limited or extensive-stage SCLC in CR after primary therapy and negative brain CT (CR = no tumor on chest X-ray or bronchoscopy) ■ Randomized to PCI versus no PCI ■ Radiation used : 24 Gy over 8 fractions ■ Neuropsychiatric assessment at 6, 18, 20, and 48 months after ■ 2-Year brain metastasis rate = 40% with PCI versus 67% without PCI ($p < 0.0001$) ■ 2-Year survival = 29% with PCI versus 21% without PCI ($p =$ NS) ■ No difference in neurocognitive changes at 2.5 years
UKCCCR/EORTC[b]	■ Prospective randomized trial ■ 314 Patients with limited-stage SCLC in CR after induction chemotherapy with or without RT ■ Randomized to PCI (dosing per MD choice) versus no PCI ■ Doses varied: 20 Gy/4, 24 Gy/8, 30 Gy/10, 36 Gy/18 (fractions) ■ Formal psychometric evaluation performed ■ 2-Year brain metastasis rate = 30% with PCI versus 54% negative PCI ($p = 0.0004$) ■ 2-Year survival = 25% positive PCI versus 19% negative PCI ($p =$ NS) ■ Larger doses (>24 Gy) have better improvement in outcome compared with ≤24 Gy ■ No neurocognitive deficit difference between groups at 2 years
Auperin meta-analysis[c]	■ 7 Trials with 987 patients between 1965 and 1995 with limited-stage SCLC ■ Trials that randomized patients after CR to chemo with or without RT to PCI versus no PCI ■ Majority (57%) got 24 Gy over 8 fractions (57%) ■ Median follow-up was 5.5 years ■ 3-Year OS = 20.7% with PCI versus 15.3% negative PCI ($p = 0.01$) (5.4% absolute OS benefit with PCI) ■ 3-Year DFS rate = 22% with PCI versus 13.5% without PCI ($p = 0.001$) ■ 3-Year brain metastasis rate = 33% with PCI versus 59% without PCI (p = 0.001) ■ No difference in extracranial metastasis rate ■ Trend to greater benefit seen: (1) with higher doses, and (2) PCI <4 months after starting chemotherapy

Table 9.19 *(continued)*

Trials	Description
EORTC[d]	■ Prospective randomized trial ■ 286 patients with extensive-stage SCLC who had any response to chemotherapy ■ Randomized to PCI versus observation ■ Primary end point: symptomatic brain metastasis ■ No baseline brain imaging; CT/MRI performed only at time of suggestive symptoms ■ Risk of brain metastasis at 1 year = 14.6% with PCI versus 40.4% without PCI ($p < 0.001$) ■ Irradiation increased median DFS = 14.7 weeks with PCI versus 12.0 weeks without PCI (p = SS) ■ 1-Year OS = 27.1% with PCI versus 13.3% without PCI (p = SS)
International PCI dose finding trial (PCI 99-01) EORTC, RTOG, IFCT[e]	■ Prospective randomized trial with (continue 720 patients with limited-stage SCLC in CR after chemotherapy and RT ■ Randomized to standard dose (25 Gy/10) versus high dose (36 Gy/2 Gy every day in 18 fractions or 36 Gy/1.5 Gy twice daily in 24 fractions) ■ Primary end point is incidence of brain metastasis at 2 years ■ Median follow-up was 39 months ■ No significant difference in 2-year incidence of brain metastasis (29% standard-dose group versus 23% high-dose group, p = 0.18) ■ 2-Year OS better in standard-dose group (42% versus 37% high-dose [p = 0.05]) due to greater chest local recurrence (40 versus 48%), extracranial metastasis (40 versus 42%), and cancer-related mortality in high-dose group ■ No imbalance in timing of RT, chemotherapy type, and other characteristics between groups ■ No details of RT data collected, but no center effect noted in the analysis ■ Slight increases in fatigue, nausea, and headache in high-dose group (not statistically significant)

[a]*Source: Arriagada R, Le Chevalier T, Borie F et al. (1995) Prophylactic cranial irradiation for patients with small-cell lung cancer in complete remission. J Natl Cancer Inst 87:183–190*
[b]*Source: Gregor A, Cull A, Stephens RJ et al. (1997) Prophylactic cranial irradiation is indicated following complete response to induction therapy in small cell lung cancer: results of a multicentre randomized trial. United Kingdom Coordinating Committee for Cancer Research (UKCCCR) and the European Organization for Research and Treatment of Cancer (EORTC). Eur J Cancer 33:1752–1758*
[c]*Source: Auperin A, Arriagada R, Pignon JP et al. (1999) Prophylactic Cranial irradiation for patients with small-cell lung cancer in complete remission. Prophylactic Cranial Irradiation Overview Collaborative Group. N Eng J Med 341:476–484*
[d]*Source: Slotman B, Faivre-Finn C, Kramer G et al. (2007) Prophylactic cranial irradiation in extensive small-cell lung cancer. N Engl J Med 16:664–672*
[e]*Source: Le Pechoux C, Dunant A, Senan S et al. (2009) Standard-dose versus higher-dose prophylactic cranial irradiation (PCI) in patients with limited-stage small-cell lung cancer in complete remission after chemotherapy and thoracic radiotherapy (PCI 99-01, EORTC 22003-08004, RTOG 0212, and IFCT 99-01): a randomized clinical trial. Lancet Oncol 10:467–474*

Consolidative chemoradiation for extensive-stage SCLC after response to chemotherapy was demonstrated to be beneficial in one randomized trial, but has not led to universal adaptation; it is being proposed in a randomized trial (Dutch Lung Cancer Study Group Trial [CREST]) (Table 9.20).

Table 9.20 Trials studying the benefit of adding consolidative radiation therapy to extensive stage SCLC after initial response to chemotherapy

Trial	Description
Jeremic et al. (Yugoslavia)[a]	■ Prospective randomized trial of 210 patients with extensive-stage SCLC treated with induction cisplatin/etoposide × 3 cycles ■ Patients with CR at both local and distant sites or PR at local site but CR at distant sites were randomized to two chemotherapy groups: A total of 109 patients with response were randomized to: (1) ACC hypofraction thoracic RT (54 Gy/1.5 Gy twice daily) plus CE and PE × 2, or (2) PE × 4 alone without radiation ■ Overall median survival and 5-year OS were 9 months and 3.4%, respectively ■ Median survival = 17 months (group 1) versus 11 months (group 2); 5-year OS = 9.1% (group 1) versus 3.7% (group 2) ($p=0.041$) ■ LC trended better in group 1, but no difference in DM control
CREST trial (proposed)	■ Prospective randomized trial of the Dutch Lung Cancer Study Group ■ Extensive-stage SCLC patients ■ Randomized to consolidation thoracic irradiation to 30 Gy in 10 fractions and PCI versus PCI alone after response to chemotherapy

[a]*Source: Jeremic B, Shibamoto Y, Nikolic N et al. (1999) Role of radiation therapy in the combined-modality treatment of patients with extensive disease small-cell lung cancer: a randomized study. J Clin Oncol 17:2092–2099*

Radiation Therapy Techniques for NSCLC

Radiation Therapy for NSCLC

Simulation

Four-dimensional (4D)-CT simulation to account for tumor motion, and individualizing target volume and margin should be considered for all patients.

Spiral CT or extended-time CT simulation (slow-CT scanning) to acquire an average image of the tumor at all phases of the respiratory cycle can be done if 4D-CT is not available. If a 4D-CT scan is performed, patients are evaluated for regularity of breathing, ability to follow instructions to feedback guidance, breath-holding ability, and suitability for implantation of fiducial markers. Based on this evaluation, one of the following treatment–delivery techniques is selected:

- Breath hold (with or without feedback guidance)
- Respiratory gating
- Free breathing (with or without feedback guidance)

The first two techniques are used in patients in whom large respiratory excursion is seen. Generally, the upper limit is 1 cm. Patients with less than 1-cm tumor excursion can be treated without breath-hold or gating techniques, but treatment planning should account for tumor motion by creating a combined image dataset of all possible respiratory positions of the target (or maximal intensity projection [MIP]).

The advantages and disadvantages of each of these techniques are summarized in Table 19.21.

Immobilization

Patients are placed in the supine position with both arms up and immobilized with a number of commercially available devices. At MDACC, a Vac-Loc bag and T-bar are used, which gives a setup uncertainty of about 7 mm. Daily imaging (kV orthogonal X-rays or cone-beam CT) can reduce this uncertainty further.

Treatment Planning

Details on treatment are given in the individual sections below; however, general planning strategies includes defining the gross tumor volume (GTV), clinical treatment volume (CTV), and planning treatment volume (PTV), based on the International Commission on Radiation Units and Measurements (ICRU) Report No. 50 guidelines. The GTV should be contoured based on CT lung or mediastinum windows. GTV includes the primary tumor and any grossly involved lymph nodes defined on CT (>1 cm in the shortest dimension) or positron-emission tomography (PET). To account for internal tumor motion for patients not planned for breath hold or gating, tumor position based on respiratory phase (0–100% at 10% interval) needs to be accounted for in contouring the GTV. This is named the *internal GTV* (iGTV). The iCTV (or ITV) is an expansion of this based on potential areas of microscopic spread of disease. At MDACC, an 8-mm margin is used, based on the most conservative estimates of micro-

Table 9.21 Simulation techniques for lung cancer patients

Technique	Commercial devices	Details of technique	Advantages	Disadvantages
Breath hold	Feedback-guided breath-hold treatment (FGBHTx), Eleckta ABC	Beam delivery occurs during patient breath holds up to 15 s using a feedback device	Highly accurate	Requires good respiratory function, compliant patient, ability to breath hold, requires regular reproducible breathing
Respiratory gating	Varian RPM	Beam delivery occurs when tumor comes to a gated position based on external surrogate marker	Compatible with patients with poor lung function	Requires regular reproducible breathing, less efficient, reliance on external surrogate for tumor position
Free breathing (motion encompassing methods)	NA	Target volume encompass the entire extent of tumor motion	Compatible in patients with poor lung function; inexpensive	Increased volume of normal tissue irradiated

NA: not applicable

scopic spread of disease not accounted for on CT imaging. The ITV expansion should respect anatomic boundaries (bone, chest wall (unless grossly involved), adjacent uninvolved organs, or structures. The PTV expansion is based on daily setup uncertainty, but can be reduced, depending on the technologies that reduce this uncertainty. If once-weekly port films are taken, a 0.5- to 1-cm PTV expansion is placed on the ITV. However, daily orthogonal kV imaging should only require a 5-mm setup uncertainty to be placed on the ITV expansion. If daily CT is obtained (using either CT-on-Rails or cone-beam CT), a 3-mm margin is adequate.

For patients not planned with the ITV approach, the respiratory-gating method or slow-CT simulation with location/size-specific tumor motion margins can be used. The slow-CT simulation method is used for patients not treated with the respiratory-gating or ITV method.

The setup uncertainty depends on tumor location and size. For upper-quadrant lesions, a 6-mm tumor motion margin may be adequate regardless of tumor size and for middle-segment tumors with tumor diameter >50 mm. For tumors <50 mm and located in the middle two quadrants of the lung, or tumor with diameter 50–80 mm in the lowest quadrants, a 13-mm tumor motion margin may be needed. For tumors <50 mm located in the lowest quadrant, an 18-mm margin might be necessary. These are *tumor motion* margins, which are added to the CTV expansion and setup uncertainty (*Liu HH, Balter P, Tutt T et al (2007) Assessing respiration-induced tumor motion and iTV using 4D-CT for radiotherapy of lung cancer. Int J Radiat Oncol Biol Phys 68:531–540*). Most tumors move more in superior–inferior directions, and individualized motion assessment even with regular X-ray fluoroscopy is recommended.

Recommendations for planning margins are summarized in Table 9.22.

Table 9.22 Treatment planning margins for various simulation and treatment devices

Technique	GTV	CTV	PTV
4D CT simulation	iGTV	ITV = iGTV + 8 mm	PTV = ITV + 7 mm[a] (setup uncertainty)
Respiratory gating	GTV at end expiration	CTV = GTV + 8 mm	PTV = CTV + 5mm (gating margin for residual motion) + 7 mm[a] (setup uncertainty)
Slow-CT simulation	GTV defined by slow CT imaging	CTV = GTV + 8 mm	PTV = CTV + 7 mm[a] (setup uncertainty) and location/size-specific "tumor motion" margin (see text)

[a]Can be reduced to 3 mm if daily CT or 5 mm if daily kV imaging is performed

Setup and Treatment Delivery

Patients are placed on the treatment couch, immobilized, and aligned, based on simulation position. Setup verification should be performed with orthogonal kV or MV films, based on bony alignment on a weekly basis. For hypofractionated irradiation that requires exquisite precision, daily CT imaging (either CT-on-Rails or cone-beam CT) for both tumor and normal anatomy visualization should be considered.

Stereotactic Body Radiotherapy

Stereotactic body radiotherapy (SBRT) is a preferred option for the management of early-stage NSCLC over conventionally fractionated external-beam radiation treatment, which yields poor local control and survival outcomes. Dosing schemes that achieve a biologically effective dose (BED) >100 Gy can be used, and dose–fractionation differ based on whether the tumor is peripherally or centrally located. Aggressive hypofractionation for central lesions may cause severe toxicities for central lesions, based on RTOG 0236 analysis. There are numerous dosing and fractionation schemes in the literature. Off-protocol, the following treatment schemes can be used:

- Peripheral lesions: 50 Gy in four continuous daily fractions, with daily on-board CT imaging (Figure 9.9)
- Central lesions: 50 Gy in four continuous daily, or 70 Gy in 10 continuous fractions, 5-days-per-week treatments with daily on-board CT imaging

Chemoradiation for Locally Advanced NSCLC

Dose and Fractionation Schemes

Although standard radiation dosing has been at 60 Gy, the local control rates are extremely poor: 34–43%. Dose escalation to 74 Gy with concurrent chemoradiation has been studied and found to be safe; however, it is also deemed a maximum tolerated dose (MTD) in one study (*Schild et al*). Therefore, achieving doses >60 Gy (60–70 Gy at 1.8–2 Gy per fraction) with concurrent chemotherapy is preferred in the off-protocol setting. For patients who cannot tolerate chemotherapy, radiation alone to 66–74 Gy should be considered.

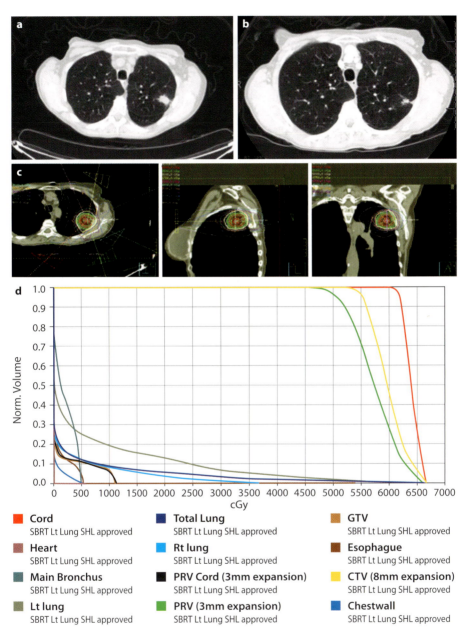

Fig. 9.9 a–d A 68-year-old lifelong smoker with a newly diagnosed T1aN0 squamous cell carcinoma of right upper lobe. **a** CT scan prior to SBRT, **b** CT scan 1 month after SBRT, and **c** six-field SBRT plan, using MIP contouring for GTV, 0.8-cm expansion for CTV, and 0.3-cm PTV expansion. Prescription to 50 Gy in four fractions using daily cone-beam CT image-guided radiation therapy (IGRT). **d** DVH analysis of the SBRT plan

Table 9.23 Target volumes in the definitive treatment of NSCLC

Target volume	Without induction chemotherapy	After induction chemotherapy
GTV	Primary tumor and all nodal disease defined by CT or PET	Should include the post-chemotherapy gross volume
CTV	As detailed in Table 9.22	As detailed in Table 9.22. CTV should include the pre-chemotherapy GTV volumes
Note	Elective nodal coverage of the contralateral mediastinum, hilum, or supraclavicular areas is not treated unless involved	For patients with a CR to induction chemotherapy, consolidative RT to areas of prior involvement should at least be 50 Gy

Target Volumes

Target volumes in the definitive treatment of NSCLC, with or without induction chemotherapy, are detailed in Table 19.23.

Radiation Modality: 3D Conformal Radiation Versus Intensity-Modulated Radiation Therapy

3D conformal radiation (3D-CRT) is probably most commonly utilized for the treatment of lung cancer patients because of great concerns that intensity-modulated radiation therapy (IMRT) delivers a higher low-dose exposure to the lungs, and because of the complex interactions between tumor motion, respiration, and IMRT dosimetry. However, IMRT may be preferred for patients with larger volumes of disease, to produce greater dose sparing of normal structures such as the heart, lung(s), esophagus, and spinal cord (see example in Figure 9.10), as when IMRT was compared to 3D-CRT in locally advanced NSCLC. Reduction of >2 Gy in the mean lung dose was achieved, with a corresponding reduction in radiation pneumonitis by 10%. However, because of the potential breakdown in dose buildup with the interplay between collimator dynamics (either with the use of sliding window or step-and-shoot) and tumor motion during an IMRT treatment delivery, it is of greater importance that motion-reduction techniques be utilized for IMRT. Proposed guidelines for the proper use of IMRT for the treatment of lung cancers are provided in Table 9.24.

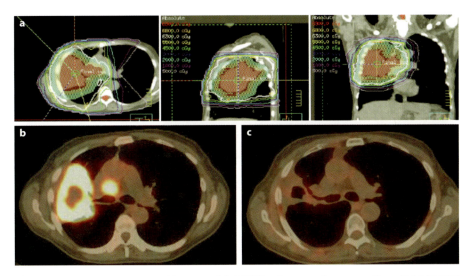

Figure 9.10 a–c **a** 58-year-old man with T3N2 adenocarcinoma. **a** Four-field IMRT plan prescribed to 63 Gy with carboplatin/Taxol. **b** FDG-PET prior to treatment. **c** Six months after chemoradiation, showing a complete response to treatment

Source: Murshed H, Liu HH, Liao Z et al. (2004) Dose and volume reduction for normal lung using intensity-modulated radiotherapy for advanced-stage non-small-cell lung cancer. Int J Radiat Oncol Biol Phys 58:1258–1267

Table 9.24 Proposed guidelines for the proper use of IMRT for the treatment of lung cancer

Guideline
4D planning is of utmost importance because of the greater conformality of IMRT
Tumor motion control and monitoring techniques must be considered and utilized for tumor motion >1 cm
Patients with larger tumors close to structures such as the brachial plexus, esophagus, and spinal cord, and those with mediastinal nodal involvement, may have greater gain from IMRT than from 3D-CRT
Tissue heterogeneity should be corrected for all IMRT plans since heterogeneity affects some beamlets greater than others do
Reducing the number of beams (5–7) may be necessary to reduce the low-dose scatter to the normal lung
Cold and hot spots must be evaluated carefully in plan evaluation
Strict IMRT quality assurance process needs to be in place to ensure mechanical and dosimetric accuracy

Endobronchial Brachytherapy

Indications and side effects of endobronchial high-dose-rate (EB-HDR) brachytherapy are detailed in Table 9.8. Techniques for EB-HDR brachytherapy are detailed in Figure 9.11.

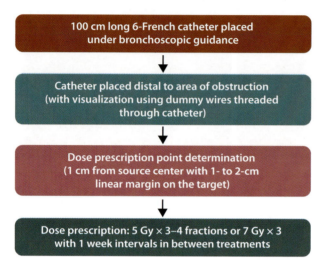

Figure 9.11 Techniques for EB-HDR brachytherapy

Postoperative Radiation Therapy

Dose and Fractionation Schemes

Dose for postoperative radiotherapy depends on amount of potential or actual residual disease (Table 9.25).

Table 9.25 Radiation dose for adjuvant treatment of NSCLC

Criteria	Total dose and fractionation
R0 resection	50 Gy in 25 daily fractions
+ECE	54 Gy in 27 daily fractions
+Margin	60 Gy in 30 daily fractions
Gross residual	66–70 Gy/33–35 fractions (consider concurrent chemotherapy)

Target Volumes

Typically, target volumes include the bronchial stump, ipsilateral hilum, ipsilateral mediastinum, and areas of positive margin/microscopic extension of disease. This should be discussed with the surgeon for the high-risk regions related to the areas of the primary disease. The CTV should not include the mediastinum or the hilum if not involved. However, if inadequate lymph node assessment is performed, the ipsilateral hilum and mediastinum should be covered empirically.

Radiation Therapy Techniques for SCLC

The current standard for definitive chemoradiation for limited-stage SCLC is derived from the Intergroup 0096 trial (the Turrisi regimen). However, dose-escalation studies and alternative fractionation schemas to reduce acute toxicities have yielded promising results (Table 9.26). The optimal radiation regimen is not yet determined, and it is being tested in the protocol CALGB 30610/RTOG 0538 (Figure 9.8).

Table 9.26 Regimens of definitive radiation therapy for SCLC

Regimen	Total dose and fractionation	
Standard (Turrisi)	45 Gy at 1.5 Gy twice daily × 30 fractions with concurrent cisplatin/etoposide	
CALGB	70 Gy at 2 Gy × 30 daily fractions with concurrent cisplatin/etoposide	
RTOG 0239	28.8 Gy at 1.8 Gy × 16 daily fractions	32.4 Gy at 1.8 Gy BID × 18 fractions

Toxicities and Normal Tissue Tolerance

Common toxicities seen in radiotherapy for lung cancers include acute effects of esophagitis, skin irritation, fatigue, and nausea/vomiting. Subacute and late toxicities include radiation pneumonitis, pericarditis, pericardial effusion, esophageal stricture/fistula, and second cancers. Effects could be reduced by observing dose–volume constraints, which are modified by whether chemotherapy is delivered concurrently or if surgery is anticipated after therapy. These are summarized in Table 9.27.

Table 9.27 DVH dose constraints for radiation treatment planning

Organ at risk	RT alone	Definitive chemoradiation	Preoperative chemoradiation
Spinal cord[a]	50 Gy	45 Gy	45 Gy
Lung[b]	MLD ≤ 20 Gy V20 ≤ 40%	MLD ≤ 20 Gy V20 ≤ 35% V10 ≤ 45% V5 ≤ 65%	MLD ≤ 20 Gy V20 ≤ 20% V10 ≤ 40% V5 ≤ 55%
Heart	V30 ≤ 45%; mean dose < 26 Gy	Same as RT alone	Same as RT alone
Esophagus[c]	D_{max} ≤ 75 Gy V70 < 20% V50 < 50%	D_{max} ≤ 75 Gy V70 < 20% V50 < 40%	D_{max} ≤ 75 Gy V70 < 20% V50 < 40%
Kidney[d]	V20 < 32% for both kidneys V20 < 15% of one kidney if the other kidney is non-functional	Same as R alone	Same as RT alone
Liver	V30 ≤ 40%; mean dose < 30 Gy	Same as RT alone	Same as RT alone

MLD: mean lung dose; D_{max}: maximum point dose; **DVH**: dose-volume histogram; **Vn**: volume of organ receiving n percent dose of Gy

[a]Treated volume size should be considered, as the chance of spinal cord damage increases with increasing RT volume. When PTV is close (<1 cm) to spinal cord, such as with vertebral invasion, spinal cord may exceed the tolerance dose but not over 60 Gy, even in a very limited volume. Higher fraction sizes reduce tolerance (e.g., 3 Gy per fraction reduce tolerance dose to 40 Gy)

[b]V20: the effective lung volume (total lung volume-gross tumor volume) receiving 20 Gy or more. For patients who undergo pneumonectomy before RT, MLD of < 8 Gy, a V20 of < 10% and V5 < 60% are recommended

[c] Mean esophageal dose < 34 Gy is used by the RTOG and recommended on the QUANTEC as well, but with little literature basis

[d] Consider a renal scan if a large volume of one kidney will be treated with high dose

Source: modified from Marks LB, Yorke ED, Jackson A et al. (2010) Use of normal tissue complication probability models in the clinic. Int J Radiat Oncol Biol Phys 76:S10-9; and Chang JY, Komaki R, Roth JA et al. (2008) Image guidance of combined modality management of NSCLC. In: Cox JD, Chang JY, Kosamaki R et al. (eds) Image-guided radiation therapy for lung cancer, Informa, pp 19–37

Follow-Up

Table 9.28 details a follow-up schedule and examinations in the treatment of lung cancer.

Table 9.28 Follow-up schedule and examinations

Schedule	Frequency
First follow-up after radiation therapy	■ 4–6 Weeks
Years 0–2	■ Every 4–6 months
Years 3+	■ Annually
Examination	
History and physical	■ Complete history and physical examination
Laboratory tests	■ If clinically indicated
Imaging	■ Contrast-enhanced chest CT ■ PET or brain MRI not routine unless clinically indicated ■ Contrast may be excluded in years 3 and beyond

Adapted from the National Comprehensive Cancer Network. NCCN guidelines for NSCLC (v. 1.2010): http://www.nccn.org/professionals/physician_gls/PDF/nscl.pdf. Cited 10 April 2010

10

Thymic Tumors

Jiade J. Lu[1], Ivan W.K. Tham[2]
and Feng-Ming (Spring) Kong[3]

Key Points

- Thymic tumours are relatively rare neoplasms with an incidence of 0.15/100,000 population per year in the United States.

- Up 40% of thymoma patients present with no symptoms. Common signs and symptoms are caused by local invasion of the disease or paraneoplastic syndrome especially myasthenia gravis: ~15% patients with myasthenia gravis has thymoma, and ~45% thymoma patients have myasthenia gravis.

- Accuracy of diagnosis and staging based on history and physical examination, laboratory and imaging studies. Tissue diagnosis by FNA or core biopsy is required before definitive treatment.

- Stage, completeness of surgical resection, and pathology are the most important prognostic factors. The Masaoka staging system is widely used.

- Thymoma usually present with an indolent behavior. Local and regional extension are the main modes of disease progression. Distant metastasis is rarely observed in thymoma, but can occur in thymic carcinoma.

- Treatment of thymoma depends on the resectability of the disease and surgery is the mainstay of therapy. Completeness of resection is prognostically significant.

- Adjuvant radiation therapy is recommended for stage II and III, as well as for residual disease (including positive margins). Radiation therapy is not necessary after complete resection for stage I cases.

- Neoadjuvant chemotherapy is indicated in unresectable cases. Chemotherapy followed by radiotherapy is recommended if surgical resection is not feasible.

- Long-term overall survival rates are 95%, 90%, 70%, and 23% for WHO type A, AB, B, and C diseases after treatment.

Epidemiology and Etiology

Thymoma is a relatively rare disease. However, it accounts for 30% of tumors and is the most common neoplasm in the anterior mediastinum. The exact cause of thymoma is largely unknown. Epidemiology statistics and risk factors are detailed in Table 10.1

[1] Jiade J. Lu, MD, MBA (✉)
Email:
mdcljj@nus.edu.sg

Ivan W.K. Tham, MD
Email:
ivan_wk_tham@nuhs.edu.sg

Feng-Ming Kong, MD, PhD, MPH
Email:
fengkong@med.umich.edu

J. J. Lu, L. W. Brady (Eds.), *Decision Making in Radiation Oncology*
DOI: 10.1007/978-3-642-13832-4_11, © Springer-Verlag Berlin Heidelberg 2011

Table 10.1 Statistics and risk factors of thymoma

Type	Description
Statistics	Thymoma is rare, with an incidence of 0.15/ 100,000 population per year in the United States
	Usually occurs in patients aged 40-60 years with a median age of 52; It is uncommon in children
	The male:female ratio of thymoma is ~1:1
Risk factors	Epstein-Barr Virus (EBV) infection
	Thymic irradiation in childhood
	Myasthenia gravis: 75% of patients has thymic disorder and 15% of them has thymoma
	Familial cytogenetic abnormalities
	MEN type I and II are associated with thymic carcinoid

Anatomy

The thymus is a temporary organ with its largest size at puberty, after which it gradually atrophies and nearly disappears. The remnant thymus is located anterior to the pericardium and the great vessels in the superior-anterior mediastinum (Figures 10.1 and 10.2).

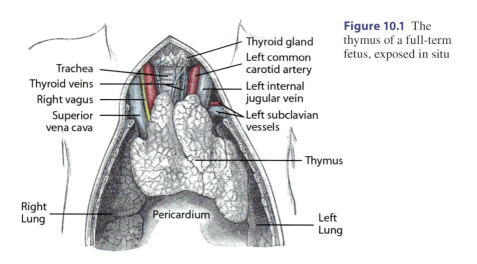

Figure 10.1 The thymus of a full-term fetus, exposed in situ

Labels: Trachea, Thyroid veins, Right vagus, Superior vena cava, Right Lung, Pericardium, Thyroid gland, Left common carotid artery, Left internal jugular vein, Left subclavian vessels, Thymus, Left Lung

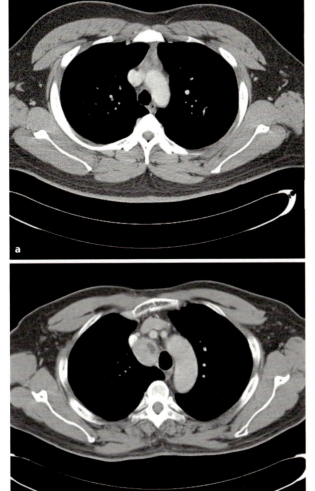

Figure 10.2 a, b a Contrast material–enhanced chest CT scan showing a normal thymus in the anterior mediastinum, **b** Chest CT scan demonstrating a rounded mass in the right paratracheal region with well-defined margins and hypoenhancing areas. Histology revealed a type AB thymoma

Pathology

Thymomas (including thymic carcinoma) arise from the thymic epithelium. A number of pathological classifications for thymomas coexist. The World Health Organization (WHO) classification is an independent prognostic factor and classifies thymoma into subtypes as listed (Table 10.2).

Table 10.2 WHO classification of the pathology of thymoma

Type	Description	5-/10-Year OS (%)
A	■ Spindle cell; medullary thymoma	100/95%
AB	■ Mixed thymoma	93/90%
B1	■ Lymphocyte rich; lymphocytic; predominantly cortical; organoid thymoma	89/85%
B2	■ Cortical thymoma	82/71%
B3	■ Epithelial; atypical; squamoid; well-differentiated thymic carcinoma	71/40%

Thymic carcinoma ≠ invasive thymoma

Thymic carcinoma accounts for 5–35% of thymic tumors

Thymic carcinomas are termed according to their differentiation (squamous cell, mucoepidermoid, etc.). All non-organotypic malignant epithelial neoplasms other than germ cell tumors are designated thymic carcinomas

Thymic carcinoid is rare: <5% of anterior mediastinum tumors

The WHO classification also includes micronodular thymoma, metaplastic thymoma, microscopic thymoma, sclerosing thymoma, and lipofibroadenoma

Source: Travis WD, Brambilla E, Müller-Hermelink HK, Harris CC (eds) (2004) Pathology and genetics: tumours of the lung, pleura, thymus and heart (WHO Classification) IARC Press, Lyon, France

Routes of Spread

Thymomas usually behave in an indolent fashion. Local and regional extensions are the major modes of progression. Spread to pleura or lung can occur, but extrathoracic metastasis is rare. Distant metastasis (either lymphogenous or hematogenous) occurs in ~30% of thymic carcinoma cases.

Diagnosis, Staging, and Prognosis

Clinical Presentation

The presenting symptoms and signs of most thymoma cases are caused by its local extension or associated paraneoplastic syndromes (Table 10.3).

Table 10.3 Commonly observed signs and symptoms in thymoma

Type	Description
General	<ul><li>Usually presents as indolent disease that progresses slowly</li><li>Most symptoms are secondary to mediastinal mass and are induced by local extension</li><li>Commonly observed symptoms include chest pain, dyspnea, dysphagia, odynophagia, cough, and superior vena cava obstruction</li><li>Weight loss and anorexia also observed</li><li>30–40% of cases asymptomatic at diagnosis</li></ul>
Paraneoplastic syndrome	<ul><li>~45% of thymoma patients has myasthesia gravis (*MG*); ~15% patients with MG have thymoma</li><li>~3% have pure red cell aplasia; ~50% patients with pure red cell aplasia have thymoma</li><li>~3% have adult-onset hypogammaglobulinemia; ~10% patients with hypogammaglobulinemia have thymoma</li><li>Rare in thymic carcinoma</li></ul>

Diagnosis and Staging

Figure 10.3 illustrates the recommended diagnostic procedures for thymoma.

Staging

There are a number of staging systems for thymoma. The commonly used Masaoka staging system is presented in Table 10.4.

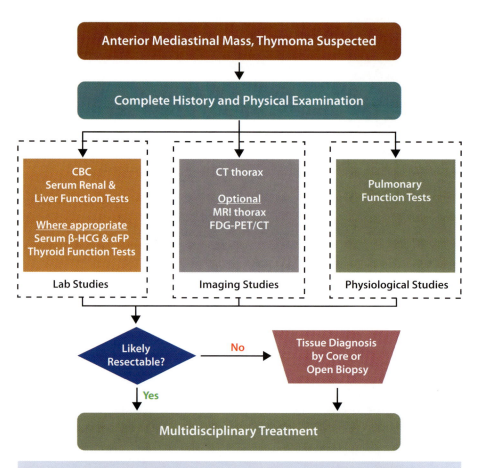

Figure 10.3 Proposed algorithm for diagnosis and staging of thymoma. *Source: Kong FM, Lu JJ (2008) Thymoma. In: Lu JJ, Brady LW (eds) Radiation oncology: an evidence-based approach. Springer, Berlin Heidelberg New York*

Table 10.4 Modified Masaoka clinical staging of thymoma

Stage	Diagnostic criteria	5-Year survival (%)
I	Macroscopically and microscopically completely encapsulated	94–100%
IIA	Microscopic transcapsular invasion	86–95%
IIB	Macroscopic invasion into surrounding fatty tissue or grossly adherent to, but not through, mediastinal pleura or pericardium	
III	Macroscopic invasion into surrounding organs such as lung, mediastinum, and great vessels	56–69%
IVA	Pleural or pericardial dissemination	11–50%
IVB	Lymphogenous or hematogenous metastasis	

Source: Masaoka A, Monden Y, Nakahara K et al (1981) Follow-up study of thymomas with special reference to their clinical stages. Cancer 48:2485–2492

Prognostic Factors

Independent prognostic factors of thymoma correlating with outcome are detailed in Table 10.5.

Table 10.5 Prognostic factors of thymoma

Type	Description
Disease related	■ **Stage (i.e., invasiveness)** of the disease ■ WHO classification of **pathology** ■ **Tumor size** (>10 cm have worse prognosis) ■ **MG** is associated with increased surgery motality rate, but is *not* an independent factor for poor survival ■ Paraneoplatic syndromes including red cell aplasia and hypogammaglobulinemia are associated with poor prognosis
Patient related	■ Gender and ethnic background (for the same pathology) are *not* prognostically significant ■ Performance status, weight loss and anemia before treatment are *not* significant in patients treated definitively
Treatment related	■ **Completeness of surgery** ■ Long-term overall survival after complete resection, partial resection, and biopsy only are 82, 72, and 27%, respectively ■ Dose of radiation

Treatment

Principles and Practice

Surgery is the main treatment modality for thymoma. Treatment modalities utilized in thymoma are detailed in Table 10.6. A proposed treatment algorithm based on the best available clinical evidence is presented in Figure 10.4.

Table 10.6 Treatment modalities for thymoma

Type	Description
Surgery	
Indications	■ Surgery is the treatment of choice for resectable thymoma; perioperative mortality is <1% ■ Completeness of resection is prognostically significant ■ Complete resection is achieved in 60–75% of cases ■ Incomplete resection leads to poor results even when adjuvant radiation is used
Techniques	■ Median sternotomy is the standard approach ■ Cervical approaches or VATS have been reported ■ Preoperative preparation (e.g., plasmapheresis) for patients with MG may be needed to avoid respiratory complications
Radiation therapy	
Indications	■ Adjuvant radiation therapy can improve local control for patients with stages II–III or residual disease after surgery ■ Mainstay treatment for unresectable disease (concurrent with chemotherapy) ■ Induction radiation can be considered if chemotherapy is contraindicated in unresectable cases
Techniques	■ 3D-CRT or IMRT to surgical bed (in adjuvant setting) or tumor (in definitive treatment) ■ AP/PA or wedge-pair (2D) technique can be used but can generate excessive dose to normal tissue
Chemotherapy	
Indications	■ Neoadjuvant chemotherapy can be used to improve resectability ■ Combined chemoradiation therapy for unresectable cases ■ Mainstay treatment in palliation
Medications	■ Cisplatin plus doxorubicin plus cyclophosphamide with or without prednisone have been tested in phase II trials with response rate of 60–77%

VATS: video-assisted thoracic surgery; **3D-CRT:** 3-dimensional conformal radiation therapy; **IMRT:** intensity-modulated radiation therapy

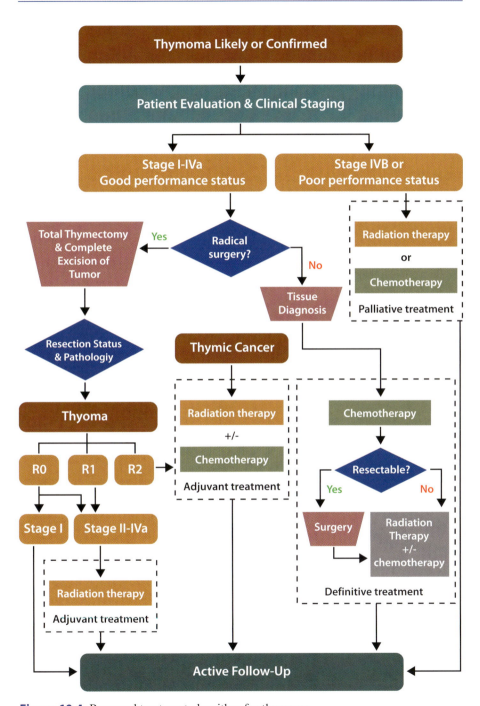

Figure 10.4 Proposed treatment algorithm for thymoma

Radiation Therapy for Resectable Thymoma

Radiation therapy (RT) is an important adjuvant treatment modality for stage II, stage III disease, as well as for residual disease post-resection. Adjuvant RT is usually not indicated after complete resection for stage I disease. There is ongoing controversy regarding the role of RT in completely resected stages II–III disease, as reported results from retrospective series vary (Table 10.7).

Table 10.7 Treatment strategies for *resectable* thymoma and supporting clinical evidence

Author	Materials and methods	Results
Curran et al[a]	■ Retrospective review of 117 patients with stages I–IV thymoma treated with surgery with or without RT	■ 5-Year OS and RFS rates of 67 and 100% (stage I), 86 and 58% (stage II), and 69 and 53% (stage III) ■ No recurrences in stage I patients after total resection without RT ■ For stages II–III, 5-year mediastinal relapse rate was 53% for surgery alone versus 0% for total resection with RT and 21% for subtotal resection/biopsy with RT ■ Poor salvage therapy results reported
Ogawa et al[b]	■ Retrospective review of 103 patients with completely resected thymoma with PORT ■ 52 treated with involved field (IF) RT, 51 treated with whole mediastinal RT with or without boost ■ Median dose 40 Gy ■ Median follow-up of was 112 months	■ 10-Year OS 100% for stage I, 90% for stage II, and 48% for stage III ■ Pleura most frequent site of first recurrence ■ No recurrences within the irradiated field ■ No dose response correlation for intrathoracic control

Table 10.7 *(continued)*

Author	Materials and methods	Results
Kondo et al[c]	■ Retrospective review of 1,320 patients with thymic epithelial tumors treated 1990–1994 ■ Stage I thymoma treated with surgery only ■ Patients with stages II and III thymoma and thymic carcinoid had surgery and RT ■ Patients with stage IV thymoma and thymic carcinoma had RT or chemotherapy	■ Total resection most important factor in treatment of thymic epithelial tumors ■ Benefit of debulking in thymoma but not thymic carcinoma ■ No evidence of benefit of adjuvant therapy for totally resected invasive thymoma and thymic carcinoma
Strobel et al[d]	■ Retrospective review of 228 patients with resected thymoma or thymic squamous cell carcinoma (*TSCC*) ■ Median follow-up of 60 months ■ 42 received adjuvant RT (mean dose, 53 Gy) ■ 33 Patients received adjuvant chemotherapy	■ Low-risk (WHO type A, AB, B1) patients had good outcome with surgery alone ■ For high-risk patients (WHO type B2, B3, TSCC, incomplete resections or ≥ stage III), recurrence rate was 34% after adjuvant treatment versus 78% with surgery alone
Forquer et al[e]	■ Retrospective review of Surveillance, Epidemiology and End Results (*SEER*) registry 1973–2005 ■ 901 Patients with surgically resected localized (stage I) or regional (stages II–III) malignant thymoma/thymic carcinoma with or without PORT	■ PORT improved 5-year overall survival rates for stages II–III (76 versus 66% for surgery alone, $p = 0.01$) but not stage I (81 versus 87% for surgery alone, $p = 0.35$) ■ PORT may potentially benefit stages II–III patients, especially after non-extirpative surgery

OS: overall survival, **RFS:** relapse-free survival, **PORT:** postoperative radiation therapy

[a] *Source: Curran WJ Jr, Kornstein MJ, Brooks JJ et al (1998) Invasive thymoma: the role of mediastinal irradiation following complete or incomplete surgical resection. J Clin Oncol 6:1722–1727*

[b] *Source: Ogawa K, Uno T, Toita T et al (2002) Postoperative radiotherapy for patients with completely resected thymoma: a multi-institutional, retrospective review of 103 patients. Cancer 94:1405–1413*

[c] *Source: Kondo K, Monden Y (2003) Therapy for thymic epithelial tumors: a clinical study of 1,320 patients from Japan. Ann Thorac Surg 76:878–884*

[d] *Source: Ströbel P, Bauer A, Puppe B et al (2004) Tumor recurrence and survival in patients treated for thymomas and thymic squamous cell carcinomas: a retrospective analysis. J Clin Oncol 22:1501–1509*

[e] *Source: Forquer JA, Rong N, Fakiris AJ et al (2010) Postoperative radiotherapy after surgical resection of thymoma: differing roles in localized and regional disease. Int J Radiat Oncol Biol Phys 76:440–445*

RT for Unresectable Thymoma

For patients with good performance status, aggressive multimodality treatment may result in satisfactory outcomes. Neoadjuvant treatment with chemotherapy (Figure 10.5) or chemoradiation (Figure 10.6) may render the tu-

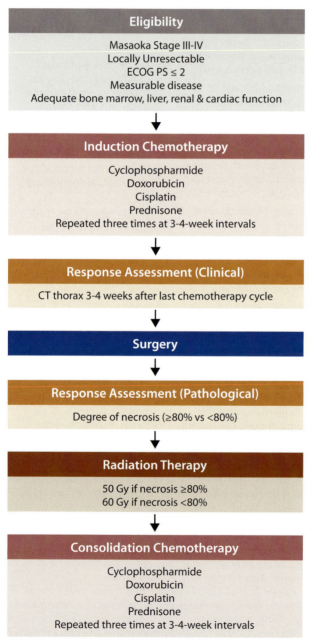

Figure 10.5 Proposed treatment algorithm for *unresectable* thymoma using neoadjuvant chemotherapy, followed by resection, radiation therapy, and consolidation chemotherapy. Alternative chemotherapy regimens may include cisplatin, epirubicin, and etoposide; cisplatin, doxorubicin, and cyclophosphamide; and cisplatin, doxorubicin, vincristine, and cyclophosphamide

Source: Kim ES, Putnam JB, Komaki R et al (2004) Phase II study of a multidisciplinary approach with induction chemotherapy, followed by surgical resection, radiation therapy, and consolidation chemotherapy for unresectable malignant thymomas: final report. Lung Cancer 44:369–379

mor resectable. Supporting evidence is discussed in Table 10.8. Alternatively, a patient may be offered definitive chemotherapy and RT (Table 10.9; Figure 10.7). Chemotherapy and RT are usually delivered sequentially to reduce the side effect profile, particularly if anthracyclines are utilized.

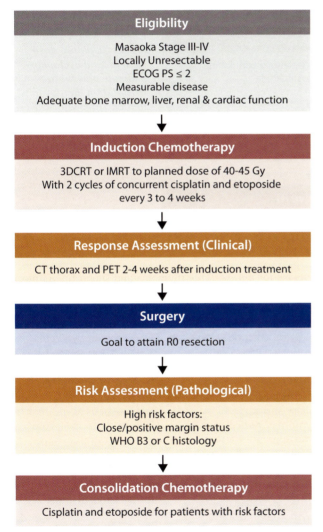

Eligibility

Masaoka Stage III-IV
Locally Unresectable
ECOG PS ≤ 2
Measurable disease
Adequate bone marrow, liver, renal & cardiac function

↓

Induction Chemotherapy

3DCRT or IMRT to planned dose of 40-45 Gy
With 2 cycles of concurrent cisplatin and etoposide
every 3 to 4 weeks

↓

Response Assessment (Clinical)

CT thorax and PET 2-4 weeks after induction treatment

↓

Surgery

Goal to attain R0 resection

↓

Risk Assessment (Pathological)

High risk factors:
Close/positive margin status
WHO B3 or C histology

↓

Consolidation Chemotherapy

Cisplatin and etoposide for patients with risk factors

Figure 10.6 Proposed treatment for *unresectable* thymoma using neoadjuvant chemoradiation, followed by surgery and consolidation chemotherapy. Preoperative radiation therapy can be used for unresectable thymoma if induction chemotherapy is contraindicated

Source: Wright CD, Choi NC, Wain JC et al (2008) Induction chemoradiotherapy followed by resection for locally advanced Masaoka stage III and IVA thymic tumors. Ann Thorac Surg 85:385–389

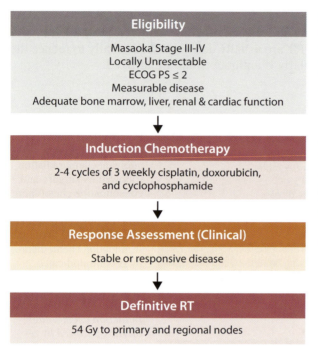

Figure 10.7 Proposed treatment algorithm of definitive treatment of *unresectable* thymoma using neoadjuvant chemotherapy, followed by radiation therapy

Source: Loehrer PJ Sr, Chen M, Kim K et al (1997) Cisplatin, doxorubicin, and cyclophosphamide plus thoracic radiation therapy for limited-stage unresectable thymoma: an Intergroup trial. J Clin Oncol 15:3093–3099

Table 10.8 Neoadjuvant strategies for *unresectable* thymoma and supporting clinical evidence

Author	Materials and methods	Results
Venuta et al[a]	■ Prospective protocol for 65 stages I–IV thymoma patients with 83 historical controls stratified to 3 risk groups for treatment ■ Group I (*n* = 18 patients), stages I–II medullary and stage I mixed thymomas; radical resection with no adjuvant therapy ■ Group II (*n* = 22), stages I and II cortical, and stage II mixed thymomas; postoperative CT and RT ■ Group III (*n* = 25), stages III–IV cortical thymomas and stage III mixed thymomas; resectable stage III lesions were removed, and highly invasive stage III and stage IV lesions had biopsy, neoadjuvant CT and surgical resection; postoperative CT and RT for all patients	■ The 8-year survival rates for patients in stages I, II, III, and IV were 95, 100, 92, and 68%, respectively ■ Group I had an 8-year survival rate of 94%; group II, 100%; and group III, 76% ■ Survival compared with that of patients operated on before 1989: differences not significant for group I; survival improved in group II (100 versus 81%, *p* = NS); and group III showed significant improvement (76 versus 43%, *p* < 0.049), suggesting potential role of multimodality treatment for high risk patients

Table 10.8 (continued)

Author	Materials and methods	Results
Kim et al[b]	■ Prospective study of 22 patients with stages III–IV invasive thymoma ■ Treated with 3 cycles of induction chemotherapy (cyclophosphamide, doxorubicin, cisplatin, and prednisone), surgical resection, and RT and 3 courses of consolidation chemotherapy	■ 77% major response rate to induction chemotherapy ■ 76% had complete resection; 24% had incomplete resection ■ With a median follow-up time of 50.3 months, 18/19 patients who completed treatment were disease free ■ Overall survival rate of 79% at 7 years
Wright et al[c]	■ Retrospective review of 10 patients with unresectable (stages III–IV) thymic tumors treated between 1997 to 2006 ■ 2 Cycles of cisplatin and etoposide with concurrent RT (33–49 Gy) delivered by 3D-CRT or IMRT prior to surgery ■ Postoperative chemotherapy given if judged to be at high risk for relapse	■ 8 Patients had a R0 resection and 2 had a R1 resection ■ 4 Patients had substantial (>90%) necrosis in resected specimen ■ No postoperative mortality ■ Median follow-up was 41 months, with 3 recurrences; 5-year overall survival of 69%

CT: chemotherapy; **NS:** not significant

[a] *Source: Venuta F, Rendina EA, Pescarmona EO et al (1997) Multimodality treatment of thymoma: a prospective study. Ann Thorac Surg 64:1585–1591*
[b] *Source: Kim ES, Putnam JB, Komaki R et al (2004) Phase II study of a multidisciplinary approach with induction chemotherapy, followed by surgical resection, radiation therapy, and consolidation chemotherapy for unresectable malignant thymomas: final report. Lung Cancer 44:369–379*
[c] *Source: Wright CD, Choi NC, Wain JC et al (2008) Induction chemoradiotherapy followed by resection for locally advanced Masaoka stage III and IVA thymic tumors. Ann Thorac Surg 85:385–389*

Table 10.9 Definitive strategies for *unresectable* thymoma and supporting clinical evidence

Author	Materials and methods	Results
Loehrer et al	■ Prospective study of 23 patients with unresectable, nonmetastatic thymoma or thymic carcinoma ■ 2–4 Cycles of neoadjuvant chemotherapy of cisplatin, doxorubicin and cyclophosphamide given 3 times weekly, followed by RT (54 Gy) to primary tumor and regional nodes for patients with stable or responsive disease	■ There were 5 complete and 11 partial responses to chemotherapy (overall response rate, 69.6%) ■ Median time to treatment failure was 93.2 months (range of 3–99.2+ months) ■ Median survival time was 93 months (range, 1–110 months) ■ 5-Year survival rate was 52.5%

Source: Loehrer PJ Sr, Chen M, Kim K et al (1997) Cisplatin, doxorubicin, and cyclophosphamide plus thoracic radiation therapy for limited-stage unresectable thymoma: an Intergroup trial. J Clin Oncol 15:3093–3099

RT Techniques

Simulation and Target Volume Delineation

A computed tomography (CT) scan with intravenous contrast should be performed from the lower neck to include the entire thorax, with arms raised above the head (in treatment position). Gated CT, 4-dimensional CT, or active breathing control (ABC) techniques are encouraged to compensate for breathing motion. Otherwise, CT can be performed at the end of natural inhalation, exhalation, or under free-breathing conditions.

Selection and delineation of gross tumor volumes (GTV), clinical target volumes (CTV), and planning target volumes (PTV) are detailed in Table 10.10.

Table 10.10 Definitions of GTV, CTV, and PTV in RT for thymoma

Target volume	Definition
GTV	■ Any gross tumor ■ Surgical clips indicative of gross residual disease should be included in postoperative cases
CTV	■ Potential residual disease and the entire thymus (if partial resection) ■ Encompassing the entire mediastinum and bilateral supraclavicular region is *not* necessary
PTV	■ CTV plus 1.5–2 cm for target motion and setup error ■ When 4D CT is used, target motion observed should be included

Dose and Treatment Delivery

Doses of adjuvant RT for thymoma depend on the status of surgical margin: 50 Gy for clear/close margins, 54 Gy for microscopically positive margins, and 60 Gy for grossly positive margins using conventional fractionation. Doses of 60–70 Gy may be needed for gross residual disease or unresected cases.

Doses lower than 50 Gy in the adjuvant setting is associated with higher local recurrence rates (*Zhu G, He S, Fu X et al (2004) Radiotherapy and prognostic factors for thymoma: a retrospective study of 175 patients. Int J Radiat Oncol Biol Phys 60:1113–1119*).

Field Arrangement and Treatment Techniques

Conventional radiation technique using anterior(AP)/posterior(PA) (anteriorly weighted) (Figure 10.8a) or wedge-pair technique (Figure 10.8b) can be considered depending on the shape of the PTV. Intensity-modulated RT (IMRT) or 3-dimensional conformal RT (3D-CRT) techniques improve the dose distribution and decrease dose to normal tissue (Figures 10.8c,d and 10.9). Figure 10.10 shows a comparison of lung dose volume histogram (DVH) treated with various techniques.

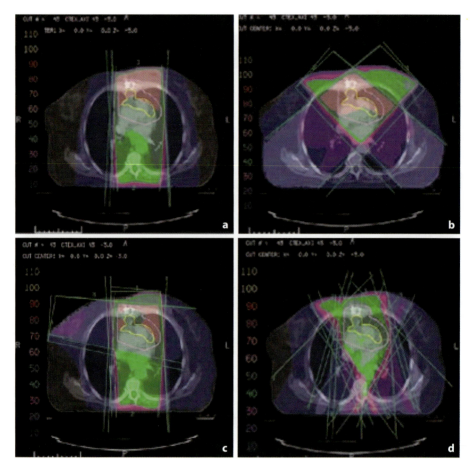

Figure 10.8 a–d Isodose distribution of **a** an AP/PA field arrangement, **b** a wedge-paired field arrangement, **c** 3D conformal radiation therapy, and **d** IMRT in postoperative case (prescription dose = 54 Gy to the International Commission of Radiation Units and Measurements [ICRU] reference point)

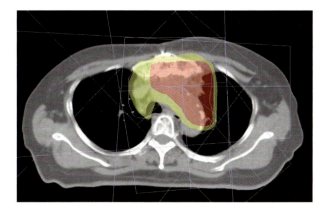

Figure 10.9 A five-field noncoplanar IMRT plan for a patient with thymic carcinoma after an R2 resection. *Red color wash* indicates 95% dose coverage of PTV to 60 Gy; *yellow color wash* indicates 95% dose coverage of PTV to 54 Gy

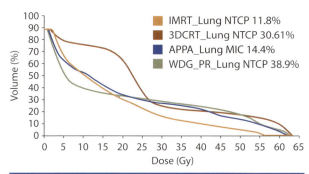

Figure 10.10 Comparison of lung dose volume histogram (DVH) treated with various techniques. *NTCP* normal tissue complication probability

Technique	Radiation Therapy (RT)	Mean Lung Dose
APPA	Anterior Posterior 2DRT	20.6 Gy
WDG	Wedge Paired 2DRT	27.8 Gy
IMRT	Intensity Modulated RT	17.2 Gy
3DCRT	3-D Conformal RT	21.4 Gy

Normal Tissue Tolerance and Side Effects

Organs at risk in the thorax for definitive RT of thymoma and their dose limitations are detailed in Chap. 9, Table 9.13.

Acute and late side effects secondary to radiation treatment are similar to those observed in lung cancer. Acute side effects may include cough, dysphagia, odynophagia, mild dyspnea, fatigue, and skin erythema. Severe long-term adverse effects are uncommon but may include radiation-induced lung and cardiac disease, and very rarely, myelopathy.

Follow-Up

Active follow-up after definitive treatment for thymoma is recommended, as late recurrences up to 12% occurring 12–20 years after surgery have been reported. Schedule and suggested examinations for follow-up are detailed in Table 10.11.

Table 10.11 Follow-up schedule and examinations

Schedule	Frequency
Years 0–2	■ Every 4–6 months
Years 2+	■ Annually
Examinations	
History and physical	■ Complete history and physical examination
Imaging studies	■ Annual CT thorax is recommended, especially for patients without adjuvant treatment ■ Other imaging tests based on clinical indication
Laboratory tests	■ Lab tests are indicated based on clinical indication

Source: National Comprehensive Cancer Network (NCCN). Clinical practice guidelines in oncology: Thymic malignancy v. 2.2009. http://www.nccn.org/professionals/physician_gls/PDF/thymic.pdf. Cited June 2009

11

Esophageal Cancer

Steven H. Lin[1] and Zhongxing Liao[2]

Key Points

- Esophageal cancer is the seventh leading cause of cancer deaths worldwide, with squamous cell responsible for 95% of all cases.
- Adenocarcinoma now accounts for over 50% of esophageal cancer in the USA, due to association with gastroesophageal reflux disease (GERD) and obesity.
- Dysphagia and weight loss are the two most common presentations in patients with esophageal cancer.
- Endoscopic ultrasound (EUS) is necessary to accompany a complete workup for proper staging and diagnosis of esophageal cancer.
- Surgery is the standard of care for early-stage esophageal cancer.
- Preoperative chemotherapy and radiation is the standard option for locally advanced esophageal cancer in surgically eligible patients.
- Pathologic complete response is around 25% after preoperative chemoradiation, which improves survival.
- Definitive chemoradiation cures some patients with esophageal cancer.
- The need to add surgical resection after chemoradiation is controversial, and may not be needed for selected patients.

Epidemiology and Etiology

Esophageal cancer is the seventh leading cause of cancer deaths worldwide. The annual incidence of esophageal cancer is as high as 30 to 800 per 100,000 people, with the highest incidences in northern Iran, southern Russia, and northern China.

Esophageal cancer accounts for 16,640 new cases in the USA annually; 14,530 people died in the USA in 2010. The epidemiology of esophageal cancer has changed drastically in the past few decades, and the absolute incidence increased from 3.8 to 23.3 per 1 million from the 1970s to 2001 in the USA.

A number of etiologic factors have been associated with esophageal cancer (Table 11.1). Targeted screening in regions (especially those with endem-

[1] Steven H. Lin, MD, PhD (✉)
Email: shlin@mdanderson.org

[2] Zhongxing Liao, MD
Email: zliao@mdanderson.org

J. J. Lu, L. W. Brady (Eds.), *Decision Making in Radiation Oncology*
DOI: 10.1007/978-3-642-13832-4_12, © Springer-Verlag Berlin Heidelberg 2011

ic gastric cancer, e.g., Japan) by using endoscopy detects cases of esophageal cancer at earlier stages, thus favoring a good outcome.

Table 11.1 Etiological factors of esophageal cancer

Type	Description
Patient related	**Lifestyle:** smoking is a known etiologic, dose-dependent risk factor. Alcohol consumption is an independent risk factor, and has a synergistic interaction with smoking. The majority of cases are squamous cell carcinoma (*SCC*)
	Dietary factors: diets rich in vegetables, fruits, fish, and poultry are protective, while typical Western diets – low in vitamins and high in red meats and processed foods – are risk factors
	Genetics: Tylosis and Plummer-Vinson syndromes are known genetic syndromes that predispose one to SCC of the esophagus
Disease related	**GERD:** associated with obesity and consumption of Western diets rich in processed and red meat. These are all risk factors for GERD and development of Barrett's esophagitis, which leads to dysplasia and invasive malignancy. The majority of cases are adenocarcinoma in the distal esophagus/GEJ
	Infectious agents: *Helicobacter pylori* is **not** known to contribute to esophageal cancers (possibly protective because of atrophic gastritis), although it is a known carcinogen for gastric cancers. HPV is a known contributing factor
	Other conditions: achalasia, esophageal diverticuli, esophageal webs, and history of squamous cell cancers of the head and neck, due to field cancerization effect
Environmental exposures	Therapeutic irradiation and injury from lye ingestion are known causative agents for SCC

GERD: gastroesophageal reflux disease; **GEJ:** gastroesophageal junction; **HPV:** human papilloma virus

Anatomy

The esophagus is an organ with an average length of 25 cm, and spans from the cricopharyngeus at the cricoid cartilage to gastroesophageal junction (GEJ). Relative to the incisors, the cervical esophagus spans from 15 to 18 cm, the upper thoracic from 18 to 24 cm, the midthoracic from 24 to 32 cm, and the lower thoracic from 32 to 40 cm (Figure 11.1).

The esophagus has four layers: mucosa with stratified squamous epithelium, submucosa, muscularis propria, and adventitia, but no serosa; hence, it has no barriers to limit locoregional spread.

Lymphatic Drainage

The esophagus is drained by a rich network of submucosal lymphatics draining to regional lymph nodes in the cervical, mediastinal, paraesophageal, left gastric, and celiac axis regions (Figure 11.1).

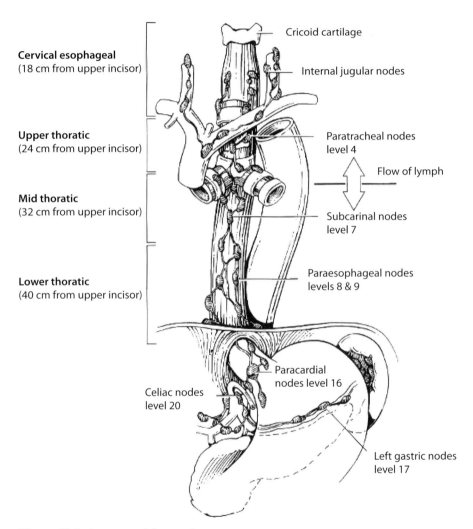

Figure 11.1 Anatomy of the esophagus

Pathology

Esophageal cancer is classified based on histologic appearance and cell of origin. Cancer of epithelial origin (squamous cell or adenocarcinoma) accounts for 95% of esophageal cancer; thus, it forms the focus of this chapter. Uncommon histologies include melanoma, choriocarcinoma, Kaposi sarcoma, and small cell carcinoma.

Until the 1970s, squamous cell carcinoma (SCC) accounted for the majority of cases of esophageal cancer in the USA, accounting for over 90–95% (worldwide, the incidence is 95%). Since then, adenocarcinoma of the distal esophagus and GEJ has the fastest-growing incidence rate of all cancers in the USA, and accounts for over 50% of all cases.

SCC usually occurs in the middle third of the esophagus (the ratio of upper:middle:lower is 15:50:35). Adenocarcinoma is most common in the lower third of the esophagus, accounting for over 65% of cases.

Routes of Spread

Local extension, regional (lymphatic), and distant (hematogenous) metastases are the three major routes of spread in esophageal cancer (Table 11.2).

Table 11.2 Routes of spread in esophageal cancer

Type	Description
Local extension	■ Lack of barrier of local extension due to lack of serosa to limit spread ■ Can spread locally to invade organs/structures such as the pericardium and heart, trachea, and vertebral bodies
Regional lymph node metastasis	■ First-echelon lymph node drainage is to the paraesophageal nodes ■ Regional lymph node spread depends on location of the primary disease ■ For cervical esophagus, regional lymph nodes include the supraclavicular and cervical nodes ■ For thoracic esophagus cancers, mediastinal nodal spread are common (paratracheal, subcarinal) ■ For the distal esophagus, the left gastric and celiac axis nodes are common sites of metastasis
Distant metastasis	■ Most common sites of distant metastasis are lung, liver, and bone ■ Much more common in adenocarcinoma

Diagnosis, Staging, and Prognosis

Clinical Presentation

The most common clinical presentation is dysphagia and weight loss, occurring in over 90% of patients. Patients with advanced disease present with symptoms related to the extent of local spread and/or areas of metastasis.

Diagnosis and Staging

Complete history, physical examination, and diagnostic imaging and laboratory tests are necessary for the proper diagnosis and staging of esophageal cancer. Figure 11.2 summarizes the workup for esophageal cancer. Table 11.3 summarizes the indications and tests for the appropriate workups of esophageal cancer.

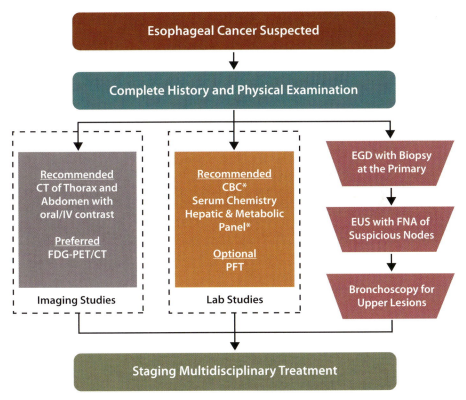

Figure 11.2 A proposed algorithm for diagnosis and staging of esophageal cancer. CBC complete blood count, PFT pulmonary function test, EGD esophagogastroduodenoscopy, EUS endoscopic ultrasound. *CBC to rule out anemia and abnormalities in preparation for chemotherapy is important, as is a complete metabolic panel for preoperative screening to determine hepatic and coagulation abnormalities

Table 11.3 Workup for diagnosis of esophageal cancer

Type	Description
Procedures	■ **Barium swallow** can visualize areas of obstruction and assess stricture. Extravasation of contrast may indicate a fistula ■ **Esophagogastroduodenoscopy** (EGD) provides direct visualization and relative location of the tumor (distance in cm from the incisors) and size of the primary tumor. Cold-forceps biopsies are obtained for pathologic diagnosis ■ **Endoscopic ultrasound** (EUS) assesses depth of invasion and involvement of adjacent lymph nodes essential for clinical staging. Suspicious lymph nodes should be biopsied with fine-needle aspiration (*FNA*) ■ **Bronchoscopy** for upper and middle thoracic esophageal lesions to exclude invasion of trachea or bronchi ■ **Laparoscopy** for GEJ/proximal stomach tumors to exclude possible intra-abdominal/peritoneal metastasis. Could also be used to place G- or J-tube for patients with complete obstruction
Imaging studies	■ **Contrast computer tomography (CT) of chest and abdomen** is useful in helping to exclude presence of metastasis to the lung and liver and locoregional spread ■ **A bone scan** maybe indicated in patients with complaints suggestive of bone metastasis or with elevated serum alkaline phosphatase (if positron-emission tomography [*PET*] is not performed) ■ **Fluorodeoxyglucose (FDG)-PET/CT** is useful for initial staging workup and monitor response to chemoradiation treatment. Detects occult metastasis in 15% of cases

Smoking cessation, and nutritional evaluation and malnutrition management (parenteral nutrition and/or gastrostomy [G-] or jejunostomy [J-] tube) may also be indicated.

Tumor, Node, and Metastasis Staging

The 7th edition of the tumor, node, and metastasis (TNM) staging and grouping system of the American Joint Committee on Cancer (AJCC) for esophageal cancer distinguishes squamous from adenocarcinoma, and also adds grade of disease as a staging factor (Tables 11.4, 11.5, and 11.6). For SCC, the location of disease is important, with the lower regions having better prognosis relative to upper and middle regions.

Table 11.4 AJCC TNM classification of carcinoma of the esophagus

Stage	Description
Primary tumor (T)	
TX	Primary tumor cannot be assessed
T0	No evidence of primary tumor
Tis	High-grade dysplasia and carcinoma in situ (*CIS*)
T1a	Lamina propria and muscularis mucosae involvement
T1b	Submucosa involvement
T2	Invasion of muscularis propria
T3	Invasion of adventitia
T4a	Pleura, pericardial, or diaphragm involvement
T4b	Other organs (aorta, vertebral body, trachea)
Regional lymph nodes (N)	
NX	Regional lymph nodes cannot be assessed
N0	No regional lymph node metastasis
N1	1–2 regional lymph node metastasis/es[a]
N2	3–6 regional lymph nodes metastases[a]
N3	≥7 Regional lymph nodes metastases[a]
Distant metastasis (M)[b]	
M0	No distant metastasis
M1	Metastasis to distant organs (retroperitoneal, paraaortic nodes, lung, liver, bone)

[a]Includes nodes previously labeled as "M1a"

[b]"M1a" designation is no longer recognized in the 7th edn. of the AJCC system

Source: Edge SB, Byrd DR, Compton CC et al (2009) American Joint Committee on Cancer, American Cancer Society. AJCC cancer staging manual, 7th edn. Springer, Berlin Heidelberg New York

Table 11.5 Stage grouping for adenocarcinoma of the esophagus

Stage Grouping							
	T1	T1	T2	T2	T3	T4a	T4b
N0	IA	IB	IB	IIA	IIB	IIIA	IIIC
N1	IIB	IIB	IIB	IIB	IIIA	IIIC	IIIC
N2	IIIA	IIIA	IIIA	IIIA	IIIB	IIIC	IIIC
N3	IIIC	IIIC	IIIC	IIIC	IIIC	IIIC	IIIC
M1	IV						

Source: Edge SB, Byrd DR, Compton CC et al (2009) American Joint Committee on Cancer, American Cancer Society. AJCC cancer staging manual, 7th edn. Springer, Berlin Heidelberg New York

Table 11.6 Stage grouping for SCC of the esophagus

Stage	TNM and grade criteria	Location
IA	T1 N0 M0 G1	Any
IB	T1 N0 M0 G2–3	Any
	T2–3 N0 M0 G1	Lower
IIA	T2–3 N0 M0 G1	Upper/middle
	T2–3 N0 M0 G2-3	Lower
IIB	T1–2 N1 M0 any G	Any
	T2–3 N0 M0 G2–3	Upper/middle
IIIA–IV	Same as adenocarcinoma	

Source: Edge SB, Byrd DR, Compton CC et al (2009) American Joint Committee on Cancer, American Cancer Society. AJCC cancer staging manual, 7th edn. Springer, Berlin Heidelberg New York

Prognostic Factors

Significant prognostic factors are detailed in Table 11.7. Table 11.8 summarizes survival by stage, and Table 11.9 ranks survival by treatment modalities from various clinical trials.

Table 11.7 Prognostic factors of esophageal cancer

Type	Description
Disease related	■ **Stage** at diagnosis is the most important prognostic factor: Depth of invasion is the most important factor for nodal and distant spread ■ **Tumor volume** is prognostically important ■ **Lymphovascular invasion** is a poor prognostic factor
Patient related	■ **Age of patients** per se is not a significant prognostic factor ■ **Performance status** may determine the feasibility of definitive therapy for patients with non-metastatic disease
Diagnostic or treatment related	■ **Incomplete pathologic response to preoperative therapy** (chemotherapy or chemoradiotherapy) is a poor prognostic factor

Table 11.8 Prognosis of esophageal cancer

Stage	5-Year OS (%)
0	100%
I	50–80%
IIA	30–40%
IIB	10–30%
III	10–15%
IV	0–5%

Table 11.9 Survival outcomes of the various treatment modalities from the clinical trials

Randomized trial[a]	1-Year OS (%)	2-Year OS (%)	3-Year OS (%)	5-Year OS (%)	MS (months)	Local failure (%)
Surgery						
U.S. Intergroup 0113	60%	37%	26%		16.1	59%
MRC OEO2 trial		34%			13.3	37%
Bosset et al					18.6	
Walsh et al	42%	26%	6%		11	
Urba et al	58%		16%		17.6	52%
Average	53%	32%	16%		15.3	49%
Radiotherapy						
RTOG 85-01	34%	10%	0%	0%	9.3	68%
ECOG	33%	12%	8%	7%	9.2	
Average	33%	11%	4%	3.5%	9.2	68%
Definitive chemoradiotherapy						
RTOG 85-01	52%	36%	30%	26%	14	46%
RTOG 85-01 (non-randomized group)	62%	35%	26%	14%	16.7	58%
ECOG	54%	27%	13%	9%	14.8	
Bedenne et al		37%			17.7	
Stahl et al		35%	24%		15	
Average	56%	34%	23%	16%	15.6	52%
Preoperative chemotherapy						
US Intergroup 0113		35%			14.9	58%
MRC OEO2 trial		43%			16.8	27%
Average		39%			15.8	42%
Preoperative chemoradiotherapy						
Walsh et al	52%	37%	32%		16	
Bosset et al					18.6	
Urba et al	72%		30%		16.9	23%
Bedenne et al		37%			19.3	
Stahl et al		39%	31%		16	
Average	62%	38%	31%		17.4	23%

OS: overall survival rate, **MS:** median survival time

[a]For specific references of each trial, please refer to specific trials listed in the tables below

Modified from Kleinberg LR, Brock MV, Jagannath SB et al (2008) Abeloff's clinical oncology, 4th edn, Chap. 78, Table 78-3, Cancer of the esophagus. Churchill Livingston, Philadelphia

Treatment

Principles and Practice

The primary goals of managing esophageal cancer are to not only to treat the underlying cancer, but also to relieve obstructive symptoms. Three main treatment modalities are used either singly or in combination for most stages of disease. A fourth modality, endoscopic mucosal resection (EMR), is mainly reserved for the earliest stage of cancer (Tis–T1aN0).

Table 11.10 summarizes each of these treatment modalities. Figure 11.3 outlines the recommended treatment pathways, based on stage of disease.

Table 11.10 Treatment modalities for esophageal cancer

Type	Description
Surgery	
Indications	■ Can be used alone for early-stage disease ■ Used in combination with chemoradiation for more locally advanced diseases ■ Occasionally used for palliation
Techniques	■ **Trans-hiatal esophagectomy** is good for distal tumors but can be used for tumors in any location with less morbidity, as compared with transthoracic approaches, but it has poorer visualization for upper/mid- thoracic tumors, with more limited nodal dissection ■ **Transthoracic approaches** includes the **Ivor Lewis** approach(right thoracotomy), which is the most common and most preferred route, since it allows exposure of all levels of the esophagus, whereas left thoracotomy provides access to only distal esophagus. More direct visualization with better exposure and nodal dissection, but with greater postoperative morbidity ■ A minimum of 15 nodes should be removed, although the optimal number after preoperative chemoradiation is not known
Outcomes	■ 5-Year OS for surgery alone is 20–25% (no significant difference between surgical techniques according to results of 2 meta-analyses) ■ Local failure rate around 19–57% when used alone ■ Surgical morbidity/mortality related to experience of the surgeons ▶

Table 11.10 *(continued)*

Type	Description
RT	
Indications	■ Outcomes are generally poor after radiation alone for definitive or adjuvant treatment ■ Adjuvant chemoradiation therapy can be used for distal esophageal/GEJ tumors ■ Preoperatively or definitive radiation with concurrent chemotherapy commonly recommended in locally advanced esophageal cancer ■ Palliative treatment for stage IV patients with obstructive symptoms due to locally advanced disease
Techniques	■ EBRT using 3D-CRT to a total dose of 50.4 Gy (1.8 Gy per daily fraction) is standard ■ IMRT is often utilized to minimize exposure to adjacent structures ■ Proton beam in combination with chemotherapy is being explored ■ Brachytherapy can be used for palliation. Its use in definitive setting is limited, however.
Outcome	■ Definitive chemoradiation provides a 5-year OS of ~20%
Chemo-/targeted therapy	
Indications	■ Used in combination with radiation for locally advanced cancers ■ Preoperative chemotherapy alone or in combination with radiotherapy for managing locally advanced GEJ esophageal cancers is controversial ■ Used as single treatment modality in stage IV disease
Medications	■ Platinum doublet is preferred over single agents ■ Cisplatin plus 5-FU or docetaxel are commonly used combinations ■ Targeted biologic agents added to standard cytotoxic chemotherapy is being explored

EBRT: external-beam radiation therapy; **IMRT:** intensity-modulated radiation therapy; **3D-CRT:** 3D-conformal radiation therapy; **GEJ:** gastroesophageal junction

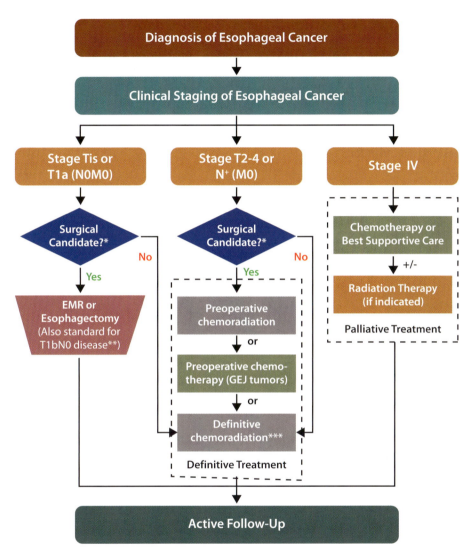

Figure 11.3 A proposed treatment algorithm for esophageal cancer. *Eligibility for surgery depends on medical operability, technical resectability, or patient preference. For many locally advanced proximal esophageal cancers, definitive chemoradiation is often advocated because of the potential morbidity of surgical resection. **Definitive chemoradiation can be considered, as evidenced by a couple of phase II trials from Japan. ***Patients are generally restaged 4–6 weeks after preoperative or definitive chemoradiation with EGD/biopsy and PET/CT. If no residual disease, patients can be observed. If persistent disease is present, salvage surgery can be considered

Treatment of Early-Stage Disease (Tis, T1a, and T1b)

Esophagectomy is standard therapy for early-stage disease. In addition, EMR can be considered for extremely early lesions (high-grade dysplasia, Tis–T1a diseases that are well to moderately differentiated, <2 cm, limited to mucosa, without ulceration or lymphovascular invasion [LVI]; Table 11.11). EMR involves submucosal injection of fluid to lift and separate the lesion from the underlying muscular layer, and resection is carried out by suction to trap the lesion in a cylinder.

Table 11.11 Results of endoscopic mucosal resection (*EMR*) for early disease

Trial	Description
Ell et al	■ Single center prospective trial of 100 consecutive cases with low risk adenocarcinoma (147 resections) ■ All lesions ≤2 cm, no lymphovascular invasion (*LVI*), G1–2, arising in Barrett's metaplasia ■ 5-Year OS = 98% (2 unrelated deaths) ■ Minor complications (e.g., minor bleeding) ■ Recurrent or metachronous lesions in 11% of cases, all successfully salvaged with repeated EMR

Source: Ell C, May A, Pech O et al (2007) Curative endoscopic resection of early esophageal adenocarcinomas (Barrett's cancer). Gastrointest Endosc 65:3–10

Treatment of Locoregionally Advanced Disease (T2, T3, T4, or N⁺)

The optimal management of locally advanced esophageal cancer is controversial. A number of management strategies have been studied in clinical trials, with mixed results.

Surgery with Preoperative (Neoadjuvant) Therapy

The role of preoperative chemotherapy alone is controversial, according to mixed results from clinical trials (Table 11.12). The efficacy of preoperative chemoradiation therapy has been demonstrated in a number of trials and meta-analyses (Table 11.13). Preoperative chemotherapy versus chemoradiation has not been tested.

Table 11.12 Clinical evidence for pre- or perioperative chemotherapy for resectable esophageal cancer: randomized trials

Trial	Description
INT 0113[a]	■ Randomized 467 cases of SCC (46%) or adenocarcinoma (54%) to surgery alone or surgery with perioperative chemotherapy ■ Chemotherapy included 3 cycles of preoperative and 2 cycles of postoperative cisplatin plus 5-FU ■ Only 71% received all 3 cycles of chemotherapy, and only 80% in the chemotherapy group received surgery (versus 96% in the surgery group) ■ No difference in resectability; R0 and R1 resections in 62 versus 59% (p = NS) and 15 versus 4% (p = 0.01), respectively ■ Pathologic complete response (CR) = 2.5% ■ 4-Year OS and MS were 26 versus 23%, and 16 versus 15 months (both p = NS), respectively ■ 5-Year disease-free survival (DFS) higher after complete resection (32%) versus incomplete resection (5%)
MRC 0E02[b]	■ Randomized 802 cases of SCC (31%) or adenocarcinoma (66%) to surgery alone or surgery with preoperative chemotherapy ■ Chemotherapy included 2 cycles of cisplatin plus 5-FU ■ 92% received surgery in chemotherapy group ■ R0 resections higher in the chemotherapy group, 60 versus 54% (p < 0.0001) ■ 2-Year OS and MS improved with preoperative chemotherapy: 43 versus 34% and 16.8 versus 13.3 months, respectively; hazard ratio (HR) = 0.79 (p = 0.004)
MRC MAGIC[c]	■ Randomized 503 cases of adenocarcinoma of the stomach (74%), GEJ (11%), or distal esophagus (15%) to surgery alone or surgery with perioperative chemotherapy ■ Chemotherapy included 3 cycles of epirubicin, cisplatin, and 5-FU (ECF) ■ Significant downstaging with chemotherapy: more T1–2 tumors in chemotherapy group (51.7 versus 36.8%) and smaller tumors (3- versus 5-cm tumors) ■ Improved survival in chemotherapy group: 5-year OS, 36 versus 23% (p < 0.009); 5-year DFS (HR for progression 0.66, p < 0.001) ■ Similar toxicity profiles between 2 groups

[a] *Source: Kelsen DP, Ginsberg R, Pajak TF et al (1998) Chemotherapy followed by surgery compared with surgery alone for localized esophageal cancer. N Engl J Med 339:1979–1984*
[b] *Source: MRC Oesophageal Working Group (2002) Surgical resection with or without preoperative chemotherapy in esophageal cancer: a randomized controlled trial. Lancet 359:1727–1733*
[c] *Source: Cunningham D, Allum WH, Stenning SP et al (2006) Perioperative chemotherapy versus surgery alone for resectable gastroesophageal cancer. N Eng J Med 355:11–20*

Table 11.13 Clinical evidence for pre- or perioperative chemoradiation therapy for resectable esophageal cancer: randomized trials and meta-analyses

Trial/meta-analysis	Description
Walsh et al (Ireland)[a]	■ Randomized 113 cases of adenocarcinoma (100%) to surgery alone or concurrent chemoradiation with surgery ■ Chemotherapy included 2 cycles of cisplatin/5-FU ■ Radiation dose of 40 Gy were delivered in 15 fractions ■ Trial discontinued because of early stopping rule ■ Pathologic complete response (pCR) = 25% ■ Improved 3-year OS and MS with chemoradiation: 32 versus 6% ($p = 0.01$) and 16 versus 11 months, respectively ■ 11 of 13 cases of pCR (85%) were alive and disease free at 2–43 months ■ Caveat: surgery-alone, historical control group had atypically poor survival
Urba et al (Michigan)[b]	■ Random 100 patients with resectable SCC (25%) and adenocarcinoma (75%) to surgery alone or concurrent chemoradiation with surgery ■ Chemotherapy used cisplatin/5-FU/vinblastine ■ Radiation dose of 45 Gy delivered in 25 fractions ■ pCR = 28% ■ Reduced local recurrence rate after trimodality treatment (19 versus 40%, $p = 0.04$) ■ Trend to improved OS by chemoradiation (30 versus 16%, $p =$ NS); however, pCR predicted for improved 3-year OS (64 versus 19%)
EORTC[c]	■ Random 282 patients with thoracic esophageal SCC to chemoradiation with surgery, or surgery ■ Chemotherapy used cisplatin ■ Split-course radiation to 37 Gy (18.5 Gy/5 days × 2, spaced with 2-week break) was used ■ pCR = 20% ■ Chemoradiation improved 5-year DFS (30 versus 25%, $p = 0.003$) and disease-specific mortality (68 versus 86%, $p = 0.002$) ■ No difference in 5-year OS (25% in both arms) ■ Postoperative mortality higher in chemoradiation (12 versus 4%)

Table 11.13 *(continued)*

Trial/meta-analysis	Description
TTROG[d]	■ Random 256 patients with SCC (37%) and adenocarcinoma (63%) to chemoradiation with surgery, or surgery ■ Chemotherapy used cisplatin/5-FU ■ Radiation dose of 35 Gy delivered in 15 fractions ■ pCR = 16%; more R0 resection in chemoradiation arm ■ No difference in PFS or OS between groups; MS of 22 versus 19.3 months ($p = 0.32$) ■ Subset analysis showed improved PFS in SCC histology for trimodality treatment (HR 0.47, $p = 0.014$)
CALGB 9781[e]	■ Randomized 56 cases (out of 475 planned cases, due to poor accrual) to chemoradiation with surgery, or surgery (75% adenocarcinoma) ■ Chemotherapy using cisplatin/5-FU in concurrent with standard radiation scheme (50.4 Gy in 28 fractions) ■ pCR = 40% ■ Chemoradiation improved MS (4.5 versus 1.8 years) and 5-year OS (39 versus 16%)
German Esophageal Cancer Study Group[f]	■ Randomized 126 cases (out of 354 planned cases, due to poor accrual) of T3-4NxM0 adenocarcinoma of GEJ or gastric cardia ■ Patients received chemotherapy (2.5× cisplatin/5-FU/and leucovorin [LV]) plus surgery or 2× chemotherapy (same regimen) then chemoradiation with surgery ■ Improved pathologic CR (15.6 versus 2%) and tumor-free lymph nodes (64.4 versus 37.7%) with chemoradiation ■ Trends to improve survival with preoperative chemoradiation (3-year OS 47.4 versus 27.7%, $p = 0.07$) ■ Postoperative mortality increased slightly in chemoradiation (10.2 versus 3.8%, $p = 0.26$) ▶

Table 11.13 (continued)

Trial/meta-analysis	Description
Meta-analysis[g]	■ Meta-analysis of 10 randomized trials comparing preoperative chemoradiation and surgery versus surgery alone ($n = 1,209$), and 8 trials compared preoperative chemotherapy and surgery alone versus surgery alone ($n = 1,724$)
	■ Chemoradiation provided improved HR (0.81) for mortality, corresponding to 13% absolute 2-year survival benefit. Both adenocarcinoma and SCC benefited equally
	■ Chemotherapy also provided improved HR (0.90, $p = 0.05$), corresponding to 7% absolute 2-year survival benefit. Only adenocarcinoma seemed to benefit

[a]*Source: Walsh T, Noonan N, Hollywood D et al (1996) A comparison of multimodal therapy and surgery for esophageal adenocarcinoma. N Engl J Med 335:462–467*
[b]*Source: Urba SG, Orringer MB, Turrisi A et al (2001) Randomized trial of preoperative chemoradiation versus surgery alone in patients with locoregional esophageal carcinoma. J Clin Oncol 19:305–313*
[c]*Source: Bosset JF, Gignoux M, Triboulet JP et al (1997) Chemoradiotherapy followed by surgery compared with surgery alone in squamous-cell cancer of the esophagus. N Engl J Med 1997; 337:161–167*
[d]*Source: Burmeister BH, Smithers BM, Gebski V et al (2005) Surgery alone versus chemoradiotherapy followed by surgery for resectable cancer of the oesophagus: a randomized controlled phase III trial. Lancet Oncol 6:659–668*
[e]*Source: Tepper J, Krasna MJ, Niedzwiecki D et al (2008) Phase III trial of trimodality therapy with cisplatin, fluorouracil, radiotherapy, and surgery compared with surgery alone for esophageal cancer: CALGB 9781. J Clin Oncol 26:1086–1092*
[f]*Source: Stahl M, Walz MK, Stuschke M et al (2009) Phase III comparison of preoperative chemotherapy compared with chemoradiotherapy in patients with locally advanced adenocarcinoma of the esophagogastric junction. J Clin Oncol 27:851–856*
[g]*Source: Gebski V, Burmeister B, Smithers BM et al (2007) Survival benefits from neoadjuvant chemoradiotherapy or chemotherapy in oesophageal carcinoma: a meta-analysis. Lancet Oncol 8:226–234*

A proposed treatment algorithm for inoperable locally advanced esophageal cancer is presented in Figure 11.4.

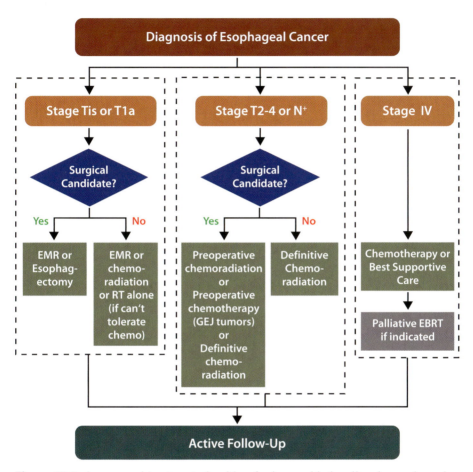

Figure 11.4 A proposed treatment algorithm for inoperable locally advanced esophageal cancer

Definitive Chemoradiation Therapy

Definitive chemoradiation is superior to radiation alone, and long-term cures (in 20–25%) have been observed for a select subset of patients (Table 11.14).

Results of clinical trials have demonstrated improved local control but not overall survival (due mostly to the offset by operative mortality) after surgical resection and chemoradiation therapy (Table 11.15; Figure 11.5).

Table 11.14 Clinical evidence for definitive chemoradiation for inoperable esophageal cancer: randomized trials

Trial	Description
RTOG 8501[a]	■ Randomized 121 unresectable cases of SCC or adenocarcinoma to CRT or radiation therapy (*RT*) alone ■ Closed early due to early stopping rule of benefit in experimental arm ■ Radiation alone arm used 64 Gy in 32 daily fractions ■ CRT arm used 50 Gy in 25 daily fractions in concurrence with cisplatin/5-FU, followed by 2 cycles of cisplatin/5-FU ■ RT field included whole esophagus to 50 Gy (RT alone arm) or 30 Gy (chemoradiation arm) followed by boost to final dose to tumor >5 cm above and below ■ Improved MS with CRT: 12.5 versus 8.9 months (*p* = 0.001) ■ 2-Year OS (38 versus 10%), local recurrence (16 versus 24%, *p*=0.01), and DM rate (22 versus 38%) all favored CRT ■ Updated results showed 5-year OS of 26% in CRT versus 0% in RT alone
INT 0123 (a.k.a. RTOG 9405)[b] (Figure 11.5)	■ Randomized 236 cases of stages T1–4, N0/1, M0 SCC or adenocarcinoma to high-dose (64.8 Gy) versus low-dose (50.4 Gy) CRT ■ Closed early due to early stopping rule of benefit in experimental arm ■ Chemotherapy used cisplatin (75 mg/m² ×1) and 5-FU (1,000 mg/m² × 4days) ■ Radiation field included superior and inferior border of 5 cm above and below the tumor to 50.4 Gy, followed by a boost to 64.8 Gy with a 2 cm margin above and below the tumor ■ No difference between high- versus low-dose arms in MS (13 versus 18.1 months), 2-year OS (31 versus 40%), or local recurrence rate (56 versus 52%) ■ 11 versus 2 treatment-related deaths in high- versus low-dose arms. But the majority of these deaths (7 of 11 cases) in the high-dose arm occurred before 50.4 Gy ■ Thus, the finding that there may be increased mortality rates in the high-dose arm is highly controversial

[a]*Sources: Herskovic A, Martz K, Al-Sarraf M et al (1992) Combined chemotherapy and radiotherapy compared with radiotherapy alone in patients with cancer of the esophagus. N Engl J Med 326:1593–1598; Cooper JS, Guo MD, Herskovic A et al (1999) Chemoradiotherapy of locally advanced esophageal cancer: long-term follow-up of a prospective randomized trial (RTOG 85-01). Radiation Therapy Oncology Group. JAMA 281:1623–1627*
[b]*Source: Minsky BD, Pajak TF, Ginsberg RJ (2002) INT0123 (Radiation Therapy Oncology Group 94-05) phase III trial of combined-modality therapy for esophageal cancer: high dose versus standard-dose radiation therapy. J Clin Oncol 20:1167–1174*

Table 11.15 Clinical evidence for surgical resection after chemoradiation therapy for esophageal cancer

Trial	Description
German[a]	■ Randomized 172 cases of locally advanced SCC to induction chemotherapy with CRT. with or without surgery ■ Identical chemotherapy regimens used in both arms included 3 cycles of bolus 5-FU/LV/cisplatin/VP-16 plus cisplatin/VP-16 in concurrence with RT ■ Radiation dose of 40 or 60 Gy delivered with or without surgery, respectively ■ pCR = 35%; improved PFS in surgery group (2-year PFS was 64.3 versus 52.1%, p = 0.03) ■ No difference in OS ■ Clinical response to chemotherapy is predictive of improved outcomes (HR + 0.3) ■ Treatment-related mortality increased in surgery group (12.8 versus 3.5%, p = 0.03)
French[b]	■ Accrued 444 cases of T3N0–1M0 SCC (89%) or adenocarcinoma (11%) to receive chemotherapy (cisplatin/5-FU) and RT ■ Initial RT dose was 46 Gy ■ Only responding patients (259 cases) were randomized to either surgery or continuation of CRT to 65 Gy ■ 2-Year local control rate improved with surgery (66.4 versus 57%, p < 0.001) ■ No difference in 2-year OS (34% after CRT plus surgery versus 40% after CRT alone, p= 0.14) ■ 3-Month mortality rate higher in surgery arm (9.3 versus 0.8%, p=0.002)

[a] *Source: Stahl M, Stuschke M, Lehmann N et al (2005) Chemoradiation with and without surgery in patients with locally advanced squamous cell carcinoma of the esophagus. J Clin Oncol 23:2310–2317*
[b] *Source: Bedenne L, Michel P, Bouche O et al (2007) Chemoradiation followed by surgery compared with chemoradiation alone in squamous cancer of the esophagus: FFCD 9102. J Clin Oncol 25:1160–1168*

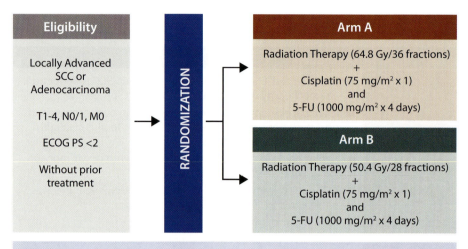

Eligibility	RANDOMIZATION	Arm A
Locally Advanced SCC or Adenocarcinoma		Radiation Therapy (64.8 Gy/36 fractions) + Cisplatin (75 mg/m² x 1) and 5-FU (1000 mg/m² x 4 days)
T1-4, N0/1, M0		Arm B
ECOG PS <2		Radiation Therapy (50.4 Gy/28 fractions) + Cisplatin (75 mg/m² x 1) and 5-FU (1000 mg/m² x 4 days)
Without prior treatment		

RESULTS
Closed early due to early stopping rule. Median survival: 13 versus 18.1 months; 2-year OS (31 versus 40%) (no significant differences between 2 arms) There may be an increased mortality rate in the high-dose arm

Figure 11.5 INT 0123 schema and results. The regimen used in the low-dose arm of INT-0123 study is considered the standard regimen for chemoradiation therapy for esophageal cancer

Adjuvant chemoradiotherapy

Postoperative radiation therapy alone is not indicated. However, adjuvant chemoradiation in proximal gastric/GEJ tumors may be indicated, based on North American Intergroup Trial 0116 (Table 11.16).

Table 11.16 Evidence support the use of adjuvant chemoradiation in tumors of gastroesophageal junction

Trial	Description
North American Intergroup 0116	■ Aimed to study the efficacy of postoperative chemoradiation in locally advanced gastric cancer ■ Random 556 patients (stages ≥Ib) with resected adenocarcinoma of stomach (80%) or GEJ (20%) to surgery alone or postoperative chemoradiation ■ Chemotherapy used 2 cycles of 5FU/LV plus 45 Gy × 2 cycles of additional 5FU/LV) ■ Median OS = 36 versus 27 months in favor of chemoradiation arm ($p = 0.005$) ■ 3-Year OS = 50% versus 41% in chemoradiation versus surgery alone arms (~10% absolute benefit)

Source: McDonald JS, Smalley SR, Benedetti J et al (2001) Chemoradiotherapy after surgery compared with surgery alone for adenocarcinoma of the stomach or gastroesophageal junction. N Engl J Med 345:725–730

Treatment for Recurrence or Palliation

Palliative radiation is often needed for symptomatic patients (especially obstruction) from primary disease with poor performance status, recurrent disease, and metastatic disease.

Individualized multidisciplinary management for recurrence after primary therapy depends on recurrent sites and patients' performance statuses (Figure 11.6). A feeding tube or stent placement is indicated for immediate relief of obstruction.

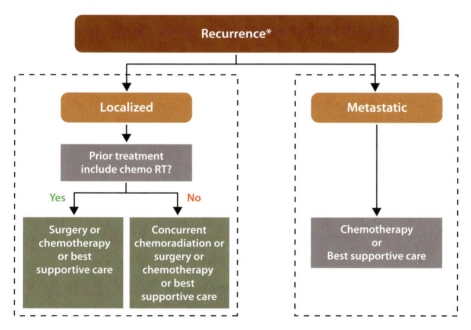

Figure 11.6 A proposed treatment algorithm for patients with recurrent esophageal cancer (ECOG performance status [PS] = 0–2). *Best supportive care is rendered for patients with ECOG PS > 2 (Karnofsky Performance Scale [KPS] < 60%)

Doses used for palliation are typically the same as in definitive treatments (50 Gy in 5 weeks), although a slightly accelerated fashion could be considered (50 Gy in 2.5-Gy fractions). Palliation after radiation or chemoradiation occurs in 2–4 weeks, and response is often durable.

The use of radiation therapy in cases with tracheoesophageal (TE) fistula due to recurrence is controversial. Clinical data have supported radiotherapy without worsening the fistula, and healing of small TE fistulas with radiation was demonstrated in some series. Hence, TE fistulas are not an absolute contraindication for radiation.

Radiation Therapy Techniques

Definitive Radiation Therapy

Immobilization and Simulation

Patients are placed in the supine position with both arms up and immobilized with a Vac-LoK bag and T-bar, which gives a setup uncertainty of about 7 mm, at our institution. Daily imaging (kV orthogonal X-rays or cone beam computed tomography [CT]) can reduce this uncertainty further.

CT imaging, preferably four-dimensional (4D)-CT simulation to account for tumor motion and individualizing target volume and margin, should be considered for all patients. Spiral CT or extended-time CT simulation (slow CT scanning) to acquire an average image of the tumor at all phases of the respiratory cycle can be done if 4D-CT is not available. Treatment planning should account for tumor motion by creating a combined image data set of all possible respiratory positions of the target (or maximal intensity projection [MIP]).

Target Definition and Delineation

In the era of CT planning and image-guided radiotherapy, margins are defined and contoured on CT scans and respect anatomic boundaries (Figure 11.7). Gross tumor volume (GTV) is contoured on MIP imaging (if 4D CT is available) to account for tumor excursion with respiratory motion.

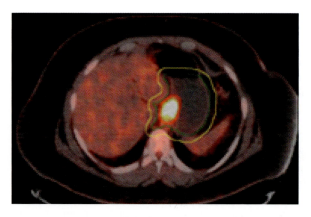

Figure 11.7 PET/CT scan image showing the FDG avid primary tumor at the GEJ. The red line indicates the GTV, the green line the CTV (notice the CTV to the stomach follows the nature anatomic structure), and the yellow line the PTV

Definitions of GTV, clinical target volumes (CTV), and planning target volumes (PTV) are detailed in Table 11.17 and Figure 11.8.

Table 11.17 Definitions of target volumes in RT for esophageal cancer

Type	Description
GTV	■ All grossly positive disease as seen on exam, EGD report, and PET/CT imaging (Figure 11.2)
CTV	■ Superiorly and inferiorly: GTV plus 4 cm for submucosal extension ■ The inferior extension of CTV at the GEJ/stomach should customized according to anatomy: May cover the lesser curvature (for paracardial and left gastric nodes) and celiac axis nodes for distal/GEJ tumors if these regions are not included as part of the GTV ■ Radially extend by 1 cm from GTV but respecting anatomic boundaries, such as the pericardial sac, vertebral body, pleura, and vessels
PTV	■ CTV plus 0.7–1 cm, or plus 0.5 cm if daily orthogonal imaging is performed

GTV is contoured on MIP imaging (if 4D-CT is available) to account for tumor excursion with respiratory motion

CTV should be delineated by attending radiation oncologists and automatic expansion from GTV is not an acceptable practice

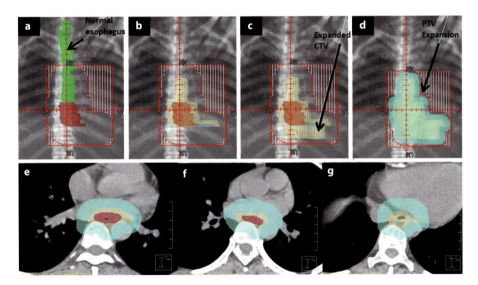

Figure 11.8 a–g Target delineation of distal esophageal cancer for 3D-CRT treatment. **a** Delineation of GTV (*red*), based on PET and EGD report. The normal esophagus is presented. **b** CTV expansion accounts for microscopic spread superiorly around 4 cm above the edge of the GTV, as well as inferiorly (**c**), to account for potential extension into the proximal stomach and regional nodes (celiac and left gastric). **d** PTV expansion by 1 cm around the CTV to account for setup error. **e–g** GTV–CTV–PTV delineation. Note the CTV expansion is manually defined to respect anatomic boundaries

Pathological examination of surgical specimens without preoperative therapy revealed that proximal and distal microscopic extension from gross tumor were 10.5 ± 13.5 and 10.6 ± 8.1 mm, respectively for SCC, and 10.3 ± 7.2 and 18.3 ± 16.3 mm, respectively, for GEJ adenocarcinoma. Thus, the minimal recommended CTV to encompass 94% of cases of microscopic spread is 3 cm, except for the distal spread of GEJ adenocarcinoma, where 5 cm is needed (*Gao XS, Qiao X, Wu F et al (2007) Pathological analysis of clinical target volume margin for radiotherapy in patients with esophageal and gastroesophageal junction carcinoma. Int J Radiat Oncol Biol Phys 67:389–96*).

Treatment Planning

Standard beam arrangement in 3D-CRT uses a three- to six-field arrangement, employing one of the following:
- A minimum anteroposterior/right posterior oblique/left posterior oblique (AP/RPO/LPO) arrangements
- AP/posteroanterior (PA)/left anterior oblique (LAO)/right anterior oblique (RAO)/ RPO/LPO fields

Intensity-modulated radiation therapy (IMRT) can further improve the conformality of the dose distribution by sparing the adjacent normal structures to help meet dose constraints (Figure 11.9; Table 11.18). Proton therapy may further improve the dosimetry, particularly for larger tumors or if adjacent nodal masses abutting critical structures.

Dose and Fractionation

Conventional daily dosing at 1.8-Gy fractions to a total dose of 45 to 50.4 Gy, using 3D-CRT (three- or four-field) or IMRT, is standard. No survival benefit with doses greater than 50.4 Gy was demonstrated in the INT 0123 study (Table 11.14).

Higher doses (approaching the same management for head and neck primaries) to 60–70 Gy should be considered for high thoracic or high cervical lesions.

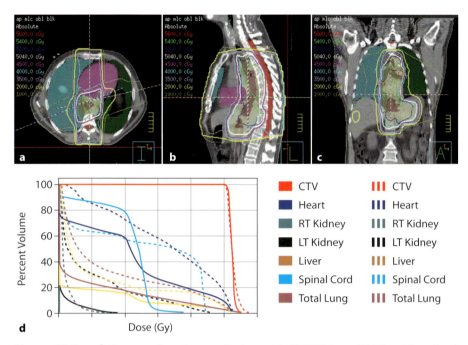

Figure 11.9 a–d Preoperative chemoradiation with IMRT for a T3N1 mid-to-distal esophageal cancer patient. **a–c** Dose distribution of IMRT plan for this case (note increased weighting for the AP/PA versus oblique fields to minimize dosing to the lungs). **d** DVH analysis of IMRT plan (*solid lines*) versus 3D-CRT (*dashed lines*)

Normal Tissue Tolerance

Acute and late toxicities can be reduced by observing dose–volume constraints, which is modified by the use of concurrent chemotherapy (Table 11.18).

Acute effects may include esophagitis, skin irritation, fatigue, and nausea/vomiting. Subacute and late toxicities include radiation pneumonitis, pericarditis, pericardial effusion, esophageal stricture/fistula, and second primary malignancy.

Table 11.18 Dose constraints to the OAR and planning OAR volumes (*PRVs*) in IMRT for esophageal cancer

OAR	RT alone	CRT	Preoperative CRT
Spinal cord	50 Gy	45 Gy	45 Gy
Lung	MLD < 20 Gy V20 < 40%	MLD < 20 Gy V20 < 35% V10 < 45% V5 < 65%	MLD < 20 Gy V20 < 20% V10 < 40% V5 < 55%
Heart	V40 < 50%	Same	Same
Esophagus	D_{max} < 75 Gy V60 < 50%	D_{max} < 75 Gy V55 < 50%	D_{max} < 75 Gy V55 < 50%
Kidney	V20 < 50% for both V20 < a third for 1 if the other is non- functional	Same	Same
Liver	V30 < 40%	Same	Same

MLD: mean lung dose; D_{max}: maximum point dose; **DVH:** dose–volume histogram; **V***n* percentage volume of organ receiving *n* Gy

Adapted from Cox JD, Chang JY, Komaki R (2007) Image-guided radiotherapy of lung cancer. Taylor and Francis, London

Follow-Up

Patients should undergo active surveillance after treatment Schedule and suggested examinations during follow-up are presented in Table 11.19.

Table 11.19 Role of FDG-PET in predicting pCR rates after preoperative chemoradiation

Trial	Description
MDACC	■ Single-center retrospective review of 83 patients with resectable esophageal cancer ■ All patients underwent preoperative chemoradiation ■ FDG-PET obtained pretreatment and 4–6 weeks after chemoradiation ■ pCR rate = 31%; posttreatment FDG-PET SUV_{max} response correlated with pCR ($p = 0.03$) ■ 2-Year OS 60 versus 33% for posttreatment SUV (SUV < 4 versus ≥ 4, $p = 0.01$) ■ Posttreatment SUV was the only preoperative factor to correlate with decreased survival. However, the FDG-PET could only predict for residual > 10% (not less)

SUV_{max}: maximum standardized uptake value

Source: Swisher SG, Erasmus J, Maish M et al (2004) 2-Fluoro-2-deoxy-D-glucose PET imaging is predictive of pathologic response and survival after preoperative CRT in patients with esophageal carcinoma. Cancer 101:1776–1185

Predictive Role of Positron-Emission Tomography for Treatment Response

Pathologic complete response to preoperative CRT ranges between 20 and 40%. Fluorodeoxyglucose–positron-emission tomography (FDG-PET) response correlated with pathologic complete response (pCR) is more superior as compared with CT or endoscopic ultrasound (EUS), but cannot be used to rule out residual disease. Thus, surgical resection is recommended after preoperative CRT (Table 11.19).

With preoperative CRT, restaging 4–6 weeks after CRT with CT or PET/CT and endoscopy (with or without biopsy) to assess for treatment response is recommended. If a patient continues to be a good surgical candidate without disease progression, surgical resection is often recommended. Observation could be considered in those with a complete clinical response to therapy, based on patient preference.

Table 11.20 Follow-up schedule and examinations

Schedule	Frequency
First follow-up after RT	■ 4–6 weeks after RT (either definitively or preoperatively)
Years 0–3	■ Every 3-6 months
Years 3–5	■ Every 6 months
Years 5+	■ Annually
Examinations	
History and physical	■ Complete history and physical examination ■ Nutrition counseling ■ EGD as clinically indicated ■ Dilatation for anastomotic stenosis if indicated
Laboratory tests	■ If clinically indicated
Imaging studies	■ CT of the chest and abdomen or PET/CT ■ Other imaging studies if clinically indicated

Adapted from the National Comprehensive Cancer Network (2010) NCCN clinical practice guidelines in oncology for esophageal cancer, ver. 1.2010. http://www.nccn. org/professionals/physician_gls/PDF/esophageal.pdf. Cited 22 April 2010

Section V
Cancers of the Gastrointestinal Tract

12

Gastric Cancer

Jeremy Tey[1] and Zhen Zhang[2]

Key Points

- Gastric cancer is the fourth most commonly diagnosed cancer and the second leading cause of cancer-related death worldwide.

- Gastric cancer is often diagnosed at an advanced stage, as early gastric cancer is asymptomatic or causes only nonspecific symptoms. Common signs and symptoms in advanced disease include fatigue, weight loss, bleeding (hematemesis, melena), anorexia, abdominal pain, and obstruction (dysphagia and/or vomiting).

- Accuracy of clinical diagnosis approaches 90%, based on history and physical examination, upper gastrointestinal radiography and endoscopy, and laboratory and imaging studies (including computed tomography [CT] and endoscopic ultrasound [EUS]). However, pathologic diagnosis is required before treatment.

- Stage at diagnosis is the most important prognostic factor and predicts the resectability of the tumor. Other prognostic factors include histological type (intestinal versus diffuse) and completeness of resection.

- Commonly observed metastatic sites include the liver, peritoneum, and distant lymph nodes. Metastasis to lung, brain, and other organs/tissues is less common.

- Treatment of gastric cancer depends on the stage of the disease. Surgery is the only curative treatment for localized diseases. Overall survival rate of patients who achieve R0 (complete) after radical D2 surgery is ~30%. However, only 15–20% cases are resectable at diagnosis, and long-term survival of patients with unresectable disease is <5%.

- As up to 70% of cases develop locoregional recurrence after surgery, adjuvant chemoradiation is recommended and is the current standard in USA. The efficacy of radiation plus fluorouracil (5-FU) regimen has been demonstrated in Intergroup-0116 (INT-0116) trial, led by the Southwest Oncology Group, and improved overall survival.

- Perioperative chemotherapy also improves overall survival rates in locoregionally advanced gastric cancer, based on level I evidence.

- Radiation therapy, with or without chemotherapy, is effective in the palliation of bleeding, pain, and obstruction.

- Palliative 5-FU based chemotherapy can be considered for metastatic gastric cancer; however, the effect of chemotherapy on prolonging survival has not been confirmed.

[1] Jeremy Tey, MD
Email: jeremy_tey@nuhs.edu.sg

[2] Zhen Zhang, MD
Email: zhenzhang6@gmail.com

J. J. Lu, L. W. Brady (Eds.), *Decision Making in Radiation Oncology*
DOI: 10.1007/978-3-642-13832-4_13, © Springer-Verlag Berlin Heidelberg 2011

Epidemiology and Etiology

Gastric cancer is the fourth most commonly diagnosed malignancy and the second most common cause of cancer deaths worldwide. It is responsible for about 800,000 deaths globally per year. In the USA, it represents roughly 2% (25,500 cases) of all new cancer cases annually. It is more common in Japan (78 per 100,000 men), Korea, China, other East Asian countries, Eastern Europe, and South America.

A number of risk factors have been identified for gastric cancer (Table 12.1). Screening is not performed in most of the world, except in Japan and Korea, where early detection has significantly improved survival.

Table 12.1 Risk factors for gastric cancer

Risk factors	Description
Patient related	**Age and gender:** Median age of diagnosis is 65; diagnosis before age 40 is rare. Male:female ratio is 1.5:1
	Lifestyle: diet thought to be primary risk factor (preserved, smoked/salted foods, lack of fresh fruit and vegetables, nitrides, nitrosoamides); cigarette smoking is associated with 1.5- to 3-fold increase of risk; low socioeconomic status; previous radiation exposure
	Race: Africans, Asians, and Hispanic Americans have a higher risk than do whites
	Past medical history: *Helicobacter pylori* infection associated with a 3- to 6-fold increase in risk, autoimmune gastritis, chronic gastritis, pernicious anemia, previous gastric resection has a 1.5- to 3-fold increase in risk, history of gastric polyps. Previous history of radiotherapy
	Genetic predisposition: Peutz-Jeghers syndrome, familial adenomatous polyposis and HNPCC syndrome (microsatellite instability gene [*MSI*]). Gene mutations include p53, *c-met, k-sam,* E-cadherin gene (*CDH1*), *bcl-2, and erb-B2.* Slightly increased risk in blood group A

HNPCC: hereditary non-polyposis colon cancer

Anatomy

The stomach begins at the gastroesophageal junction and ends at the pylorus. The greater curvature forms the left and convex border of the stomach, and the lesser curvature forms the right and concave border of the stomach. It is divided into four parts: the cardia, fundus, body, and antrum. Its wall is divided into five layers: mucosa, submucosa, muscularis externa, subserosa, and serosa (Figure 12.1). It is covered with peritoneum and is closely related to the left lobe of the liver, spleen, left adrenal gland, superior portion of the left kidney, pancreas, transverse colon, and major blood vessels including the celiac axis and superior mesenteric artery (Figure 12.2).

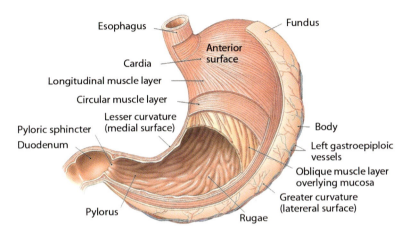

Figure 12.1 Regions of stomach and the probability of gastric carcinoma, according to the primary location: tumors arising from gastroesophageal junction, cardia, and fundus account for ~35%; from the body, ~25%; from antrum and distal stomach, ~40%

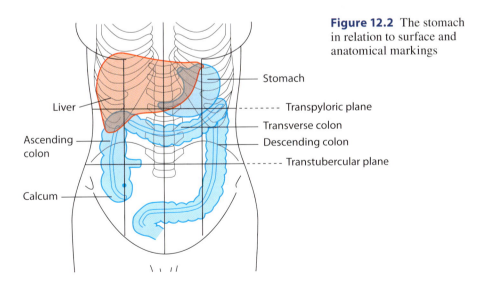

Figure 12.2 The stomach in relation to surface and anatomical markings

Pathology

Adenocarcinoma accounts for >90% of all gastric cancers, and thus is the focus of this chapter. Adenocarcinomas are further subclassified into *intestinal* versus *diffuse* type (Lauren's classification) (Table 12.2). Borrmann's classification describes the gross pathologic findings of gastric cancer, and is associated with the aggressiveness of the disease (Table 12.3).

Table 12.2 Lauren's classification and characteristic factors of gastric cancer (adenocarcinomas)

Type	Description
Intestinal	■ Occurs in older population ■ More common in men ■ Occurs usually in body and distal stomach ■ Associated with H. pylori infection ■ Often preceded by precancerous lesions ■ Prone to hepatic metastases ■ Associated with a better prognosis
Diffuse	■ Occurs in younger population ■ More common in women ■ Occurs usually in the proximal stomach ■ Associated with hereditary factors ■ Not associated with precancerous lesions ■ Prone to peritoneal metastases ■ Associated with a poorer prognosis

Table 12.3 Borrmann's classification of gastric cancer

Type	Description
I	Polypoid or fungating
II	Ulcerating lesions surrounded by elevated borders
III	Ulcerating lesions with invasion of the gastric wall
IV	Diffusely infiltrating (linitis plastica)
V	Not classifiable

Other histologies include lymphomas (~4%), carcinoid tumors (~3%), malignant stromal cell tumors (~2%), and squamous cell carcinomas (~1%). Gastric lymphoma including mucosa-associated lymphatic tissue (MALT) is the second most commonly diagnosed malignancy of the stomach, and is mentioned in Chap. 25, "Non-Hodgkin's Lymphoma."

Routes of Spread

Local extension, regional (lymphatic), and hematogenous metastases are the three major routes of spread in gastric cancer (Table 12.4).

Table 12.4 Routes of spread in gastric cancer

Route	Description
Local extension	■ Direct involvement of liver, duodenum, pancreas, transverse colon, omentum, diaphragm ■ Proximal tumors may spread upward to involve the esophagus ■ Perineural invasion can occur
Regional lymph node metastasis	■ Lymph node involvement is seen in up to 80% of cases at diagnosis ■ Lymph node involvement depends on the origin of the primary disease ■ Proximal/gastroesophageal junction tumors may spread to lower paraesophageal lymph nodes ■ Tumors of the body can involve all nodal sites ■ Tumors of the distal stomach/antrum may involve periduodenal, and porta hepatic nodes ■ Lymph nodes other than direct draining regions are usually involved in advanced disease
Distant metastasis	■ Distant metastases occurs in ~30% of cases at diagnosis ■ The most common route of hematogenous metastasis is the via the portal vein to the liver (30%) ■ Metastases to other organs and tissues such as lung and brain are less common ■ Peritonea dissemination occurs in ~25% of cases of advanced gastric cancer and is considered metastatic disease ■ Bilateral ovarian metastases can occur (Krukenberg tumors)

Lymph Node Metastasis

Pattern of lymphatic spread depends on the location of the primary tumor (gastroesophageal junction/cardia versus greater/lesser curvature versus pylorus/antrum) of the stomach. Commonly involved lymph nodes in cancer of the stomach are illustrated in Figures 12.3 (on CT scan) and 12.4. The corresponding lymph node stations are listed in Table 12.5.

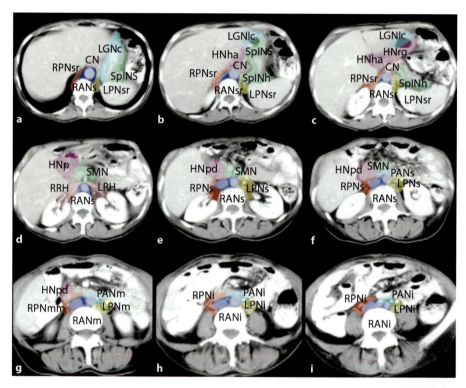

Figure 12.3 a–i Lymph node groups commonly involved in gastric cancer on CT images. **CN:** Coeliac; **SMN:** Superior Mesenteric; **RRH:** Right Renal Hilum; **LRH:** Left Renal Hilum; **HNpd:** Hepatic Nodes (pancreatico duodenum); **HNp:** Hepatic Nodes (pyloric); **HNha:** Hepatic Nodes (hepatic artery); **HNrg:** Hepatic Nodes (right gastroepiploic); **LPN:** Left Paraaortic Nodes; **RPN:** Right Paraaortiic Nodes; **RAN:** Retroaortic Nodes, **PAN:** Preaortic Nodes; **SpINs:** Splenic Nodes; **SpINh:** Splenic Nodes (hilar); **LGN:** Left Gastric Nodes; **LGNIc:** Left Gastric Nodes(gastropancreatic) **sr:** suprarenal; **s:** superior; **m:** middle; **i:** inferior

(Adapted from Martinez-Monge R, Fernandez PS, Gupta N, et al. (1999) Cross-sectional Nodal Atlas: A Tool for the Definition of Clinical Target Volumes in Three-dimensional Radiation Therapy Planning. Radiology, 211:815-82 . Used with permission from RSNA)

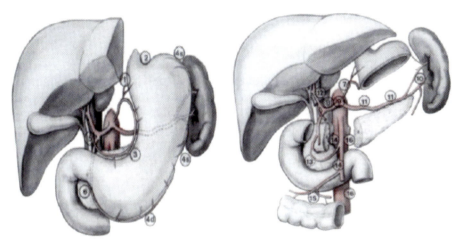

Figure 12.4 Lymph node groups surrounding the stomach

Table 12.5 Lymph node stations commonly involved in gastric cancer (Japanese Research Society for the Study of Gastric Cancer)

Station	Nodes	Station	Nodes
1	Right cardial	9	Along the celiac axis
2	Left cardial	10	At the splenic hilus
3	Along the lesser curvature	11	Along the splenic artery
4	Along the greater curvature	12	At the hepatoduodenal ligament
5	Suprapyloric	13	At the posterior aspect of pancreatic head
6	Infrapyloric	14	At the root of the mesenterium
7	Along the left gastric artery	15	In the mesocolon of the transverse colon
8	Along the common hepatic artery	16	Para-aortic lymph nodes

Figure and table adapted from Hartgrink HH, van de Velde CJ (2005) Status of extended lymph node dissection. J Surg Oncol 90:153–165. Used with permission from Wiley, Inc.

Diagnosis, Staging, and Prognosis

Clinical Presentation

Stomach cancer is often asymptomatic or causes only nonspecific symptoms in its early stages. Commonly observed symptoms include abdominal pain, weight loss, anorexia, etc., and are detailed in Table 12.6. The average interval between onset of symptoms and diagnosis is approximately 3 months in 40% of patients and longer than 1 year in approximately 20% of patients.

Table 12.6 Commonly observed signs and symptoms in gastric cancer

Type	Description
General	■ Usually lack of specific symptoms in the early stage ■ Indigestion or burning sensation (heartburn) ■ Anorexia ■ Weight loss ■ Lethargy
Locoregional disease	■ Abdominal pain or discomfort in upper abdomen ■ Nausea or vomiting (secondary to gastric outlet obstruction ■ Postprandial fullness ■ Diarrhea or constipation ■ Dysphagia ■ Bleeding (hematemesis/melena)
Distant disease	■ Lymphadenopathy at supraclavicular fossa (**Virchow's node**), is considered distant metastases ■ **Blumer's shelf** (palpable mass on rectal examination) suggests implants to the pelvis ■ Palpable ovarian mass (**Krukenburg tumor**) suggests ovarian involvement from drop metastasis ■ Hepatomegaly with disease extension to the liver

Diagnosis and Staging

Figure 12.5 illustrates the diagnostic procedure of gastric cancer, including suggested examination and tests.

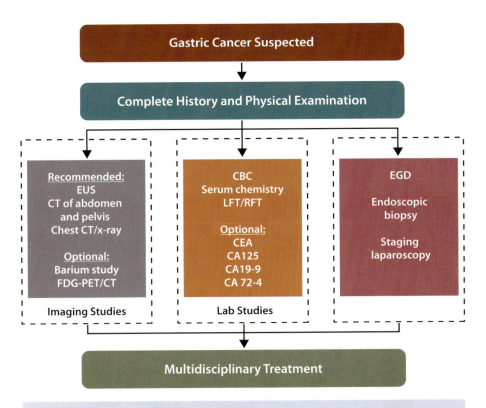

- EUS accuracy for tumor T-classification ranges from 77 - 93% and accuracy for nodal N-classification is 65 - 90%
- Accuracy of CT scan for T-classification is 43–70% and sensitivity and specificity for nodal staging range from 65 - 97%, and 49 - 90%
- Staging laparoscopy is used to rule out peritoneal spread if neoadjuvant chemotherapy, chemoradiation, or surgery is planned
- Chest CT or x-ray is used to rule out pulmonary metastases
- Accuracy of clinical diagnosis approaches 90%
- CEA, CA125, CA19-9, and CA72-4 may be elevated in 44% of patients; however, sensitivity and specificity is low (ranging from 6 - 31%)

Figure 12.5 Proposed algorithm for diagnosis and staging of gastric cancer

Tumor, Node, and Metastasis Staging

Diagnosis and clinical staging depends on findings from history and physical examination, imaging, endoscopy, biopsy, and laboratory tests. Pathological diagnosis is required for all gastric cancer patients.

Pathological staging depends on findings after surgical resection and pathological examination, in addition to those required in clinical staging.

The 7th edition of the tumor, node, metastasis (TNM) staging and grouping system of American Joint Committee on Cancer (AJCC) is presented in Tables 12.7 and 12.8.

Table 12.7 AJCC TNM classification of gastric cancer

Stage	Description
Primary tumor (T)	
TX	Primary tumor cannot be assessed
T0	No evidence of primary tumor
Tis	Carcinoma in situ: intraepithelial tumor without invasion of the lamina propria
T1a	Tumor invades lamina propria or muscularis mucosae
T1b	Tumor invades submucosa
T2	Tumor invades muscularis propria[a]
T3	Tumor penetrates subserosal connective tissue without invasion of visceral peritoneum[b] or adjacent structures (including spleen, transverse colon, liver, diaphragm, pancreas, abdominal wall, adrenal gland, kidney, small intestine, and retroperitoneum)
T4a	Tumor invades serosa (visceral peritoneum)
T4b	Tumor invades adjacent structures
Regional lymph nodes (N)	
NX	Regional lymph nodes cannot be assessed
N0	No regional lymph node metastasis (pN0 denotes negative finding in all examined lymph nodes, regardless of the total number removed and examined)
N1	Metastasis in 1–2 regional lymph nodes
N2	Metastasis in 3–6 regional lymph nodes
N3a	Metastasis in 7–15 regional lymph nodes
N3b	Metastasis in ≥16 regional lymph nodes

Table 12.7 *(continued)*

Stage	Description
Distant metastasis (M)	
M0	No distant metastasis
M1	Distant metastasis (including seeding of the peritoneum and positive peritoneal cytology)

[a]Penetration to the muscularis propria with extension into the gastrocolic or gastrohepatic ligaments, or into the greater or lesser omentum, without perforation of the visceral peritoneum covering these structures is categorized as T3; perforation of the visceral peritoneum covering the gastric ligaments or the omentum is categorized as T4

[b]Intramural extension to the duodenum or esophagus is classified by the depth of the greatest invasion in any of these sites including stomach

Source: Edge SB, Byrd DR, Compton CC et al (2009) American Joint Committee on Cancer, American Cancer Society. AJCC cancer staging manual, 7th edn. Springer, Berlin Heidelberg New York

Table 12.8 AJCC stage grouping of gastric cancer

Stage Grouping					
	T1	T2	T3	T4a	T4b
N0	IA	IB	IIA	IIB	IIIB
N1	IB	IIA	IIB	IIIA	IIIB
N2	IIA	IIB	IIIA	IIIB	IIIC
N3	IIB	IIIA	IIIB	IIIC	IIIC
M1	IV				

Source: Edge SB, Byrd DR, Compton CC et al (2009) American Joint Committee on Cancer, American Cancer Society. AJCC cancer staging manual, 7th edn. Springer, Berlin Heidelberg New York

Prognosis

The most important prognostic factors of gastric cancer include staging at diagnosis (especially the N category), patients' performance status, and treatment modality. The overall survival of patients according to treatment is shown in Table 12.9.

Prognosis of patients treated without surgery is particularly poor. Pertinent prognostic factors after complete resection include location of the tumor, differentiation, and lymphovascular invasion (LVI).

Table 12.9 Overall survival (*OS*) according to treatment based on results of prospective trials

Survival time	T1N0M0 radical surgery (%)	Localized disease			Advanced disease
		Radical surgery (%)	Adjuvant chemo--radiation therapy (%)	Perioperative chemo-therapy (%)	Palliation only
3 Years	–	41%	50%	–	<5%
5 Years	~90%	10–30%	–	~36%	<5%
MS	–	27%	35%	–	~6 Months

MS: median survival

Source: results from trials including the INT0116/MAGIC trial

Treatment

Principles and Practice

Surgery is the only curative treatment modality for gastric cancer; however, radiation with concurrent chemotherapy should be considered for patients with inoperable disease.

Surgery alone is sufficient for T1N0M0 tumors. As locoregional recurrence occurs in 40–65% of cases after radical surgery in locoregionally advanced disease, adjuvant therapy is usually recommended after radical surgery (Table 12.10).

Table 12.10 Treatment modalities used in gastric cancer

Type	Description
Surgery	
Indications	■ Surgery is the mainstay curative treatment option ■ Subtotal gastrectomy with gastrojejunostomy alone is the treatment of choice for Tis–T2N0M0 disease ■ Total gastrectomy is not indicated if 5-cm clear margin and reconstruction can be achieved ■ Palliative gastrectomy may be performed for palliation of local symptoms
Facts	■ Removal of at least 15 lymph nodes is recommended ■ ≥5-cm proximal and distal margins whenever possible
Radiation therapy	
Indications	■ Adjuvant treatment after complete resection in T2–T4 and/or N^+ diseases ■ Definitive treatment (with chemotherapy) for inoperable disease ■ Palliative treatment to primary or metastatic foci
Techniques	■ EBRT using 3D-CRT or IMRT ■ IORT may further improve local control
Chemo-/targeted therapy	
Indications	■ Adjuvant treatment with chemoradiation after surgery ■ Perioperative chemotherapy given before and after surgery ■ Adjuvant chemotherapy alone after surgery is controversial ■ Used concurrently with EBRT for inoperable disease ■ Mainstay treatment for palliative therapy
Medications	■ 5-FU is the mainstay medication for chemotherapy in gastric cancer ■ Other agents used in combination with 5-FU include cisplatin, docetaxel, epirubicin, oxaliplatin, paclitaxel, and irinotecan ■ Anti-Her2 target therapies used in Her2-positive advanced–gastric cancer patients in conjunction with 5-FU/cisplatin-based chemotherapy

EBRT: external-beam radiation therapy; **IORT**: intraoperative radiotherapy

A proposed treatment algorithm based on the best available clinical evidence is presented in Figure 12.6.

The extent of lymphadenectomy is both diagnostic and therapeutic. More extensive lymph node dissection improves the accuracy of gastric cancer staging and reduces locoregional recurrences. However, impact on survival is debatable.

Table 12.11 shows the types of lymph node dissections performed during surgery.

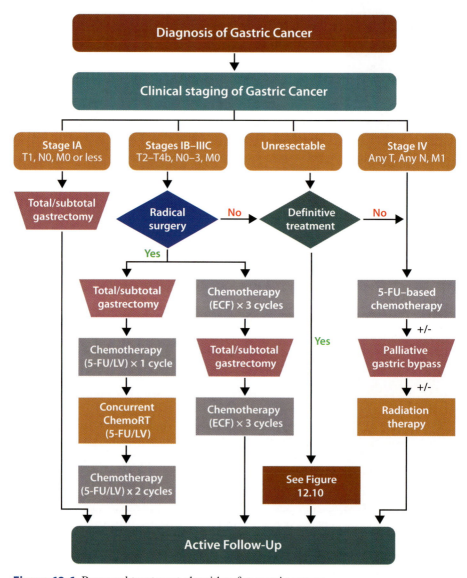

Figure 12.6 Proposed treatment algorithm for gastric cancer

Table 12.11 Types of lymph node dissections

Type	Description
D0	No lymph node dissection
D1	Removal of stomach and greater and lesser omentum with perigastric lymph nodes within 3 cm of the stomach (lymph node stations 1–6)
D2	D1 dissection plus dissection of lymph node stations 7–11. Typically includes a splenectomy and distal pancreatectomy
D3	D2 dissection plus dissection of lymph node stations 12–16

Treatment of Early-Stage Disease (Tis-2, N0, M0)

Surgery is the mainstay curative treatment modality. Tis, T1, and T2 diseases are curable with surgery alone. Overall survival rates after surgery alone for stage IA and IB disease are ~90 and ~60%, respectively.

Adjuvant treatment is not indicated for T1N0M0 disease after complete resection. However, adjuvant chemoradiation may be considered for some patients with T2N0M0 gastric cancer.

Treatment of Locoregionally Advanced Gastric Cancer (T3–4, N0–3, M0)

Neoadjuvant Treatment

Neoadjuvant therapy including chemotherapy, radiation therapy, or chemoradiation has been studied in prospective clinical trials (Table 12.12; Figure 12.7).

Table 12.12 Treatment strategies for locoregionally advanced gastric cancer and supporting clinical evidence

Randomized trial	Description
MRC MAGIC[a]	■ Randomized 503 cases of resectable stomach (74%), gastroesophageal junction (GEJ) (11%), or distal esophagus (15%) to perioperative chemotherapy and surgery versus surgery alone ■ Chemotherapy was 3 preoperative and 3 postoperative cycles of epirubicin (50 mg/m^2), cisplatin (60 mg/m^2) on D1, and continuous intravenous 5-FU (200 mg/m^2) for 21 days ■ 5-Year OS were 36 versus 23% in favor of perioperative chemotherapy ■ Significant downstaging in chemotherapy group ▶

Table 12.12 *(continued)*

Randomized trial	Description
Zhang et al (China)[b]	■ Randomized 370 patients with resectable gastric cardia disease to preoperative RT (40 Gy in 20 fractions), followed by surgery versus surgery alone ■ Significant improvement in survival and locoregional disease control was observed with the preoperative RT arm to surgery alone arm ■ 5-Year survival rate was 30 versus 20%, $p = 0.0094$, with local relapse rates of 39 versus 52%, $p < 0.025$, in favor of preoperative RT ■ Only patients with adenocarcinoma of gastric cardia were included
Walsh et al[c]	■ Randomized 113 cases of esophageal and gastric cardia cancer to preoperative chemoradiation therapy (chemoRT) and surgery versus surgery alone ■ ChemoRT was 5-FU ($15 g/m^2$, days 1–6)/cisplatin ($75 \ mg/m^2$ on day 7) for 2 cycles every 6 weeks. RT dose was 40 Gy in 15 daily fractions ■ Significant improvement in 3-year survival (32 versus 6%) and median survival (16 versus 11 months) in favor of preoperative chemoRT ■ 25% of patients in chemoRT arm had complete pathological response
RTOG 9904[d]	■ Prospective phase II trial ■ 49 Patients with localized gastric adenocarcinoma received two cycles of induction 5-FU/leucovorin and cisplatin, followed by concurrent chemoRT with IV 5-FU and weekly paclitaxel ■ Radiotherapy dose was 45 Gy in 25 daily fractions ■ Pathological complete response rates were 26% and R0 resection rates were 77%

[a] *Source: Cunningham D, Allum WH, Stenning SP et al (2006) Perioperative chemotherapy versus surgery alone for resectable gastroesophageal cancer. N Engl J Med 355:1–20*
[b] *Source: Zhang ZX, Gu XZ, Yin WB et al (1998) Randomized clinical trial on the combination of preoperative irradiation and surgery in the treatment of adenocarcinoma of gastric cardia (AGC)—report on 370 patients. Int J Radiat Oncol Biol Phys 42:929–934*
[c] *Source:Walsh TN, Noonau N, Hollywood D et al (1996) A comparison of multimodal therapy and surgery to esophageal adenocarcinoma. N Engl J Med 335:462–467*
[d] *Source: Ajani JA, Winter K, Okawara GS et al (2006) Phase II trial of preoperative chemoradiation in patients with localized gastric adenocarcinoma (RTOG 9904): quality of combined modality therapy and pathologic response. J Clin Oncol 24:3953–3958*

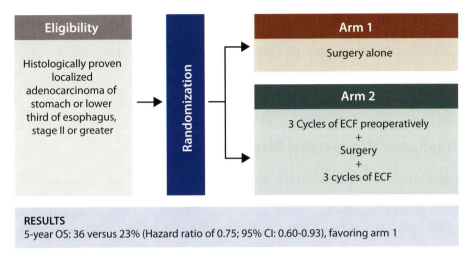

Figure 12.7 UK Medical Research Council (*MRC*) Adjuvant Gastric Infusional Chemotherapy (*MAGIC*) trial protocol schema and results

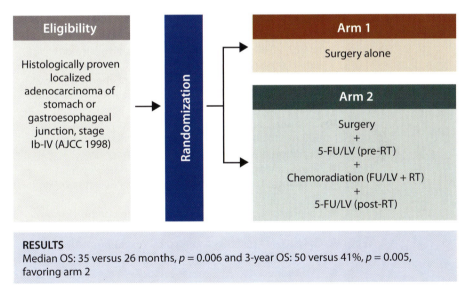

Figure 12.8 Southwest Oncology Group/Intergroup study (*SWOG 9008/INT 0116*) schema and results

Adjuvant Treatment

Clinical evidence for adjuvant chemoradiation therapy or chemotherapy after surgical resection is presented and illustrated in Table 12.13 and Figure 12.8.

A proposed treatment algorithm for nonmetastatic and resected gastric cancer, based on the INT 0116 trial, is detailed in Figure 12.9.

Treatment of Inoperable Disease

For patients with nonmetastatic but inoperable gastric cancer, high-dose radiation therapy with concurrent chemotherapy is indicated. Clinical evidence for combined chemoradiation is presented in Table 12.14. A proposed algorithm for treatment of nonmetastatic and inoperable disease is detailed in Figure 12.10.

Table 12.13 Treatment strategies for locoregionally advanced gastric cancer and supporting clinical evidence

Randomized trial/ analysis	Description
INT 0116[a]	■ Randomized 556 patients with resected stomach (80%) or GEJ (20%) stage ≥IB (1988 AJCC) to surgery alone versus postoperative chemoradiation ■ Adjuvant treatment included 1 cycle of chemotherapy then concurrent chemotherapy for 2 cycles with RT and chemotherapy × 2 cycles ■ Chemotherapy used was 5-FU (425 mg/m^2 reduced to 400 mg/m^2/day with RT) and leucovorin (20 mg/m^2) ■ Radiation dose was 45 Gy in 25 daily fractions ■ Significant improvement in median OS of 35 versus 26 months ($p = 0.006$) and 3-year OS of 50 versus 41% ($p = 0.005$) ■ Local and regional failure decreased in chemoRT group (19 versus 29%, and 65 versus 72%) ■ Only 10% of patients received D2 resection (surgery style is not required in the protocol) ■ 41% Grade 3 and 30% grade 4 toxicity in the chemoRT arm
Meta-analysis[b]	■ 4,919 Gastric cancer patients treated with surgery and adjuvant chemotherapy in 23 randomized trials were analyzed ■ Adjuvant chemotherapy improved OS and DFS ■ Pooled relative risk of death was 0.85 (95% confidence interval [CI]: 080–0.90)

[a] *Source: Macdonald JS, Smalley S, Benedetti J et al (2001) Chemoradiotherapy after surgery compared with surgery alone for adenocarcinoma of the stomach or gastro-esophageal junction. N Engl J Med 345:725–730*
[b] *Source: Liu TS, Wang Y, Chen SY et al (2008) An updated meta-analysis of adjuvant chemotherapy after curative resection for gastric cancer. Eur J Surg Oncol 34:1208–1216*

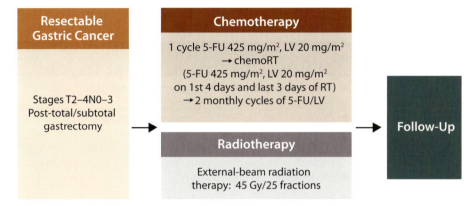

Figure 12.9 Proposed treatment algorithm of adjuvant treatment of locoregionally advanced gastric cancer with combined chemoradiation therapy based in INT0116 protocol. A dose of radiation should be escalated to 50.4–54 Gy if positive margin or gross residual disease is discovered on pathology

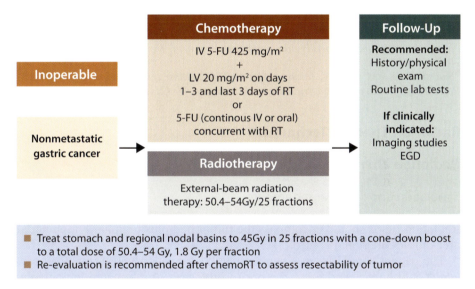

Figure 12.10 Proposed treatment algorithm for definitive chemoradiation therapy for nonmetastatic but inoperable gastric cancer

Recurrence and Palliation for Metastasis

Advanced gastric cancer includes patients with metastatic or locoregionally advanced disease not fit for definitive treatment. External-beam radiation with or without chemotherapy can be used to palliate local symptoms. Clinical evidence for palliation is detailed in Table 12.14.

Table 12.14 Clinical evidence for palliative treatment of inoperable or metastatic gastric cancer for disease/symptomatic control

Retrospective study	Description
Tey et al (NCI Singapore)[a]	▪ Retrospective study of 33 patients with advanced and inoperable or metastatic gastric cancer ▪ Palliative EBRT delivered with a median dose of 30 Gy in 10 fractions ▪ Symptom palliation achieved in 54.3, 25, and 25% of patients with bleeding, pain, and obstruction, respectively ▪ Median survival was 145 days
Kim et al (MDACC)[b]	▪ Retrospective study of 37 patients with locally advanced cancer ▪ Palliative EBRT delivered with a median dose of 35 Gy in 14 fractions with or without chemotherapy. ▪ Symptom palliative achieved in 70, 81, and 86% of patients with bleeding, pain, and obstruction, respectively ▪ Patients receiving chemoRT had trend toward better survival (6.7 versus 2.4 months, $p = 0.08$)

[a] *Source: Tey J, Back MF, Shakespeare TP et al (2007) The role of palliative radiation therapy in symptomatic locally advanced gastric cancer. Int J Radiat Oncol Biol Phys 2007 67:385–388*
[b] *Source: Kim MM, Rana V, Janjan NA et al (2008) Clinical benefit of palliative radiation therapy in advanced gastric cancer. Acta Oncol 47:421–427*

Radiation Therapy Techniques

Radiation Therapy for Adjuvant Therapy

Simulation and Field Arrangements

Radiation fields should encompass the tumor bed plus regional lymph nodal areas for locoregional control.

The patient should be in a supine treatment position with arms overhead, and should have fasted for 2–3 h prior to the scan. A computed tomography (CT) scan (3- to 5-mm cut) should be performed from the top of diaphragm to the bottom of L4. For a gastroesophageal junction/cardiac tumor, the CT scan should be started from the carina. Intravenous contrast is preferred. Organs at risk (OARs) should be delineated. Field setup is illustrated in Figure 12.11, and

Figure 12.11 a–f Postoperative radiation fields of a patient with T4aN1 gastric cancer of the antral primary. **a–c** Gastric remnant, tumor bed (*red*); celiac artery (*light yellow*); porta hepatis (*light blue*); right kidney (*light orange*); pancreatic head (*orange*). DRR (**d, e**) and DVH (**f**) of 3D conformal plan. (*Zhang Z. Gastric cancer. In: Lu JJ, Brady LW (eds) (2008) Radiation oncology: an evidence-based approach. Springer, Berlin Heidelberg New York*

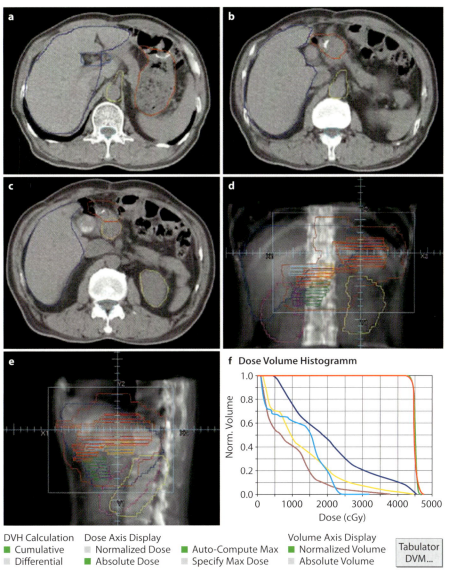

f Dose Volume Histogramm

DVH Calculation   Dose Axis Display   Volume Axis Display
■ Cumulative   ▨ Normalized Dose ■ Auto-Compute Max   ■ Normalized Volume   Tabulator
▨ Differential   ■ Absolute Dose   ▨ Specify Max Dose   ▨ Absolute Volume   DVM…

ROI Statistics

Line Type	ROI	Trial	Min	Max	Mean	Std. Cev	% Out- side crid	% > Max	Generalized EUD
	CTV	Treat	3627.7	4787.3	4497.4	98.1	0.00%	0.00%	4497.41
	L-Kidney	Treat	171.3	4510.5	1250.4	982.0	0.00%	0.00%	1260.2
	Liver	Treat	287.0	4675.8	2041.8	1162.5	0.00%	0.00%	2042.39
	R-Kidney	Treat	123.5	4304.3	913.5	768.7	0.00%	0.00%	914.177
	SC	Treat	100.0	3202.8	1176.8	813.9	4.09%	0.00%	1212.77
	Duodenum	Treat	4240.5	4609.2	4504.1	60.6	0.00%	0.00%	4502.64
	Tumor bed	Treat	4201.1	4754.1	4502.2	68.7	0.00%	0.00%	4501.52

the setup should consider surgical clips and pre- and postoperative surgery CT scans of the abdomen.

The suggested nodal coverage depends on the location of the primary disease and the status of lymph node involvement (Tables 12.15 and 12.16).

Three-dimensional (3D) conformal radiotherapy planning has been shown to produce superior dose distributions and reduced radiation doses to the kidneys and spinal cord, compared with anterior–posterior (AP-PA) techniques.

Dose and Treatment Delivery

Conventional fractionation to a total dose of 45–50.4 Gy is recommended for adjuvant radiation therapy with concurrent chemotherapy, using high-energy (≥6 MVx) photons. Boosts to 50.4–54 Gy for positive margins or residual disease should be given if doses of surrounding critical organs are within their tolerance.

Intensity-Modulated Radiation Therapy in the Adjuvant Setting

The benefit of intensity-modulated radiation therapy (IMRT) and the delineation of clinical target volume (CTV) in adjuvant treatment have been suggested by many publications; however, this needs to be further confirmed by the clinical outcome.

If used, tumor bed and subclinical target volumes including lymphatic draining regions (depends on the site of the primary tumor, as described in Tables 12.15 and 12.16) should be delineated as CTV.

Radiation Therapy for Unresectable Disease or Palliation

Simulation and Target Volume Delineation

In the definitive setting, the clinical target volume should include the tumor (stomach plus perigastric tumor extension) and draining lymph nodes in all cases.

Definitions of gross target volume (GTV), CTV, and planning target volume (PTV) in definitive radiation therapy or palliation for local symptoms for gastric cancer are suggested as follow:

■ GTV: tumor for preoperative RT
■ CTV: tumor or tumor bed, residual stomach, and regional lymph nodes
■ PTV: CTV plus margin considering organ motion and setup uncertainties

Table 12.15 Recommended nodal coverage depending on site of primary tumor in the stomach: cardia/proximal third of stomach (*prox*) and antrum/pylorus/distal third of stomach (*distal*)

Origin and stage (AJCC 7th edn)	Remaining stomach	Tumor bed volumes[a]	Nodal volume
Cardial/prox third of stomach	Preferred, but spare 2/3 of one kidney (usually right)	T category dependent	N classification dependent
Antrum/distal third of stomach	Yes, but spare 2/3 of one kidney (usually left)		
T3N0	Variable, dependent on surgical pathological findings[b]	■ Prox: medial left hemidiaphragm, adjacent body of pancreas (with or without tail) ■ Distal: head of pancreas (with or without body), 1st and 2nd part of duodenum	■ Prox: none or PG[c] ■ Distal: none or PG ■ Optional: CN, HNpd, PHN, SpINs[c]
T4aN0	Variable, dependent on surgical pathological findings[b]	■ Prox: Medial left hemidiaphragm, adjacent body of pancreas (with or without tail) ■ Distal: head of pancreas (with or without body), 1st and 2nd part of duodenum	■ Prox: none or PG; ■ Optional: PEN, MN, CN[c] ■ Distal: none or PG; ■ Optional: CN, HNpd, PHN, SpINs[c]
T4bN0	Prox: variable, dependent on surgical pathological findings[b] Distal: preferable, dependent on surgical pathological findings[b]	As for T4aN0 plus sites of adherence with 3- to 5-cm margin	■ Prox: nodes related to sites of adherence with or without PG,PEN, MN, CN ■ Distal: nodes related to sites of adherence with or without PG, HNpd, CN, PHN, SpINs

▶

Table 12.15 *(continued)*

Origin and stage (AJCC 7th edn)	Remaining stomach	Tumor bed volumes[a]	Nodal volume
T1–3N+	Preferable	Not indicated for T1–2, as above for T3	■ Prox: PG, CN, SplN, SplNs, with or without PEN, MN, HNpd, PHN[d] ■ Distal: PG, CN, HNpd, PHN, SPINs. Optional: splenic hilum
T4a/bN+	Preferable	As for T4a/bN0	As for T1–3N+ and T4bN0

PG: perigastric; **CN**: celiac; **SplN**: splenic; **SplNs**: suprapancreatic; **PHN**: porta hepatic; **HNpd**: pancreaticoduodenal; **PEN**: periesophageal; **MN**: mediastinal

[a] Use preoperative imaging (CT, barium swallow), surgical clips, and postoperative imaging (CT, barium swallow)

[b] For tumors with >5-cm margins confirmed pathologically, treatment of residual stomach is not necessary, especially if this would result in substantial increase in normal tissue morbidity

[c] Optional node inclusion for T3–4a N0 lesions if adequate surgical node dissection (D2) and at least 10–15 nodes are examined pathologically

[d] Pancreaticoduodenal and porta hepatic nodes are at low risk of nodal positivity is minimal (1–2 positive nodes, with 10–15 examined) and this region does not need to be irradiated Periesophageal and mediastinal nodes are at risk if there is esophageal extension.

Modified from Gunderson LL, Tepper JE (eds) (2007) Clinical radiation oncology, 2nd edn. Churchill Livingstone, Philadelphia; Gunderson LL, Tepper JE (2002) Radiation treatment parameters in the adjuvant postoperative therapy of gastric cancer. Semin in Radiat Oncol 12:187–195

Table 12.16 Recommended nodal coverage depending on site of primary tumor in stomach: body/middle third of stomach

Origin and stage (AJCC 7th edn)	Remaining stomach	Tumor bed volumes[a]	Nodal volume
Body/mid-third of stomach	Yes, but spare 2/3 one kidney	T category dependent	N category dependent, spare 2/3 of one kidney
T3N0, especially posterior wall	Yes	Body of pancreas (with or without tail)	▪ None or PG ▪ Optional: CN, SplN, SplNs, HNpd, PHN[b]
T4aN0	Yes	Body of pancreas (with or without tail)	▪ None or perigastric ▪ Optional: CN, SplN, SplNs, HNpd, PHN[b]
T4bN0	Yes	As for T4aN0 plus sites of adherence with 3- to 5-cm margin	Nodes related to sites of adherence with or without PG, SplNs, SplN, HNpd, CN, PHN
T1–3N+	Yes	Not indicated for T1-2, as above for T3	PG, CN, SplN, SplNs, HNpd, PHN
T4a/bN+	Yes	As for T4a/bN0	As for T1–3N+ and T4bN0

PG: perigastric; **CN**: celiac; **SplN**: splenic; **SplNs**: suprapancreatic; **PHN**: porta hepatic; **HNpd**: pancreaticoduodenal; **PEN**: periesophageal; **MN**: mediastinal

[a]Use preoperative imaging (CT, barium swallow), surgical clips, and postoperative imaging (CT, barium swallow)

[b]Optional node inclusion for T3—4a N0 lesions if adequate surgical node dissection (D2) and at least 10–15 nodes are examined pathologically

Modified from Gunderson LL, Tepper JE (eds) (2007) Clinical radiation oncology, 2nd edn. Churchill Livingstone, Philadelphia

Dose and Treatment Delivery

A dose of 45 Gy in 25 daily fractions is administered for treatment of inoperable disease, followed by a 5.4- to 9-Gy cone-down boost to GTV plus 1.5 cm to a total dose of 50.4–54 Gy with concurrent chemotherapy.

The optimal dose of effective palliation for gastric cancer has not been established. External-beam radiotherapy to a dose to a total of 30 Gy in ten fractions has been shown to provide relief of symptoms in 54, 25, and 25% of patients with bleeding, pain, and obstruction, respectively (*Tey J, Back MF, Shakespeare TP et al (2007) The role of palliative radiation therapy in symptomatic locally advanced gastric cancer. Int J Radiat Oncol Biol Phys 67:385–388*).

Normal Tissue Tolerance

OARs in radiation therapy of gastric cancer, in both adjuvant and definitive settings, include small bowel, liver, kidneys, stomach, and spinal cord (Table 12.17).

Table 12.17 Dose limitation of OARs in radiation therapy for upper abdominal malignancies

OAR	Dose limitations (Gy)	Endpoint	Rate (%)
Spinal cord	$D_{max} = 50$		0.2%
	$D_{max} = 60$	Myelopathy	6%
	$D_{max} = 69$		50%
Entire liver[a]	Mean dose: 30–32	Classical RILD	<5%
	Mean dose <42		<50%
Small intestine[b]	V45 < 195 ml (entire potential space within peritoneal cavity)	Grade ≥3 acute toxicity	<10%
Heart	Mean dose < 26 (pericardium)	Pericarditis	<15%
	V30 < 46% (pericardium)	Pericarditis	<15%
	V25 < 10% (entire heart)	Long term cardiac mortality	<1%
Bilateral entire kidneys	Mean dose < 15–18	Clinically relevant renal dysfunction	<5%
	Mean dose < 28		<50%

D_{max}: maximum dose; **RILD**: radiation-induced liver dysfunction; Vn: volume receiving n Gy

[a]Patients with no preexisting liver disease or hepatocellular carcinoma

[b]Entire potential space within the peritoneal cavity

Source: Marks LB, Yorke ED, Jackson A et al (2010) Use of normal tissue complication probability models in the clinic. Int J Radiat Oncol Biol Phys 76:S10–S19

Follow-Up

Active follow-up is recommended for gastric cancer patients after definitive or palliative treatment. Schedule and suggested examinations during follow-up are presented in Table 12.18.

Side Effects and Complications

Toxicities and complications depend on the site and volume of irradiation. Acute side effects include gastritis, fatigue, nausea, vomiting, skin reaction, bone marrow toxicity, abdominal colic, and/or diarrhea.

Long-term side effects include radiation induced kidney dysfunction, (and associated risk of renovascular hypertension), small bowel stricture/perforation, liver dysfunction, and spinal cord dysfunction.

Table 12.18 Follow-up schedule and examinations

Schedule	Frequency
First follow-up	■ 4–6 Weeks after radiation therapy
Years 0–3	■ Every 3–6 months
Years 3–5	■ Every 6 months
Years 5+	■ Annually
Examination	
History and physical	■ Complete history and physical examination
Laboratory tests	■ Full blood count and renal function if clinically indicated
Imaging studies	■ Chest X-ray (if clinically indicated) ■ CT of the abdomen and pelvis (if clinically indicated)

13 Pancreatic Cancer

Jiade J. Lu[1] and Vivek K. Mehta[2]

Key Points

- Pancreatic cancer is the ninth most commonly diagnosed cancer and the fourth leading cause of cancer deaths in industrialized countries.

- Early-stage pancreatic cancer usually has no specific symptoms. Common signs and symptoms in advanced diseases include fatigue, weight loss, jaundice, anorexia, diabetes mellitus, and abdominal/back pain.

- Accuracy of clinical diagnosis based on history and physical examination, laboratory and imaging studies (including computed tomography [CT] and endoscopic ultrasound [EUS]) approaches 90%. Tissue diagnosis in unresectable cases is needed before treatment, but its use is controversial in patients slated for surgical resection.

- Stage at diagnosis is the most important prognostic factor and predicts the resectability of a tumor. Overall survival (OS) of patients achieving R0 (complete) resection after radical surgery is ~20%. However, only 15–20% of cases are resectable at diagnosis, and long-term survival of patients with unresectable disease is less than 5%.

- Commonly observed metastatic sites include liver, peritoneum, and lung. Metastasis to bone, brain, and other organs/tissues is uncommon.

- Treatment of pancreatic cancer depends on the stage of disease. Surgery is the only curative treatment for localized diseases. T1, T2, and some T3 pancreatic cancers are resectable. Completeness of resection (R0 versus R1 versus R2 resection) is prognostically important.

- As 80% of cases develop locoregional recurrence after surgery, adjuvant chemoradiation is recommended and is the current standard in the USA. The efficacy of the gemcitabine (GEM) → 5-FU plus radiation therapy → GEM regimen has been demonstrated in the Radiation Therapy Oncology Group (RTOG) 9704 Trial.

- Radiation therapy (with concurrent chemotherapy) plays a major role in locoregionally advanced disease. An optimal treatment regimen is yet to be determined. Results from phase II trials indicated that full-dose GEM concurrent with three-dimensional conformal radiotherapy (3D-CRT) or intensity-modulated radiation therapy (IMRT) is well tolerated and efficacious, with 1-year OS rate approaching 60%.

- GEM-based chemotherapy is the mainstay treatment for metastatic pancreatic cancer. Erlotinib in concurrent with GEM further improves median survival time and OS rate.

[1] Jiade J. Lu, MD, MBA (✉)
Email: mdcljj@nus.edu.sg

[2] Vivek K. Mehta, MD
Email: vivek.mehta@swedish.org

J. J. Lu, L. W. Brady (Eds.), *Decision Making in Radiation Oncology*
DOI: 10.1007/978-3-642-13832-4_14, © Springer-Verlag Berlin Heidelberg 2011

Epidemiology and Etiology

The incidence of pancreatic cancer is 7.6 per 100,000 people worldwide. In 2010, approximately 43,140 new cases of pancreatic cancer were diagnosed in the USA. It is the ninth most commonly diagnosed malignancy and the fourth most common cause of cancer death in industrialized countries.

A number of risk factors have been identified for pancreatic cancer (Table 13.1). However, screening in high-risk patients by using imaging or laboratory tests (including carbohydrate antigen [CA] 19-9, computed tomography [CT], ultrasound, etc.) is not supported by clinical evidence.

Table 13.1 Risk factors of pancreatic cancer

Stage	Risk Factors
Patient Related Factors	**Age and Gender:** ~70% of pancreatic cancer are diagnosed after age 65; Diagnosis before age 45 is rare. Male:female ratio is 1.3:1
	Lifestyle: cigarette smoking and high calorie/fat diet are associated with 1.5-fold increase of risk, respectively; The significance of coffee drinking and alcohol consumption are not confirmed
	Family medical history: ~10% are familial (i.e., pancreatic cancer diagnosed in 2 or more first-degree relatives) with 18-fold of increase of risk as compared to those with no or 1 diagnosis of pancreatic cancer in first-degree relatives
	Past medical history: peptic ulcer surgery, abdominal irradiation, diabetes mellitus, and chronic pancreatitis
	Genetic predisposition: associated with activation of *K-ras* (oncogene), and abnormalities in *BRCA-2* (familial breast, ovarian, pancreas cancer syndrome), *TP16* (familial pancreas cancer syndrome), *LKB1/STK11* (Peutz-Jeghers polyposis GI malignancy syndrome), and HNPCC syndrome
Environmental Factors	**Industrial chemicals:** workers in manufacturing 2-naphthylamine, benzidine, gasoline derivatives have ~5-fold increased risk

HNPCC: hereditary non-polyposis colon cancer

Anatomy

The human pancreas is an elongated, retroperitoneal organ, 15–25 cm long. The pancreas has four regions: head, neck, body, and tail (Figure 13.1). It lies at the level of L1–L2, behind the stomach, and near the duodenum, kidneys, and major blood vessels including the celiac axis and superior mesenteric artery (Figure 13.2).

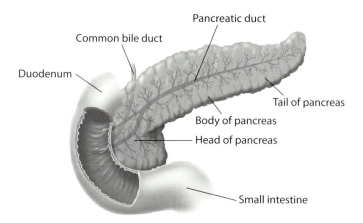

Figure 13.1 Regions of pancreas and the probability of pancreatic carcinoma according to the primary origin. (Pancreatic head tumors arise to the right of the superior mesenteric-portal vein confluence [~75%]; pancreatic body tumors arise between the superior mesenteric-portal vein confluence and left border of the aorta [~15%], and tail tumors arise between left border of the aorta and the splenic hilum [~5%], multicentric disease accounts for ~10% of cases)

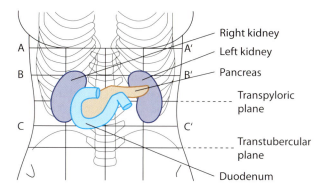

Figure 13.2 Pancreas, kidneys, and duodenum in relation to surface and anatomical markings

Pathology

Malignant neoplasms of the pancreas can arise from either endocrine (95%) or exocrine (5%) components of the pancreas. Certain types of pancreatic cancer may carry a different biological behavior: Cystadenocarcinoma, intraductal carcinoma, and solid and cystic papillary neoplasms (Hamoudi tumors) carry better prognosis; acinar cell cancer and giant cell tumors are usually aggressive.

Adenocarcinoma of ductal origin accounts for ~75% of all pancreatic cancers, thus is the focus of this chapter.

Routes of Spread

Local extension, regional (lymphatic), and distant (hematogenous) metastases are the three major routes of spread in pancreatic cancer (Table 13.2).

Table 13.2 Routes of spread in pancreatic cancer

Routes	Descriptions
Local Extension	■ Direct involvement of liver, duodenum, and major blood vessels such as celiac axis, superior mesenteric artery, porta hepatis, from tumors of pancreatic head or body is common
	■ Body/tail tumor extension to the stomach, intestine, and spleen may occur in advanced stages. Obstruction of the bile duct is relatively uncommon in body/tail tumors
	■ ~90% have perineural invasion; Peritoneal seeding is common, even in resectable disease (as high as 40%)
Regional Lymph Node Metastasis	■ Lymph node involvement is seen in ~75% of cases at diagnosis
	■ Lymphatic drainage depends on the origin of the primary disease (Figure 13.3 and Table 13.3)
	■ Lymph nodes other than direct draining regions are usually involved in advanced disease
Distant Metastasis	■ The most common route of hematogenous metastasis is through the main venous drainage of pancreas via portal vein to the liver, then lung
	■ Common sites of metastasis include liver (~ 65%), peritoneum (~ 40%) , and lung (~ 30%)
	■ Metastasis to other organs and tissues is relatively uncommon; Abdominal metastais without locoregional failure after treatment is <20%

Lymph Node Metastasis

Pattern of lymphatic spread depends on the location of the primary tumor (head versus body/tail) of the pancreas. Commonly involved lymph nodes in cancer of the pancreatic head and body/tail are illustrated in Figure 13.3 and Figure 12.3 (Chapter 12, "Gastric Cancer"). In addition, the corresponding lymph node stations are listed in Table 13.3.

Early lymph nodal involvement in multiple sites is common in pancreatic cancer, and communication between nodes on the posterior surface of the pancreatic head and nodes around the celiac artery is commonly observed.

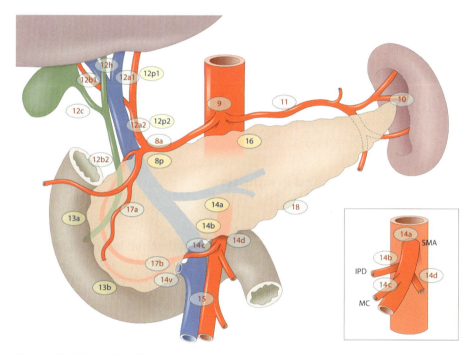

Figure 13.3 Lymph node groups commonly involved in pancreatic cancer

Table 13.3 Lymph node groups commonly involved in pancreatic cancer (Japan Pancreas Society Classification)

Classi-fication	Lymph node location	Classi-fication	Lymph node location
6	Infrapyloric	13	In hepatoduodenal ligament
7	Along left gastric artery	14	On posterior surface of pancreatic head
8	Along common hepatic artery	15	Along superior mesenteric artery
9	Around the celiac artery	16	Along middle colic artery
10	At the splenic hilum	17	Around abdominal aorta
11	Along the splenic artery	18	On anterior surface of pancreatic head
12	Along inferior margin of pancreatic body/tail		

Source: Matsuno S, Egawa S, Fukuyama S et al (2004) Pancreatic Cancer Registry in Japan: 20 years of experience. Pancreas; 28:219–230. Used with permission from Lippincott Williams & Wilkins

Diagnosis, Staging, and Prognosis

Clinical Presentation

Signs and symptoms of pancreatic cancer depend on the location of the primary tumor. Commonly observed symptoms include pain, weight loss, jaundice, anorexia, etc., and are detailed in Table 13.4. The average interval between onset of symptoms and diagnosis is approximately 3 months.

Table 13.4 Commonly observed signs and symptoms in pancreatic cancer

Origin of Tumor	Symptoms
General	■ Pain, jaundice and weight loss form the classic triad ■ Epigastric/abdominal pain (~90%) ■ Anorexia, nausea, vomiting, or other GI symptoms (~80%) which may further cause malnutrition ■ Weight loss (~90%) secondary to malnutrition, hypermetabolism, pain, or fever ■ ~20% present with new diagnosis of diabetes ■ Fatigue (full recovery after rest is uncommon) ■ Migratory thrombophlebitis (Trousseau' sign) and palpable gallbladder (Courvoisier's sign) are uncommon
Body/ Tail of Pancreas	■ Onset of symptoms usually delayed until invasion of adjacent organs/tissues occur ■ Persistent and dull pain of abdomen and/or upper back, worse in supine position ■ Invasion or occlusion of splenic vein can cause thrombosis, splenomegaly, and gastric varices ■ Jaundice is uncommon at early stage
Head of Pancreas	■ Earlier onset of symptoms as compared to tumors from pancreatic body or tail ■ ~90% have jaundice; Painless jaundice is seen in 10–30% ■ Jaundice, pain, and infection secondary to obstruction of the bile duct ■ Swelling of the pancreas, reduction in pancreatic fluid excretion, and digestive dysfunction from obstruction of pancreatic duct, which may cause malnutrition, diabetes mellitus (~15%), and weight loss

Diagnosis and Staging

Figure 13.4 illustrates a proposed diagnostic procedure of pancreatic cancer, including suggested examination and tests.

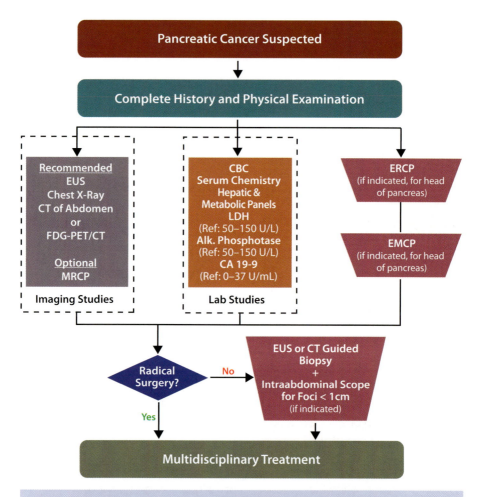

Pancreatic Cancer Suspected

Complete History and Physical Examination

Recommended
EUS
Chest X-Ray
CT of Abdomen
or
FDG-PET/CT

Optional
MRCP

Imaging Studies

CBC
Serum Chemistry
Hepatic &
Metabolic Panels
LDH
(Ref: 50–150 U/L)
Alk. Phosphotase
(Ref: 50–150 U/L)
CA 19-9
(Ref: 0–37 U/mL)

Lab Studies

ERCP
(if indicated, for head
of pancreas)

EMCP
(if indicated, for head
of pancreas)

Radical Surgery?   No

EUS or CT Guided Biopsy
+
Intraabdominal Scope
for Foci < 1cm
(if indicated)

Yes

Multidisciplinary Treatment

- EUS is more sensitive than enhanced CT for small (2-5 mm) lesions
  ERCP is used to decompress biliary tree and obtain tissue in pancreatic head cancer;
  Its use in body/tail disease is limited
- Pathological diagnosis before surgical resection is controversial, but is recommended in
  unresectable cases before treatment
- Accuracy of clinical diagnosis approaches 90%
- CA19-9 value before/after treatment are prognostically important

Figure 13.4 A proposed algorithm for diagnosis and staging of pancreatic cancer

Tumor, Node, and Metastasis Staging

Diagnosis and clinical staging depend on findings from the history and physical examination, imaging, and laboratory tests. Pathological staging depends on findings during surgical resection and pathological examination, in addition to those required in clinical staging. The 7th edition of the tumor, node, and metastasis (TNM) staging systems and groupings of the American Joint Committee on Cancer (AJCC) for pancreatic cancer is presented in Tables 13.5 and 13.6.

Table 13.5 AJCC TNM classification of carcinoma of exocrine pancreas (clinical or pathological)

Stage	Descriptions
Primary Tumor (T)	
TX	Primary tumor cannot be assessed
T0	No evidence of primary tumor
Tis	Carcinoma in situ
T1	Tumor limited to the pancreas, 2 cm or less in greatest dimension (resectable primary tumor)
T2	Tumor limited to the pancreas, more than 2 cm in greatest dimension (resectable primary tumor)
T3	Tumor extends beyond the pancreas but without involvement of the celiac axis or superior mesenteric artery (potentially resectable primary tumor)
T4	Tumor involves the celiac axis or the superior mesenteric artery (unresectable primary tumor)
Regional Lymph Nodes (N)	
NX	Regional lymph nodes cannot be assessed
N0	No regional lymph node metastasis
N1	Regional lymph node metastasis. Regional lymph node sampling from nodes around common hepatic artery, celiac artery, splenic hilum, infrapyloric nodes are required duirng Whipple's procedure in pathological staging. Ideally, ≥10 lymph nodes should be sampled during surgery.
Distant Metastasis (M)	
MX	DIstant metastasis cannot be assessed
M0	No distant metastasis
M1	Distant metastasis (including seeding of the peritoneum and positive peritoneal cytology)

Table 13.5 *(continued)*

Stage Grouping				
	T1	T2	T3	T4
N0	IA	IB	IIA	III
N1	IIB	IIB	IIB	III
M1	IV	IV	IV	IV

Source: Edge SB, Byrd DR, Compton CC et al (2010) American Joint Committee on Cancer, American Cancer Society. AJCC Cancer Staging Manual, 7th edn. Berlin Heidelberg New York, Springer-Verlag

Prognosis

The prognosis of pancreatic cancer is usually dismal, regardless of treatment. The most important prognostic factors include staging at diagnosis, a patient's performance status, and treatment modality (Table 13.6).

For patients undergoing R0 (complete) resection, pertinent prognostic factors include the number of lymph nodes involved, differentiation, size of the tumor, tumor location (head versus other), and postoperative CA 19-9.

Table 13.6 Overall survival (OS) according to treatment based on results of prospective trials published after 2005

	Localized Disease		Advanced Disease
	Radical Surgery*	CRT	Palliation Only**
1-year	>60% (DFS)	40%-63%	18%-23%
3-year	23%-31%	20%-30%	<5%
5-year	16%-23%	<5%	<5%
MS	~20 months	~11 months	~6 months

*No improvement in prognosis can be observed in patients undergo R2 resection (with gross residual disease) as compared with those without surgery.
**With gemcitabine-based chemotherapy; The medial survival of untreated cases is approximately 4 months
MS: medial survival; **DFS:** Disease-free survival; **CRT:** chemoradiation therapy

Source: Results from trials including CONKO-001, RTOG 9704, ECOG E4201, NCIC PA.3, and by Burris et al, and Hong et al detailed in the next section

Treatment

Principles and Practice

Surgery is the only curative treatment modality for pancreatic cancer; however, locoregional recurrence takes place in ~80% of cases after radical surgery. Therefore, adjuvant chemoradiation therapy is usually recommended after radical surgery (Table 13.7). The dismal outcome in patients with locoregionally advanced pancreatic cancer requires multimodality treatment.

Table 13.7 Treatment modalities used in pancreatic cancer

Type	Description
Pancreaticoduodenectomy (Whipple Surgery)	
Indications	■ The only curative treatment modality ■ For T1, T2, and some T3 disease ■ ~85% of pancreatic cancers are not resectable due to involvement of the major blood vessels or distant metastasis
Facts	■ Mortality is 1–3% in experienced hands ■ Locoregional recurrence after surgical resection approximates 80%, including 40% intra-abdominal and 60% hepatic recurrence ■ Completeness of resection (R0 vs. R1/R2) is a strong prognostic indicator
Radiation Therapy	
Indications	■ Adjuvant treatment after complete resection ■ Definitive treatment (with chemotherapy) for unresectable disease ■ Palliative treatment to primary or metastatic foci
Techniques	■ EBRT using 3D-CRT or IMRT ■ IORT may improve local control but has not shown a survival advantage, as part of either adjuvant or definitive treatment ■ Interstitial brachytherapy has no proven role in the treatment of pancreatic cancer
Chemo/Targeted Therapy	
Indications	■ Adjuvant treatment after surgery (with EBRT) ■ Adjuvant treatment with concurrent EBRT for unresectable disease ■ Mainstay treatment for palliative therapy
Medications	■ GEM is the mainstay medication for chemotherapy in pancreatic cancer. It significantly improves treatment outcome in patients with advanced pancreatic cancer, as compared to 5-FU ■ Erlotinib used with concurrent GEM further improves median survival and overall survival

EBRT: external beam radiation therapy; **IORT:** intra-operative radiation therapy; **GEM:** gemcitabine

A proposed treatment algorithm based on the best available clinical evidence is presented in Figure 13.5.

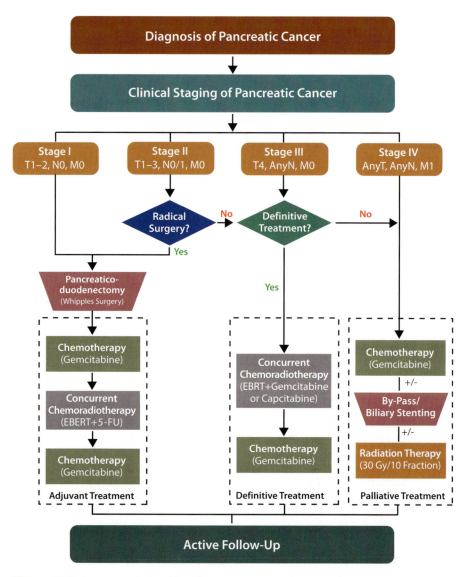

Figure 13.5 A proposed algorithm for management of pancreatic cancer

Treatment of Resectable Pancreatic Cancer (T1-3, N0-1, and M0)

Surgery is the mainstay curative treatment modality, and T1, T2, and some of T3 diseases are resectable. However, locoregional recurrence occurs in ~80% of cases after surgery including R0 resection; thus, adjuvant therapy is usually necessary.

Adjuvant Treatment

Clinical evidence for adjuvant therapy in resectable pancreatic cancer is illustrated and presented in Figure 13.6 and Table 13.8.

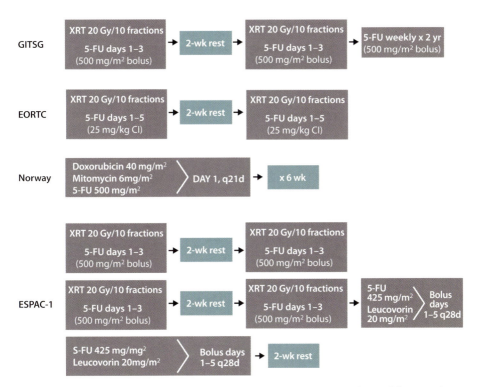

Figure 13.6 Key adjuvant therapy trials in pancreatic cancer. Designs of four randomized landmark trials evaluating adjuvant therapy in pancreatic cancer

Source: Berlin JD (2007) Adjuvant therapy for pancreatic cancer: To treat or not to treat? Oncology 21[6]: 712-718. Used with permission.

Table 13.8 Adjuvant treatment strategies for resectable pancreatic cancer and supporting clinical evidence

Randomized trial	Description
GITSG 9173[a]	■ Randomized 42 cases of pancreatic cancer after radical resection (R0) to observation or adjuvant CRT ■ Adjuvant-CRT regimen used RT (40 Gy in 2 split courses spaced 2 weeks apart) plus 5-FU (500 mg/m^2 on first and last 3 days of RT) → 5-FU × 2 years ■ MS (20 versus 11 months; $p = 0.035$); 2-year OS (42 versus 18%), and 5-year OS (19 versus 5%) favored adjuvant-CRT arm ■ GITSG continued the adjuvant-CRT arm in 30 more patients after R0 resection, and confirmed the benefit of adjuvant CRT with a 2-year OS of 46%
EORTC 40891[b]	■ Randomized 114 cases of pancreatic head cancer, except for T3 disease after radical resection to adjuvant CRT or observation ■ Used GITSG regimen without adjuvant 5-FU after CRT (~20% failed to receive planned adjuvant CRT) ■ ~20% of cases did not receive adjuvant CRT as planned ■ For pancreatic head cancer, MS (17.1 versus 12.6 months), 2-year OS (34 versus 26%), and 5-year OS (20 versus 10%) favored adjuvant-CRT arm, but not with statistical significance
ESPAC-1[c]	■ Randomized trial (2 × 2 design) intended to study 2-year OS in observation, adjuvant chemotherapy, adjuvant CRT, and adjuvant CRT → chemotherapy after R0 surgery ■ Reported 289 cases of pancreatic cancer after resection (R0 not required in accrual) ■ Intended primary end point never reported ■ 2- and 5-year OS rates were 40 and 21% after chemotherapy or adjuvant CRT → chemotherapy, versus 30 and 8% after observation or adjuvant CRT ■ 5-year OS for control, adjuvant RT, adjuvant CRT, and adjuvant CRT → chemotherapy were 10.7, 7.3, 29, and 13.2%, respectively ■ Criticized for its design and accrual process, as well as various doses of RT, although 40 Gy in split courses required by the protocol
RTOG 9704[d]	■ Randomized 451 cases of pancreatic cancer after complete gross total resection (R0 or R1) to 3 and 12 weeks of GEM versus 5-FU treatment before and after adjuvant CRT, respectively ■ Same adjuvant CRT regimen (50.4 Gy/1.8 Gy/day) for both arms ■ Study design and regimens are detailed in Figure 13.7 ■ MS (20.5 versus 16.9 months), 3-year OS (31 versus 22%) favored GEM arm ($p = 0.09$) ■ Trend of survival benefits were only demonstrated in pancreatic head tumors ($n = 388$)

Table 13.8 *(continued)*

Randomized trial	Description
CONKO-001[e]	■ Randomized 368 cases of pancreatic cancer after surgery to GEM treatment versus observation after R0 or R1 resection ■ Same adjuvant regimen (1,000 mg/m^2, day[s] 1, 8, 15 of every 4-week cycle) for 6 months ■ Median DFS time were 13.4 versus 6.9 months ($p < 0.001$); median OS were 22.1 versus 20.2 months ($p = 0.005$) ■ 3- and 5-year DFS were 23.5 versus 8.5%, and 16 versus 6.5%; 3- and 5-year OS were 36.5 versus 19.5%, and 21 versus 9%. Both favored GEM arm

GEM: gemcitabine; **OS:** overall survival; **GITSG:** Gastrointestinal Tumor Study Group; **EORTC:** European Organization for Research and Treatment of Cancer; **ESPAC:** European Study Group for Pancreatic Cancer; **RT:** radiation therapy; **CRT:** chemoradiation therapy

[a] *Sources: Kalser MH, Ellenberg SS. (1985) Pancreatic cancer. Adjuvant combined radiation and chemotherapy following curative resection. Arch Surg; 120:899-903. Gastrointestinal Tumor Study Group. (1987) Further evidence of effective adjuvant combined radiation and chemotherapy following curative resection of pancreatic cancer. Cancer; 59:2006–2010*

[b] *Source: Klinkenbijl JH, Jeekel J, Sahmoud T et al (1999) Adjuvant radiotherapy and 5-fluorouracil after curative resection of cancer of the pancreas and periampullary region: phase III trial of the EORTC gastrointestinal tract cancer cooperative group. Ann Surg; 230:76–84*

[c] *Source: Neoptolemos JP, Stocken DD, Friess H et al (2004) A randomized trial of chemoradiotherapy and chemotherapy after resection of pancreatic cancer. N Engl J Med, 350:1200–1210*

[d] *Source: Regine WF, Winter KA, Abrams RA et al (2008) Fluorouracil vs gemcitabine chemotherapy before and after fluorouracil-based chemoradiation following resection of pancreatic adenocarcinoma: a randomized controlled trial. JAMA; 299:1019–1026*

[e] *Source: Neuhaus P, Riess H, Post S et al (2008) CONKO-001: final results of the randomized, prospective, multicenter phase III trial of adjuvant chemotherapy with gemcitabine versus observation in patients with resected pancreatic cancer. J Clin Oncol; 26[Suppl]:Abstract 4504*

Figure 13.7 details Radiation Therapy Oncology Group (RTOG) 9704 Trial protocols and results. A proposed treatment algorithm for resectable pancreatic cancer based on RTOG 9704 protocol is detailed in Figure 13.8.

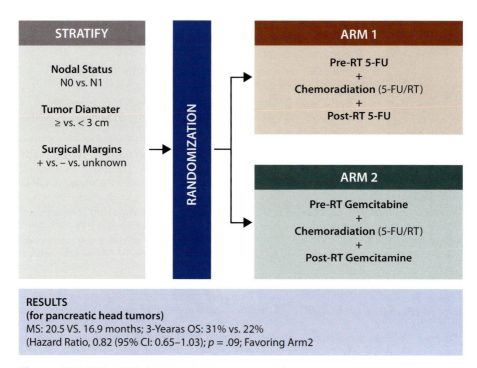

Figure 13.7 RTOG 9704 protocol schema and results

Neoadjuvant Treatment

Although neoadjuvant chemotherapy or chemoradiation may benefit marginally resectable pancreatic cancer, its use in resectable disease has not demonstrated survival benefits in prospective trials.

Adjuvant Treatment

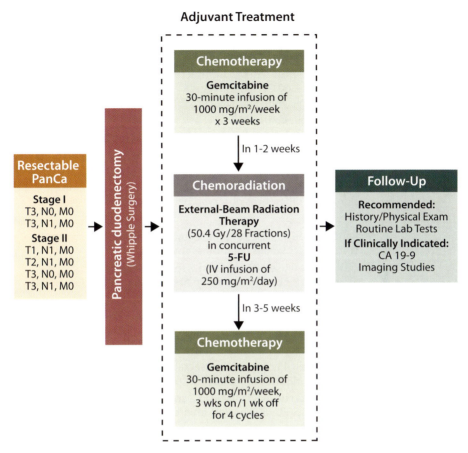

Figure 13.8 A proposed treatment algorithm for adjuvant chemoradiation therapy for resectable pancreatic cancer, based on RTOG 9704 protocol

Treatment of Nonmetastatic but Unresectable Pancreatic Cancer (T4, N0-1, and M0)

Most patients with locoregionally advanced pancreatic cancer are unresectable. The efficacy of combined chemoradiation therapy has been demonstrated repeatedly in randomized trials (Tables 13.9 and 13.10, Figure 13.9), and is the mainstay treatment strategy. By-pass surgery and stenting is important and commonly used in patients with bile duct obstruction to obtain relief of acute symptoms.

Table 13.9 Clinical evidence for the treatment of unresectable locoregionally advanced pancreatic cancer: prospective trials based on 5-FU chemotherapy

Trial	Description
GITSG 9273[a]	■ Randomized 194 cases of unresectable pancreatic cancer to compare RT (60 Gy) alone versus RT (60 Gy or 40 Gy) plus 5-FU in unresectable pancreatic cancer ■ RT only regimen used 60 Gy ■ 2 CRT arms used 5-FU plus either 60 or 40 RT (split course) ■ MS (40.3 versus 42.3 versus 20.9 weeks) for RT (40 Gy) plus 5-FU, RT (60 Gy) plus 5-FU, and RT (60 Gy) only, respectively ■ 1-year OS (40 versus 10%) favored CRT arms over RT alone. No significant differences observed between 60 Gy versus 40 Gy in CRT arms
ECOG[b]	■ Randomized 91 cases of unresectable pancreatic cancer to compare CRT versus chemotherapy alone ■ CRT regimen used RT (40 Gy in 2 split courses spaced 2 weeks apart) plus 5-FU (600 mg/m^2 on first 3 days of RT cycle) → 5-FU at 600 mg/m^2/week ■ Chemotherapy alone arm used 5-FU at 600 mg/m^2/week ■ MS of 8.2 versus 8.3 months; there was no difference between 2 arms
GITSG 9283[c]	■ Randomized 43 cases of unresectable pancreatic cancer to compare SMF chemotherapy versus RT plus 5-FU ■ CRT regimen used RT (40 Gy in 2 split courses spaced 2 weeks apart) plus 5-FU (500 mg/m^2 on first and last 3 days of RT) → 5-FU × 2 years ■ Chemotherapy regimen used SMF ■ MS (42 versus 32 weeks) and 1-year OS (41 versus 19%) favored CRT arm ($p < 0.02$)

SMF: streptozocin, mitomycin, and 5-FU; **ECOG:** Eastern Cooperative Oncology Group; **GITSG:** Gastrointestinal Tumor Study Group

[a] *Source: Moertel CG, Frytak S, Hahn RG et al (1981) Therapy of locally unresectable pancreatic carcinoma: a randomized comparison of high dose [6,000 rads] radiation alone, moderate dose radiation [4,000 rads + 5-FU], and high dose radiation + 5-FU: the GITSG. Cancer; 48:1705–1710*
[b] *Source: Klaassen DJ, MacIntyre JM, Catton GE et al (1985) Treatment of locally unresectable cancer of the stomach and pancreas: a randomized comparison of 5-FU alone with radiation plus concurrent and maintenance 5-FU–an ECOG study. J Clin Oncol; 3:373–378*
[c] *Source: Gastrointestinal Tumor Study Group. (1988) Treatment of locally unresectable carcinoma of the pancreas: comparison of combined-modality therapy [chemotherapy plus radiotherapy] to chemotherapy alone. J Natl Cancer Inst; 80:751–755*

Table 13.10 Clinical evidence for the treatment of unresectable locoregionally advanced pancreatic cancer: prospective trials based on GEM chemotherapy

Trial	Description
ECOG E4201[a] (Figure 13.9)	■ Randomized trial studied GEM versus GEM plus RT ■ 69 of 316 planned cases of LAPC (closed early due to slow accrual) ■ CRT regimen used RT (50.4 Gy/1.8 Gy/day) plus GEM (600 mg/m^2/week for 6 cycles) followed by GEM (1,000 mg/m^2, day[s] 1, 8, 15 of every 4-week cycle) for 5 cycles ■ Chemotherapy alone arm used GEM (1,000 mg/m^2/week every 3 of 4-week cycle) × 7 cycles ■ MS (11 versus 9.2 months; $p = 0.044$) favored GEM plus RT
FFCD/SFRO 2000-01[b]	■ Randomized 119 cases of LAPC to CRT group (60 Gy, 2 Gy per fraction; concomitant 5-FU infusion, 300 mg/m^2/day, day[s] 1–5 for 6 weeks; cisplatin, 20 mg/m^2/day, day[s] 1–5 during weeks 1 and 5) or GEM (1,000 mg/m^2/week × 7 weeks) group ■ Maintenance GEM (1,000 mg/m^2/week, 3/4 weeks) was given in both arms until disease progression or toxicity ■ MS (8.6 versus 13 months; $p = 0.03$) and 1-year OS (32% versus 53%) favored GEM only arm
Li et al (Taiwan)[c]	■ Randomized 34 cases of LAPC to GEM (600 mg/m^2/week for 6 weeks) or 5-FU (500 mg/m^2/day for 3 days every 2 weeks for 6 weeks) with concurrent 3D-CRT (50.4-61.2 Gy at 1.8 Gy/day) ■ All received GEM (1,000 mg/m^2 weekly, 3/4 weeks) after CRT ■ Complete plus partial response rates (50 versus 13%; $p = 0.005$), MS (14.5 versus 6.7 months; $p = 0.027$) and median time to progresssion (7.1 versus 2.7 months; $p = 0.019$) favored GEM arm ■ Grades 3 or 4 adverse effects were not significantly different between 2 arms
NCCTG N9942[d]	■ Multicenter phase II trial with 47 cases of nonmetastatic unresectable pancreatic cancer ■ Weekly low dose GEM (30 mg/m^2 twice a week) and cisplatin (10 mg/m^2 in 1st 3 weeks) were used with concurrent RT ■ 3D-CRT (50.4 Gy to tumor bed) was used ■ All patients received GEM (1,000 mg/m^2/week, 3/4 weeks) × 3 cycles ■ MS and 1-year OS were 10.2 months and 40%, respectively. No significant improvement was detected, compared with historical data ▶

Table 13.10 (continued)

Trial	Description
Hong et al (Korea)[e]	■ Phase II trial with 41 cases of nonmetastatic unresectable pancreatic cancer ■ Weekly standard dose of GEM (1,000 mg/m^2/week × 5 weeks) and 2 doses of cisplatin (70 mg/m^2 on days 1 and 29) and were used with concurrent RT ■ 3D-CRT (45 Gy in 25 daily fractions) was used ■ MS, 1- and 2-year OS rates were 16.7 months, 63.3 and 27.9%, respectively
Small et al (US multi-center)[f]	■ Multicenter phase II trial with 39 cases of nonmetastatic pancreatic cancer of various stages ■ Standard dose of GEM (1,000 mg/m^2/week × 2 followed by 1-week break in cycles 1 and 3 [21-day cycles]; 1,000 mg/m^2/week × 3 weeks followed by 1-week break in cycle 2 [28-day cycle]) was used with concurrent 3D-CRT ■ 3D-CRT (36 Gy in 3 weeks, i.e., 2.4 Gy/day × 15 days) was used with a BED of 44 Gy ■ 1-year OS rates were 94, 76, and 47% for patients after complete resection, marginally resectable, and unresectable cases
Chang et al (Stanford)[g]	■ Single institutional phase II trial of 77 patients (including 19% with metastasis and 8% with local recurrence) with unresectable pancreatic cancer treated with SBRT ■ SBRT used 25 Gy in 1 fraction (21% of cases also received EBRT to 45–54 Gy) ■ 96% of cases received GEM-based chemotherapy (various regimens) ■ FFLP and local recurrence rates at 6 and 12 months were 91 versus 84%, and 5 versus 5%, respectively ■ The PFS and OS rates at 6 and 12 months were 26 versus 9%, and 56 versus 21%, respectively ■ Toxicity (≥2) were 11 and 25% at 6 and 12 months, respectively

LAPC: locally advanced pancreatic cancer, **PFS:** progression-free survival, **NCCTG:** North Central Cancer Treatment Group, **BED:** biologic effective dose, **SBRT:** stereotactic body radiotherapy **FFLP:** freedom from local progression

[a] Source: Loehrer PJ, Powell ME, Cardenes HR et al (2008) A randomized phase II study of gemcitabine in combination with radiation therapy versus gemcitabine alone in patients with localized, unresectable pancreatic cancer: E4201. J Clin Oncol; 26:Abstract 4506

[b] Source: Chauffert B, Mornex F, Bonnetain F et al (2008) Phase III trial comparing intensive induction chemoradiotherapy [60 Gy, infusional 5-FU and intermittent cisplatin] followed by maintenance GEM with GEM alone for locally advanced unresectable pancreatic cancer. Definitive results of the 2000-01 FFCD/SFRO study. Ann Oncol; 19:1592–1599

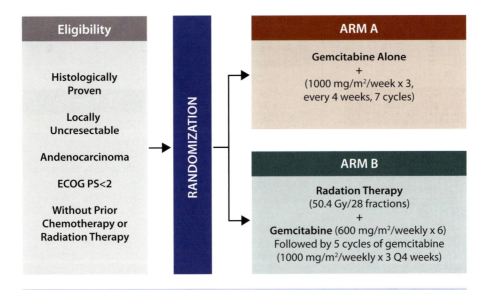

Figure 13.9 ECOG E4201 schema and results

Table 13.10 *(continued)*

[c] *Source: Li CP, Chao Y, Chi KH et al (2003) Concurrent chemoradiotherapy treatment of locally advanced pancreatic cancer: GEM versus 5-FU, a randomized controlled study. Int J Radiat Oncol Biol Phys; 57:98–104*

[d] *Source: Haddock MG, Swaminathan R, Foster NR et al (2007) GEM, cisplatin, and radiotherapy for patients with locally advanced pancreatic adenocarcinoma: results of the NCCTG Phase II Study N9942. J Clin Oncol; 25:2567–2572*

[e] *Source: Hong SP, Park JY, Jeon TJ et al (2008) Weekly full-dose gemcitabine and single-dose cisplatin with concurrent radiotherapy in patients with locally advanced pancreatic cancer. Br J Cancer; 98:881–887*

[f] *Source: Small W Jr, Berlin J, Freedman GM et al (2008) Full-dose GEM with concurrent radiation therapy in patients with non-metastatic pancreatic cancer: a multicenter phase II trial. J Clin Oncol; 26:942–947*

[g] *Source: Chang DT, Schellenberg D, Shen J et al (2009) Stereotactic radiotherapy for unresectable adenocarcinoma of the pancreas. Cancer; 115:468–472*

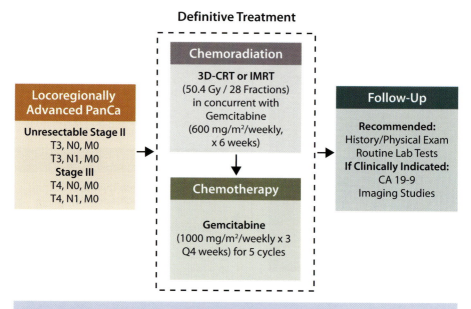

Figure 13.10 A proposed treatment for definitive treatment of unresectable pancreatic cancer by using GEM-based chemotherapy

A proposed treatment algorithm for nonmetastatic and unresectable pancreatic cancer, based on the ECOG E4201 Trial, is detailed in Figure 13.10.

If concurrent gemcitabine is contraindicated, intolerable, or patients decline gemcitabine, capecitabine with concurrent radiation therapy can be recommended (Figure 13.11).

Definitive Treatment

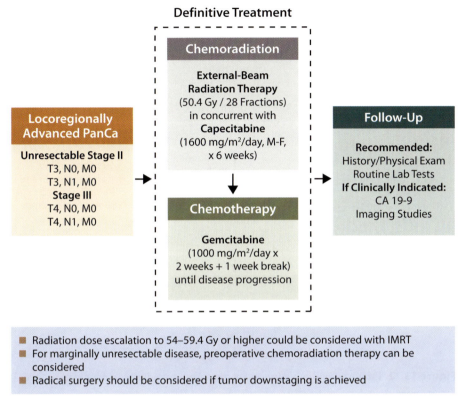

Figure 13.11 A proposed treatment algorithm for definitive treatment of unresectable pancreatic cancer by using capecitabine-based chemotherapy

Source: Ben-Josef E, Shields AF, Vaishampayan U et al (2004) IMRT and concurrent capecitabine for pancreatic cancer. Int J Radiat Oncol Biol Phys 59: 454-459.

Advanced Pancreatic Cancer (T1-4, N0-1, and M1)

Advanced pancreatic cancers include metastatic or locoregionally advanced disease in which definitive treatment is not feasible. A proposed algorithm for palliation are detailed in Figure 13.12.

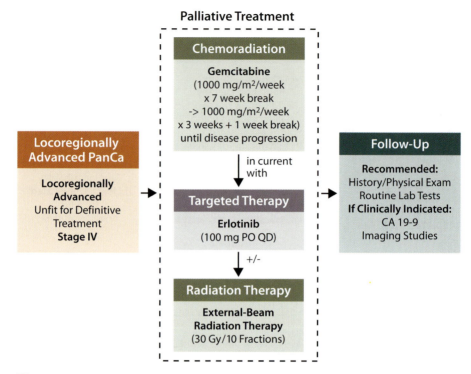

Figure 13.12 Proposed palliative treatment algorithm for advanced pancreatic cancer

Table 13.11 Treatment fields used in the RTOG 9704 protocol for adjuvant radiotherapy

Field	Borders
AP/PA (head of pancreas)	■ Superior: top of T11 ■ Inferior: bottom of L3 ■ Right: C-loop of duodenum or 2–3 cm right of the tumor ■ Left: 2–3 cm left of the tumor
AP/PA (body/tail of pancreas)	■ Superior: top of T11 ■ Inferior: bottom of L3 ■ Right: 2–3 cm right of the tumor ■ Left: 2–3 cm right of the tumor
Lateral	■ Superior/inferior: as AP/PA fields ■ Anterior: 2–3 cm anterior to the tumor ■ Posterior: half of the vertebral body (to avoid spinal cord)
■ All fields should be irradiated on daily basis ■ Irradiation to the entire pancreas is unnecessary ■ Because the lateral fields encompass most of the liver and bilateral kidneys, the AP/PA versus lateral field weighting should be roughly 2:1	

Radiation Therapy Techniques

Radiation Therapy for Adjuvant Therapy

Simulation and Field Arrangements

Radiation fields should encompass the tumor bed and regional lymph nodal areas for locoregional control.

A CT scan (3- to 5-mm cut) with oral contrast should be performed from the top of the diaphragm to the bottom of L4. Organs at risk (OARs; Table 12.17) should be delineated. Field setup is illustrated in Figure 13.13 and Table 13.11, and should consider surgical clips and pre- and postsurgical CT scans of the abdomen.

There is no benefit to using 5 or 6 fields, as compared with a four-field (anterior–posterior and posterior–anterior [AP/PA] and opposed lateral) setting, if 18-MV x-rays are used *(Source: van der Geld YG, van Triest B, Verbakel WF et al (2008) Evaluation of four-dimensional computed tomography-based intensity-modulated and respiratory-gated radiotherapy techniques for pancreatic carcinoma. Int J Radiat Oncol Biol Phys 72:1215–1220).*

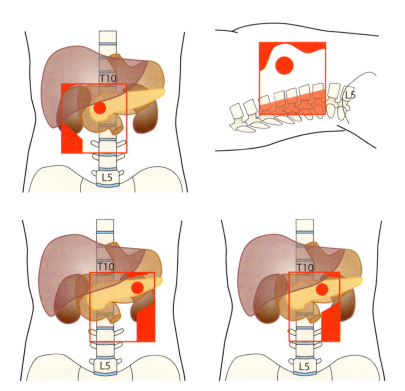

Figure 13.13 Radiation fields (AP/PA and lateral) for adjuvant treatment of carcinoma of the head of the pancreas

Dose and Treatment Delivery

Conventional fractionation to a total dose of 45 Gy–50.4 Gy is recommended after R0 resection, using high-energy ($\geq$10 MVX) photon therapy. A boost to 54 Gy to residual tumor with a 2-cm-margin (surgical clips) is recommended after R1 or R2 resection.

Intensity-Modulated Radiation Therapy in an Adjuvant Setting

The benefit of intensity-modulated radiation therapy (IMRT) and the delineation of clinical target volume (CTV) in adjuvant treatment have not been fully addressed. If used, tumor bed and subclinical target volumes, including lymphatic draining regions (depends on the site of the primary tumor [head versus body/tail], as described in Figure 13.3), should be delineated as CTV *(Sun W, Leong CN, Zhang Z et al (2010) Proposing the lymphatic target volume for elective radiation therapy for pancreatic cancer: a pooled analysis of clinical evidence. Radiat Oncol 5: 28).*

Radiation Therapy for Unresectable Disease

Simulation and Target Volume Delineation

High-dose irradiation of subclinical disease in nonresected pancreatic cancer has no clinical relevance if control of gross disease cannot be achieved. In addition, most of the first-echelon nodes can be encompassed within the margin of gross disease. Thus, it is reasonable to irradiate gross disease without regional lymph nodes in a definitive setting.

A CT scan (3- to 5-mm cut) should be performed with oral and intravenous (i.v.) contrast from the top of the diaphragm to the bottom of L4. OARs should be delineated.

Compared with conventional technique, three-dimensional conformal radiotherapy (3D-CRT) or IMRT directed to the gross tumor volume (GTV) with a margin can reduce the dose to the OARs, thereby improving the therapeutic ratio and facilitating dose escalation *(Source: Taremi M, Ringash J, Dawson LA (2007) Upper abdominal malignancies: intensity-modulated radiation therapy. Front Radiat Ther Oncol 40:272–288).*

Definitions of GTV, CTV, and planning target volume (PTV) in 3D-CRT and IMRT are as follows:
- GTV: gross tumor on imaging studies
- CTV: GTV plus 0.5 cm
- PTV: CTV plus 0.5–1 cm, or internal target volume (ITV) plus 0.5 cm

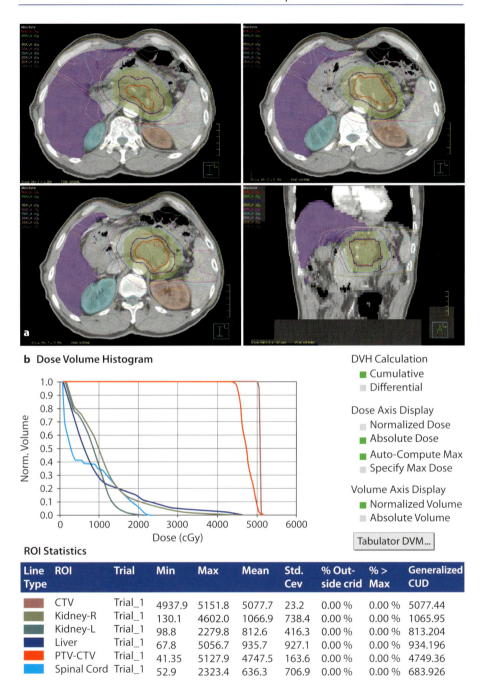

b Dose Volume Histogram

DVH Calculation
- Cumulative
- Differential

Dose Axis Display
- Normalized Dose
- Absolute Dose
- Auto-Compute Max
- Specify Max Dose

Volume Axis Display
- Normalized Volume
- Absolute Volume

Tabulator DVM...

ROI Statistics

Line Type	ROI	Trial	Min	Max	Mean	Std. Cev	% Outside crid	% > Max	Generalized CUD
	CTV	Trial_1	4937.9	5151.8	5077.7	23.2	0.00 %	0.00 %	5077.44
	Kidney-R	Trial_1	130.1	4602.0	1066.9	738.4	0.00 %	0.00 %	1065.95
	Kidney-L	Trial_1	98.8	2279.8	812.6	416.3	0.00 %	0.00 %	813.204
	Liver	Trial_1	67.8	5056.7	935.7	927.1	0.00 %	0.00 %	934.196
	PTV-CTV	Trial_1	41.35	5127.9	4747.5	163.6	0.00 %	0.00 %	4749.36
	Spinal Cord	Trial_1	52.9	2323.4	636.3	706.9	0.00 %	0.00 %	683.926

Figure 13.14 a, b a IMRT for a patient with pancreatic cancer in the head of the pancreas. The 7 coplanar fields used were 128°, 96°, 64°, 32°, 0°, 328°, and 296° to avoid excessive dose to liver, kidneys, and small intestine. Prescribed dose to the PTV was 50.4 Gy. *Red line* GTV, *blue line* PTV. **b** Dose volume histogram (*DVH*) of the same plan

Dose and Treatment Delivery

A total dose of 50.4 Gy–59.4 Gy in 30–33 fractions with seven to nine co-planar fields can be used according to the shape of the PTV (Figure 13.14).

Normal Tissue Tolerance

OARs in radiation therapy for pancreatic cancer, in both adjuvant and definitive settings, include small bowel, liver, kidneys, and spinal cord (Dose limitations of OARs in radiation therapy for upper abdominal malignancies are detailed in Table 12.17).

Follow-Up

The dismal prognosis of pancreatic cancer requires close follow-up after completion of treatment. Schedule and suggested examinations during follow-up are presented in Table 13.12.

Common radiation-induced adverse effects include nausea, vomiting, abdominal discomfort/pain, radiation-induced liver disease, etc. Due to the poor prognosis, reports on long-term complications after pancreatic cancer treatment are rare.

Table 13.12 Follow-up schedule and examinations

Schedule	Frequency
First follow-up	■ 4–6 weeks after radiation therapy
Year 0–1	■ Every 3–4 months
Years 2–5	■ Every 6 months
Year 5+	■ Annually
Examinations	
History and physical	■ Complete history and physical examination
Laboratory tests	■ Complete blood count and serum chemistry ■ Liver and renal function tests ■ CA 19-9 (if clinically indicated)
Imaging studies	■ Chest X-ray (if clinically indicated) ■ CT of the abdomen and pelvis (if clinically indicated)

Source: Mehta VK. Pancreatic Cancer. In: Lu JJ, Brady LW. Radiation oncology: an evidence-based approach. Springer, Berlin Heidelberg New York 2008

14

Hepatocellular Carcinoma

Sarah E. Hoffe[1]

Key Points

- Hepatocellular carcinoma (HCC) is the 5th most common cancer worldwide, with the third highest incidence of cancer-related death. In Asia and Africa, chronic hepatitis B viral infection is the leading cause of HCC, while hepatitis C viral infection predominates in Europe, Japan, and North America.

- Common sites of metastasis include other parts of the liver, abdominal lymph nodes, peritoneum, bone, and lung.

- Approximately 60–80% of patients with HCC have underlying cirrhosis of the liver. High-risk patients are screened with liver ultrasound and alpha-fetoprotein (AFP) levels for 6–12 months.

- HCC patients are often asymptomatic; when symptoms develop, they often include upper abdominal pain, weight loss, malaise, jaundice, and anorexia.

- Imaging studies can often confirm the diagnosis of HCC, without a tissue biopsy, because these lesions are hypervascular and will demonstrate a classic pattern with intense uptake on arterial phase scanning, followed by contrast washout in the delayed venous phase.

- A nodule in the 1- to 2-cm range can meet criteria for HCC if it demonstrates classic arterial enhancement on two imaging modalities such as triphasic computed tomography/magnetic resonance imaging (CT/MRI). If a lesion >2 cm shows classic enhancement on one modality, that is sufficient. A tissue biopsy should be considered if there are no classic imaging findings.

- At least 12 staging systems exist for HCC (e.g., tumor, node, metastasis [TNM], Okuda, Barcelona).

- Surgical resection or transplantation offers the best chance of cure for HCC, but most patients are not eligible. Transplant series show 4-year recurrence-free survival rates in the range of 92%; resection series show 5-year survival rates up to 70%, but most patients develop recurrence.

- Strategies for bridge to transplant or palliation include embolization (chemo-/radio-/or bland), radiation therapy (3D-conformal radiation including image-guided intensity-modulated radiation therapy, stereotactic body radiosurgery, or protons/charged particles) and targeted therapies (sorafenib).

[1] Sarah E. Hoffe, MD
E-Mail: sarah.hoffe@moffitt.org

J. J. Lu, L. W. Brady (Eds.), *Decision Making in Radiation Oncology*
DOI: 10.1007/978-3-642-13832-4_15, © Springer-Verlag Berlin Heidelberg 2011

Epidemiology and Etiology

Hepatocellular carcinoma (HCC) is the 5th most commonly diagnosed cancer worldwide, with the 3rd highest incidence for cancer-related death. The incidence of HCC is rising in the USA, and in 2009, approximately 22,620 new cases of HCC were diagnosed; 18,160 patients died from the disease.

A number of risk factors have been identified for HCC (Table 14.1). Screening high-risk patients consists of liver ultrasound and serum alpha-fetoprotein (AFP) testing every 6–12 months according to the American Association for the Study of Liver Disease (AASLD) guidelines.

Table 14.1 Risk factors of hepatocellular cancer

Factor	Description
Patient Related	**Age and gender:** average age at diagnosis is 64 years in the USA; younger age at diagnosis is more common in patients in Africa and Southeast Asia, due to hepatitis B virus carriage. HCC is more common in men than in women
	Lifestyle: excessive alcohol intake, obesity, long-term anabolic steroid use, and behaviors increasing infection with hepatitis B and C. Increasing cases are being reported with non-alcoholic steatohepatitis (*NASH*) in the setting of metabolic syndrome or diabetes mellitus
	Family medical history: hereditary hemochromatosis is associated to HCC
	Past medical history: porphyria cutanea tarda, alpha1-antitrypsin deficiency, Wilson's disease, autoimmune hepatitis, primary biliary cirrhosis, hepatitis B virus infection, hepatitis C virus infection, obesity, diabetes mellitus, tyrosinemia
	Genetic predisposition: genetic predisposition: inherited metabolic diseases that increase the risk of cirrhosis such as hemochromatosis
Environmental	**Environment exposures:** aflatoxin (a natural product of the *Aspergillus* fungus) commonly found in grains is a significant causative agent of HCC. Exposure to vinyl chloride and thorium dioxide is related. Chronic exposure to arsenic such as found in wells can increase the risk of primary liver cancer

Anatomy

The human liver is the largest internal organ in the body, and weighs approximately 3 pounds. A non-cirrhotic liver can function even if 75% of it is removed, due to its capacity for regeneration.

Surgeons and anatomists have established subdivisions of the liver, and a number of hepatic terminologies were proposed. The Scientific Committee of the International Hepato-Pancreato-Biliary Association formulated a new system, the Brisbane 2000 Terminology of Liver Anatomy and Resections, and has become accepted as the surgical gold standard (Figure 14.1). The liver is divided into three functional livers: the right, the left, and the caudate, in the Brisbane system (Table 14.2).

Anatomical Term	Couinaud segments referred to	Term for surgical resection	Diagram (pertinent area is shaded)
Right Hemiliver or Right Liver	Sg 5-8 (+/- Sg1)	Right Hepatectomy or Right Hemihepatectomy (stipulate +/- segment 1)	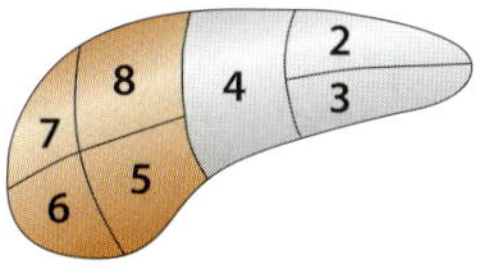
Left Hemiliver or Left Liver	Sg 2-4 (+/- Sg1)	Left Hepatectomy or Left Hemihepatectomy (stipulate +/- segment 1)	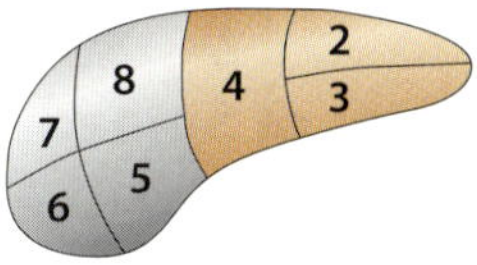

Border or watershed: The border or watershed of the first order division which separates the two hemilivers is a plane which intersects the gallbladder fossa and the fossa for the IVC and is called the midplane of the liver.

Figure 14.1 Brisbane 2000 System of liver anatomy and resections.

Source: Strasberg SM (2005) Nomenclature of hepatic anatomy and resections: a review of the Brisbane 2000 system. J Hepatobiliary Pancreat Surg 12:351–355. Used with permission from Springer, Berlin Heidelberg New York

Table 14.2 Liver anatomy as defined by the Brisbane System

Section	Description
Right hemiliver	■ Further divided into 2 sections ■ Each of which contains 2 segments based on blood supply and bile drainage
Left hemiliver	■ Further divided into 2 sections as well ■ The left medial section contains segment 4A and 4B, known as the *quadrate lobe* ■ The left lateral section contains segments 2 and 3
Caudate hemiliver (segment 1)	■ Is considered separately because of its blood supply and venous/biliary drainage

Pathology

Primary malignant neoplasms of the hepatocytes rather than biliary ductal epithelial cells are termed HCC. They have also been known as *liver cell carcinomas* or *hepatomas.*

Histologically, these malignancies are predominantly adenocarcinomas. Rarely, some of these cancers may have characteristics of both primary liver and biliary ductal cells and can be termed *hepatic cholangiocarcinomas.* Grossly, these cancers can appear unifocal, multifocal, or diffusely infiltrative. Under the microscope, they can range from well differentiated to highly anaplastic. One variant of the well- to moderately well-differentiated HCC is called the *clear cell type* because of the high content of glycogen in the cell's cytoplasm. A variant with a more favorable prognosis is the *fibrolamellar type,* which is usually seen in the absence of cirrhosis. Poorly differentiated types can be seen as pleomorphic giant cells or as small completely undifferentiated cells.

Routes of Spread

HCC have a strong tendency to invade vascular channels. They can involve major vessels by local extension, which can be assessed either radiographically or pathologically. Major vascular invasion indicates that the tumor has invaded branches of the main portal vein (right or left) or one or more of the three hepatic veins (right, middle, or left).

HCC can also disseminate within the liver via the portal veins. Regional node involvement is uncommon in HCC until later in the course of disease. Distant (hematogenous) metastases are less frequent until later in the course of disease (Table 14.3).

Table 14.3 Routes of spread in HCC

Route	Characteristics
Local extension	■ Strong propensity for vascular invasion ■ Cause invasion of major vessels such as the inferior vena cava and portal vein ■ Can directly invade other adjacent organs, such as the diaphragm, adrenal gland, or intestine
Regional lymph node metastasis	■ The regional nodes include hilar, hepatoduodenal ligament nodes, inferior phrenic, and caval nodes ■ Incidence approximates 10–15% in early stages. In the fibrolamellar variant of HCC, rates of regional lymph node involvement are higher ■ Late in the course of disease, lymph node involvement to distant abdominal sites can occur ■ Inferior phrenic nodes were previously classified as distant, but now regional ■ In the 7th edition of the AJCC staging manual, patients with positive nodes are classified as having stage IV disease because they have the same prognosis as patients with distant metastasis
Distant metastasis	■ The main mechanism is dissemination via the portal veins (intrahepatic) and hepatic veins ■ With invasion through the liver capsule or rupture, there can be peritoneal metastasis ■ Hematogenous metastases are less frequent with HCC than with cholangiocarcinoma ■ Late in the disease course, blood borne metastases often occur to the lungs and bone

Diagnosis, Staging, and Prognosis

Clinical Presentation

Most patients with HCC are asymptomatic until advanced stages of disease (Table 14.4). In early stages of HCC, the patients may have no clinical symptoms but may have an elevated AFP or a nodule seen on ultrasound. In advanced stages, patients may develop jaundice, weight loss, anorexia, malaise, and abdominal pain.

Table 14.4 Commonly observed signs and symptoms in HCC

Category	Presentation
Symptoms	■ Jaundice ■ Malaise ■ Anorexia ■ Abdominal pain or discomfort ■ Weight loss
Signs	■ Abdominal mass and tenderness ■ Splenomegaly ■ Ascites ■ Muscle wasting ■ Spider nevi
Neoplastic syndromes	■ Hypercholesterolemia ■ Erythrocytosis ■ Hypercalcemia ■ Hypoglycemia

Diagnosis and Staging

Figures 14.2 and 14.3 illustrate the screening and diagnostic procedure of HCC, including suggested examination and tests.

Once a diagnosis of HCC is made, a multidisciplinary evaluation is needed not only to confirm whether the cancer is localized, but also to evaluate important parameters of liver function and comorbidity.

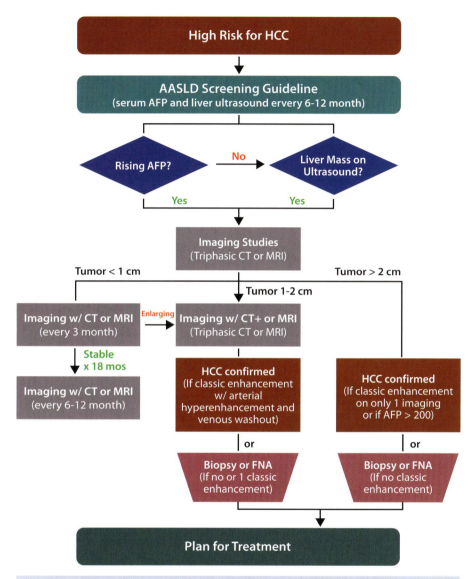

Figure 14.2 Proposed algorithm for screening of HCC in high-risk patients

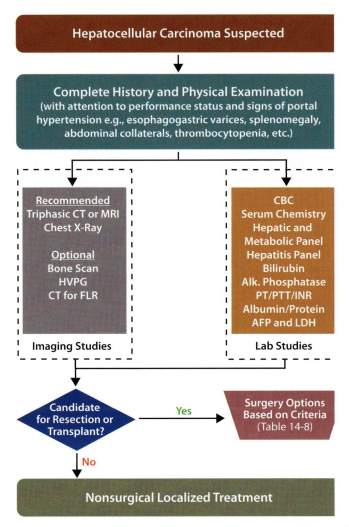

Figure 14.3 A proposed algorithm for diagnosis and staging of HCC. Consider hepatic venous pressure gradient (*HVPG*) study to evaluate for portal hypertension. A bone scan is indicated for potential transplant candidates or if bone metastasis is suspected. Future liver remnant (*FLR*) by CT calculation is recommended if resection is indicated. If FLR is insufficient, a strategy of portal vein embolization (PVE) may be considered. This procedure redirects blood flow toward the portion of the liver that will remain after resection so that it hypertrophies while the embolized segments atrophy

Tumor, Nodule, and Metastasis Staging

At least 12 staging systems have been proposed and used for HCC. Some of these staging systems incorporate aspects of liver function as liver cirrhosis in the background liver and the subsequent degree of liver damage affects outcome, other systems (e.g., tumor, nodule, and metastasis [TNM] staging system) incorporate tumor characteristics only, and some systems incorporate both liver function and tumor stage.

A detailed discussion of the staging systems is out of the scope of this chapter. The commonly used Barcelona Clinic Liver Cancer (BCLC) and 7th edition of American Joint Committee on Cancer (AJCC) staging systems for HCC are provided in Tables 14.5 and 14.6, and Figure 14.4.

Table 14.5 AJCC TNM classification of HCC

Stage	Description
Primary tumor (T)	
TX	Primary tumor cannot be assessed
T0	No evidence of primary tumor
TX	Primary tumor cannot be assessed
T1	Solitary tumor without vascular invasion
T2	Solitary tumor with vascular invasion or with multiple tumors ≤5 cm
T3a	Multiple tumors >5 cm in largest dimension
T3b	Single tumor or multiple tumors of any size involving a major branch of the portal vein or hepatic vein
T4	Tumor(s) with direct invasion or adjacent organs other than the gallbladder or with perforation of visceral peritoneum
Regional lymph nodes (N)	
NX	Regional lymph nodes cannot be assessed
N0	No regional lymph node metastasis
N1	Regional lymph node metastasis
Distant metastasis (M)	
MX	Distant metastasis cannot be assessed
M0	No distant metastasis
M1	Distant metastasis

Source: Edge SB, Byrd DR, Compton ML et al (2009) American Joint Committee on Cancer, American Cancer Society. AJCC cancer staging manual, 7th edn. Springer, Berlin Heidelberg New York

Table 14.6 Stage grouping of HCC

Stage Grouping				
	T1	**T2**	**T3a/b**	**T4**
N0	I	II	IIIA/B	IIIC
N1	IVA	IVA	IVA	IVA
M1	IVB	IVB	IVB	IVB

Source: Edge SB, Byrd DR, Compton ML et al (2009) American Joint Committee on Cancer, American Cancer Society. AJCC cancer staging manual, 7th edn. Springer, Berlin Heidelberg New York

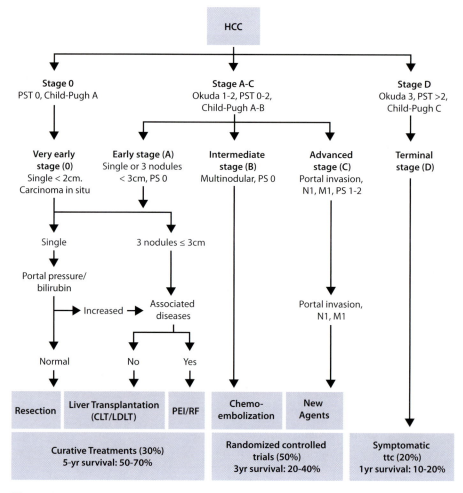

Figure 14.4 BCLC staging and treatment schedule.

Source: Pons F, Varela M, Llovet M (2005) Staging systems in hepatocellular carcinoma. HPB (Oxford) 7:35–41

In addition to tumor staging, the Child-Pugh score is useful to predict the operative risk for HCC patients. It places patients into one of three categories by evaluating clinical as well as laboratory parameters. Patients with compensated cirrhosis are categorized as Child-Pugh class A, while patients with decompensated cirrhosis are classes B and C. See Table 14.7.

Table 14.7 Child-Pugh score

Parameter	Points[a] for increasing abnormality		
	I	II	III
Encephalopathy (grade)	None	1–2	3–4
Ascites	None	Slight	Moderate
Albumin	>3.5	2.8–3.5	<2.8
Prothrombin time (s)	1–4	4–6	>6
Bilirubin (mg/dl)	1–2	2–3	>3
For primary biliary cirrhosis	1–4	4–10	>10

[a]Class A = 5–6 points, good operative risk; class B = 7–9 points, moderate operative risk; class C = 10–15 points, poor operative risk

Prognoses

Once the diagnosis of HCC is established and the work-ups to establish extent of disease are completed, the patient is classified as having one of the following:
- Potentially resectable or transplantable disease which is medically operable
- Unresectable disease
- Medically inoperable but otherwise localized disease
- Metastatic disease

Prognosis of HCC is related to the stage at diagnosis and whether the patient can undergo surgery or transplantation. The 5-year overall survival after surgery for early stage HCC is presented in Table 14.8.

General health of the patient, the liver function of the patient, and the growth rate of the tumor are important considerations as well. Prognostic factors should be analyzed for each patient also include: the AFP level, hepatitis serology, creatinine, bilirubin, prothrombin time international normalized ratio (INR), and fibrosis score (F0 value if the fibrosis is none to moderate, and F1 if the fibrosis is severe or if there is cirrhosis).

Table 14.8 5-Year overall survival (*OS*) after surgery for early stage HCC

Procedure	Recurrence-free survival (%)	Recurrence rate (%)	5-year OS (%)
Resection[a]		≥70%	50–70%
Transplant[b]	61–83%	<15%	64–75%

[a]*Sources: Llovet JM, Fuster J, Bruix J (1999) Intention-to-treat analysis of surgical treatment for early hepatocellular carcinoma: resection versus transplantation. Hepatology 30:1434–1440; Poon RT, Fan ST, Lo CM et al (2002) Long-term survival and pattern of recurrence after resection of small hepatocellular carcinoma in patients with preserved liver function: implications for a strategy of salvage transplantation. Ann Surg 235:373–382; Kianmanesh R Regimbeau JM, Belghiti J (2003) Selective approach to major hepatic resection for hepatocellular carcinoma in chronic liver disease. Surg Oncol Clin N Am 12:51–63*
[b]*Sources: Vauthey JN, Ribero D, Abdalla EK et al (2007) Outcomes of liver transplantation in 490 patients with hepatocellular carcinoma: validation of a uniform staging after surgical treatment. J Am Coll Surg 204:1016–1027; Yao FY, Ferrell L, Bass NM et al (1996) Liver transplantation for hepatocellular carcinoma: expansion of the tumor size limits does not adversely impact survival. N Engl J Med 11:693–699. Zhu A, El-Khoueiry A, Llovet JM (2009) Accomplishments in 2008 in the management of hepatobiliary cancers. Gastrointest Cancer Res 3:S28–S36*

Treatment

Principles and Practice

Surgery (resection/transplant) is the gold standard curative treatment modality for HCC. Since the majority of patients are not ideal candidates for surgery, nonsurgical treatment modalities for localized disease have been widely used for both early-stage and locally advanced HCC.

Targeted therapy with sorafenib has been demonstrated to improve survival in patients with advanced HCC.

Treatment of Early-Stage HCC

Surgical Treatment

Resection is generally favored in the setting of a non-cirrhotic patient with early-stage disease or a cirrhotic patient with a solitary tumor and Child-Pugh A status, without portal hypertension. A patient with more advanced localized disease or a less favorable Child-Pugh statuses may consider liver transplant. Patient and tumor criteria for surgery are listed in Table 14.9.

Tumor size, number of tumors, and the presence of vascular invasion are major independent predictors of survival.

Table 14.9 Surgery modalities used in early-stage HCC

Method	Particulars
Surgical resection	
Patient criteria	■ Medically fit patients with adequate hepatic reserve, generally Child-Pugh A ■ In highly selected cases, Child-Pugh B may be considered for limited resection ■ Must have an adequate future liver remnant (*FLR*) after surgery ■ If no cirrhosis, at least 20% FLR, but if Child-Pugh A cirrhosis, at least 30–40% FLR with adequate vascular and biliary inflow/outflow ■ No evidence of portal venous hypertension
Tumor criteria	■ Optimal resection candidates have a solitary lesion ■ No extrahepatic metastasis ■ No major vascular invasion preferred: presence of vascular invasion correlates with recurrence ■ Selected patients with multifocal disease and/or evidence of major vascular invasion may be considered but is controversial
Facts/issues	■ Perioperative mortality is <3% in experienced hands ■ Outcome after resection detailed in Table 14.8
Liver transplant	
Patient criteria	■ Must be medically fit ■ Generally considered for Child-Pugh B and C patients ■ MELD score is measured and has been adopted by UNOS to stratify patients on the transplant list according to their risk of death within 3 months ▶

Table 14.9 *(continued)*

Method	Particulars
Liver transplant	
Tumor criteria	■ UNOS/Milan criteria: single lesion ≤5 cm, or 1–3 lesions all ≤3 cm ■ UCSF criteria: solitary lesion ≤6.5 cm or up to 3 lesions with the largest <4.5 cm and total tumor diameter <8 cm ■ No evidence of extrahepatic disease ■ No evidence of macrovascular involvement
Facts/issues	■ 5-Year OS rate approaches 70% with a recurrence rate of <15% ■ Up to 20% of patients drop out from the waiting list before transplantation ■ Whether resection or transplant is preferred for Child-Pugh A ■ A patient who fits UNOS criteria is controversial ■ Patients with small multinodular tumors or those with advanced liver dysfunction, transplant is preferred

UNOS: United Network for Organ Sharing; **UCSF:** University of California San Francisco; **MELD:** model for end-stage liver disease

Sources: Pawlik TM, Poon RT, Abdalla EK et al (2005) Critical appraisal of the clinical and pathologic predictors of survival after resection of large hepatocellular carcinoma. Arch Surg 140:450–458; Abdalla EK, Denys A, Hasegawa K et al (2008) Treatment of large and advanced hepatocellular carcinoma. Ann Surg Oncol 15:979–985

Neoadjuvant Treatment

The role of liver-directed therapies prior to surgery has potential downstaging effect for resection or transplantation and is being actively explored. In addition, since there is the potential for tumor progression while patients are awaiting transplant, there is interest in optimizing "bridge" to transplant options.

A detailed discussion on down staging strategies is out of the scope of this chapter. Preliminary results for stereotactic body radiosurgery (SBRT), one of the modalities in the neoadjuvant setting, is presented in Table 14.10.

Table 14.10 Clinical evidence for neoadjuvant treatment for early-stage HCC using SBRT

Trial	Description
Baylor University	▪ Preliminary data from 6 HCC patients treated with SBRT, followed by surgery ▪ Medial dose of SBRT was 48 Gy in 3 fractions ▪ Pathological study revealed 2/6 tumors had no viable disease (pCR), 3/6 reduced in size (PR), and 1/6 had progression.

Source: O'Connor JK, Goldstein RM, Berger BD et al (2008) Stereotactic body radiation therapy as a bridge to transplant in hepatocellular carcinoma: acute toxicity and explant pathology. Int J Radiat Oncol Biol Phys 72:S128

Adjuvant Treatment

No standard treatment has been proven to show benefit in the adjuvant setting. As the multikinase inhibitor sorafenib has been shown to prolong overall survival in advanced HCC patients not suitable for curative therapy, studies are ongoing to test its efficacy in an adjuvant setting.

Nonsurgical Localized Treatment

For patients who are not candidates for resection or liver transplant, a number of nonsurgical liver-targeted treatment modalities, including percutaneous ethanol injection (PEI), radiofrequency ablation (RFA), and SBRT can be used.

Overall survival after PEI or RFA ranges between 30 and 50% for early-stage HCC, and depends on conditions of the patients or tumor. A detailed discussion on PEI and RFA as primary treatment is out of the scope of this chapter, and clinical evidence of SBRT for primary treatment of early stage HCC is presented in Table 14.11.

Table 14.11 Clinical evidence for neoadjuvant treatment for early-stage HCC using SBRT

Trial	Description
Princess Margaret Hospital (Canada)[a]	■ 31 HCC patients with Child-Pugh A and median tumor size of 173 ml treated with SBRT ■ Median dose of SBRT was 36 Gy (range 24–54 Gy) in 6 fractions ■ Contoured GTV on triphasic CT or MRI and added 8 mm to contour CTV ■ Two PTVs created a PTV primary, which is GTV plus individualized margin and PTV secondary which is CTV plus individualized margin ■ Median survival time for all patients were 11.7 months
Takeda et al (Japan)[b]	■ 16 patients with solitary HCC (tumor volume <100 ml) treated with SBRT with or without transarterial chemoembolization ■ 14 of 16 patients, a total dose of 35–50 Gy was delivered in 5–7 fractions over 5–9 days ■ All patients were alive at ~2-year follow-up. 8 of 16 patients had CR, and 7 had stable disease ■ 1 Patient developed local recurrence after 489 days ■ 6 Patients had intrahepatic recurrences outside the treated volume ■ No serious treatment-related toxic manifestations developed

[a]*Source: Tse RV, Hawkins M, Lockwood G et al (2008) Phase I study of individualized SBRT for HCC and intrahepatic cholangiocarcinoma. J Clin Oncol 26:657–664*
[b]*Source: Takeda A, Takahashi M, Kunieda E et al (2008) Hypofractionated stereotactic radiotherapy with and without transarterial chemoembolization for small HCC not eligible for other ablation therapies: preliminary results for efficacy and toxicity. Hepatol Res 38:60–69*

Treatment of Advanced HCC

Most patients with HCC are not ideal surgical candidates, secondary to widespread multifocal tumor within the liver, extensive macrovascular tumor invasion, or medical comorbidities.

A number of nonsurgical treatment options are available for these patients. Historically, RFA and transarterial chemoembolization (TACE) formed the mainstay of liver directed therapies in this setting. More recently, new options with radioembolization and high-dose partial liver irradiation have emerged (Table 14.12).

Table 14.12 Nonsurgical treatment modalities in advanced HCC

Particular/trial	
RFA alone	
Mechanism(s)/ indication(s)	■ RFA is achieved by exposing the tumor to heat ■ RFA candidate must have a tumor located away from major intrahepatic vessels which could absorb some of the heat, thus limiting effective delivery ■ Optimally, the tumor should be <3 cm for RFA alone
Technique(s)/ outcome(s)	■ Can be performed by laparoscopic, open, or percutaneous approaches ■ Complete necrosis has been observed in ~60% of tumors <3 cm in diameter treated with RFA
RFA in combination with embolization	
Mechanism(s)/ indication(s)	■ Arterial embolization therapy targets the arterial branch of the hepatic artery supplying the tumor ■ Combination therapy is recommended for patients with HCC tumor sizes from 3 to 5 cm
Technique(s)/ outcome(s)	■ Treatment is based on selectively infusing particles coated with chemotherapy, radioactivity with yttrium-90, or with bland particles. Retrospective data suggests that 5-year survival rates in the 50% range may be possible with this approach
Bland embolization (TAE) and TACE	
Mechanism(s)/ indication(s)	■ Take advantage of the liver's dual blood supply. Since hepatocellular cancers are hypervascular, they preferentially receive flow from the hepatic artery ■ Contraindications to TAE or TACE include: ■ Portal vein occlusion ■ Child-Pugh class C ■ Total bilirubin > 3mg/ml (unless a segmental rather than lobar injection)
Mechanism(s)/ indication(s)	■ With bland embolization, reduction in blood flow to the tumor caused by the radiologist injecting bland particles (such as gelatin sponge particles, alcohol particles, or microspheres) results in tumor ischemia and necrosis ■ With TACE, a concentrated dose of chemotherapy (with doxorubicin, cisplatin, or irinotecan) is injected, as well as the embolic particles
Radioembolization	
Indications and utilization	■ Indicated for patients who have portal vein thrombus ■ The procedure can be directed to treat the entire lobe or a segment/subsegment, depending on the patient's clinical status ■ In bilobar HCC, one lobe will be treated first, and then the second lobe 4–6 weeks later ▶

Table 14.12 *(continued)*

Particular/trial	
Radioembolization	
Techniques	■ Millions of microspheres of 20–30 μm in diameter embedded with radioactive yttrium-90 can be delivered in HCC through catheter placed through the femoral artery further into the hepatic artery ■ The radioactive half-life of this beta emitter is 64.1 h ■ Requires an extensive angiographic workup prior to the actual outpatient procedure to ensure the arterial anatomy of the tumor location, and no flow to other organs, which would allow aberrant distribution of radioactivity ■ A nuclear medicine scan after the injection of diagnostic imaging spheres similar in size and shape to the yttrium-90 microspheres to ensure no excessive flow to the lungs
Chemo-/targeted therapy	
Indications	■ Targeted therapy with sorafenib is indicated in patients with advanced HCC ■ Efficacy of cytotoxic chemotherapy agents has not been confirmed
Medications	■ Most cytotoxic agents have not demonstrated efficacy for HCC if used systemically ■ Potential benefit from doxorubicin on survival in advanced HCC, but meta-analysis not showing survival improvement ■ Small phase II studies have suggested response rates of 15–20% with combinations of gemcitabine and oxaliplatin ■ Targeted therapy with sorafenib, a multikinase inhibitor, holds the most promise by results of phase III randomized clinical trials
External-beam radiation therapy	
Indications	■ Unresectable HCC with preserved liver function as detailed in the "Radiation Therapy Technique" section ■ Used with other treatment modalities such as TACE as residual HCC cells may be observed after "definitive" dose of RT alone

Table 14.12 *(continued)*

Particular/trial	
External-beam radiation therapy	
Techniques	■ Data in the 1990s emerged for efficacy with 3D conformal radiation strategies ■ More evidence has accumulated regarding not only 3D conformal treatment but Intensity modulated radiation therapy (IMRT) and stereotactic body radiation therapy (SBRT) ■ Multiple different strategies of either radiation alone or combined with other modalities has been investigated
RILD	■ Extensive work on partial liver radiation techniques and avoidance of RILD by investigators at the University of Michigan ■ RILD is a clinical syndrome with anicteric hepatomegaly, ascites and elevated liver enzymes occurring from 2 weeks to 4 months after radiation therapy
Early evidence on the use of EBRT for HCC and RILD	
University of Michigan[a]	■ A total of 36 patients have been entered onto this study ■ Prescription depended on the ability to perform, on a routine basis, 3D treatment planning with dose–volume histogram generation ■ 21 of 25 patients (84%) with disease that could be delineated on CT scan were eligible for boost treatment ■ Dose given to the tumor depended on the volume of normal liver that could be excluded from the boost field: 45 Gy if more than 50% of the normal liver could be excluded and 60 Gy if more than 75% of the normal liver could be excluded dose ■ These results show that intrahepatic tumors can be safely treated with high doses of radiation when dose prescription is guided by the dose–volume histogram of the normal liver
Dawson et al[b]	■ 203 Patients treated with conformal liver radiotherapy and concurrent hepatic arterial chemotherapy were prospectively followed for RILD ■ 19 of the 203 patients treated with focal liver irradiation developed RILD ■ No cases of RILD were observed when the mean liver dose was <31 Gy ■ Tolerance dose for 50% complication risk for whole organ irradiated uniformly [TD50 (1)] = 45.8 Gy for patients with liver metastases, and TD50 (1) = 39.8 Gy for patients with primary hepatobiliary cancer ▶

Table 14.12 *(continued)*

Particular/trial	
Early evidence on the use of EBRT for HCC and RILD	
Dawson et al[c]	■ Review based on analyses of over 180 patients received partial irradiation of the liver ■ Liver exhibits a large volume effect ■ No cases of RILD have been reported in patients with a mean liver dose of less than 31 Gy ■ Estimates of the liver doses associated with a 5% risk of RILD for uniform irradiation of one third, two thirds, and the whole liver are 90, 47, and 31 Gy, respectively

TAE: trans-arterial embolization; **TACE**: trans-arterial chemo-embolization; **RILD**: radiation-induced liver disease

[a]*Source: Lawrence TS, Tesser RJ, Ten Haken RK et al (1990) An application of dose volume histograms to the treatment of intrahepatic malignancies with radiation therapy. Int J Radiat Oncol Biol Phys 19:1041–1047*
[b]*Source: Dawson LA, Normolle D, Balter JM et al (2002) Analysis of RILD using the Lyman NTCP model. Int J Radiation Oncol Biol Phys 53:810–821*
[c]*Source : Dawson LA, Ten Haken RK, Lawrence TS et al (2001) Partial irradiation of the liver. Semin Radiat Oncol 11:240–246*

Clinical evidences support the use of external-beam radiation therapy (including three-dimensional conformational radiation therapy [3D-CRT] and SBRT) for HCC is presented in Tables 14.13 and 14.14.

Radiation Therapy Techniques

Simulation and Target Volume Delineation

A diagnostic triphasic computed tomography (CT) scan should be done to guide treatment planning. With modern CT scanners, a bolus of 100–150 ml of contrast can be injected rapidly, and the patient can be imaged in the arterial and portal phase of enhancement. Magnetic resonance imaging (MRI) with contrast also is helpful to delineate the extent of primary liver disease, but positron-emission tomography (PET) has a high false-negative rate.

Percutaneously implanted fiducial markers adjacent to the tumor for image-guided radiation (IGRT), or real-time tumor tracking or the use of daily cone-beam CT can be used.

At simulation, immobilization in the supine position with arms overhead can be facilitated with a body cradle. Some centers prefer a full-body mold if SBRT is delivered versus a half-body mold for 3D-CRT. If abdominal compression will be used, the patient should be simulated using the same technique.

Table 14.13 Clinical evidences supporting the use of 3D-CRT in combination with or without other liver-targeted therapies

Modality	Patient number and characteristics	Dose	Outcome
3D-CRT alone[a]	n = 25, Child-Pugh A/B	66 Gy i n 33 fractions	CR: 80%, PR 12% Grade 4 toxicities: 22% CP score : B 22% Infield LR, 41% out-of-field recurrence
3D-CRT with or without TACE[b]	n = 276 TACE; n = 64 TACE then 3DCRT	1.8–2.0; up to 66 Gy if constraints could be met	MS: 19 months TACE versus 17 months TACE plus RT
3D-CRT with or without TACE[c]		1.8–2.0 Gy per fractions; mean dose 46.9 Gy	2-Year progression-free survival rate, TACE plus RT = 36 versus 100% TACE alone
3D-CRT to PVTT/IVC TT (tumor thrombus of portal vein or IVC) plus T[d]	n = 158; 44 EBRT and 114 no EBRT	Median: 50 Gy	MS 8 months, 1-year survival of 34.8%, EBRT group versus MS of 4 months and 1 year 11.4% non-EBRT
TACE followed by 3D-CRT Lipiodol/doxorubicin Then 3D CRT 7–10 days later[e]	n = 30	Mean dose: 44 Gy at 1.8 Gy	63.3% response rate; MS = 17 months

3D-CRT: three-dimensional conformal radiation therapy; **F/U**: follow-up; **MS**: medial survival; **PVTT**: portal vein tumor thrombosis

[a] *Source: Mornex F, Girard N, Beziat C et al (2006) Feasibility and efficacy of high-dose three-dimensional-conformal radiotherapy in cirrhotic patients with small-size hepatocellular carcinoma non-eligible for curative therapies – mature results of the French Phase II RTF-1 trial. Int J Radiat Oncol Biol Phys 66:1152–1158*

[b] *Source : Chung YL, Jian JJ-M, Cheng SH et al (2006) Sublethal irradiation induces vascular endothelial growth factor and promotes growth of hepatoma cells: implications for radiotherapy of hepatocellular carcinoma. Clin Cancer Res 12:2706–2715*

[c] *Source: Chia-Hsien Cheng J, Chuang VP, Cheng SH et al (2001) Unresectable hepatocellular carcinoma treated with radiotherapy and/ or chemoembolization. Int J Cancer 96:243–252*

[d] *Source: Zeng ZC, Fan J, Tang ZY et al (2008) Prognostic factors for patients with hepatocellular carcinoma with macroscopic portal vein or inferior vena cava tumor thrombi receiving external-beam radiation therapy. Cancer Sci 99:2510–2517*

[e] *Source: Seong J, Keum KC, Han KH et al (1999) Combined transcatheter arterial chemoembolization and local radiotherapy of unresectable hepatocellular carcinoma. Int J Radiat Oncol Biol Phys 43:393–397*

Table 14.14 Clinical evidences support the use of SBRT in more advanced HCC

Study	Patient number and characteristics	Dose	Outcome
Mendez et al (Netherlands)[a]	n = 11 Child-Pugh A/B	Varied: 37.5 Gy/3; 25 Gy in 5 fractions 30 Gy in 10 fractions	1-Year local control: 75% OS 1 year: 75% OS 2 year: 40%
Wulf et al (Switzerland)[b]	n = 5	30 Gy/10 in 3 patients; 37.5 Gy/3 in 1 patient; 26 Gy/1 in 1 patient	Median follow-up = 15 months, no local failure, no toxicity > RTOG 2
Indiana University Phase I Dose Escalation Trial (USA)[c]	n = 17, Child-Pugh A/B	Phase I: 36 Gy/3 and reached 48 Gy/3	48 Gy/3 no DLT in CPA; 2 patients with CPB grade 3 toxicity at 42 Gy/3 10 Patients alive without progression at median follow-up at 24 months
SBRT/TACE (Korea)[d]	n = 31, 32 lesions	Median: 36 Gy/3 fractions with range of 30–39 Gy	23 Lesions, SBRT alone; 9 lesions targeted PVTT with SBRT and TACE to follow; median survival small HCC: 12 months MS advanced HCC with PVTT: 8 months

SBRT: stereotactic body radiation therapy; **MS:** medial survival; **DLT:** dose-limiting toxicity; **CPA:** cyclophosphamide; **PVTT:** portal vein tumor thrombosis

[a] Source: Méndez Romero A, Wunderink W, Hussain SM et al (2006) Stereotactic body radiation therapy for primary and metastatic liver tumors: A single institution phase I–II study. Acta Oncol 45:831–837
[b] Source: Henderson MA, Azzous F, Breen T et al (2007) Preliminary toxicity analysis of a phase I/II trial evaluating stereotactic body radiotherapy for the treatment of hepatocellular carcinoma. Poster presentation, ASTRO 2007. Int J Radiat Oncol Biol Phys 69:S297; Wulf J, Hädinger U, Oppitz U et al (2001) Stereotactic radiotherapy of targets in the lung and liver. Strahlenther Onkol 177:645–655
[c] Source: Henderson MA, Azzous F, Breen T et al (2007) Preliminary toxicity analysis of a phase I/II trial evaluating stereotactic body radiotherapy for the treatment of hepatocellular carcinoma. Poster presentation, ASTRO 2007. Int J Radiat Oncol Biol Phys 69:S297
[d] Source: Choi BO, Choi IB, Jang HS et al (2008) Stereotactic body radiation therapy with or without transarterial chemoembolization for patients with primary hepatocellular carcinoma: preliminary analysis. BMC Cancer 8:351

A CT scan (3- to 5-mm cut) with intravenous and oral contrast should be performed from top of the lungs to the iliac crest to capture all organs necessary for dose–volume histogram analysis. Once the isocenter is tattooed on the patient, a 4D scan will be done to delineate the tumor in all phases of respiration. If gating is the preferred strategy, the CT data may be acquired in the exhale phase only. Organs at risk (OARs) (Tables 14.15 and 12.1) should be delineated. Field setup is illustrated in Table 14.15.

Table 14.15 Treatment planning considerations

Aim	Method
Targets	■ Identify GTV as enhancing region on CT. Target for HCC is gross disease without elective nodal irradiation ■ Proceed with 4D scan to determine motion ■ Techniques to consider for physiological movement from breathing including abdominal compression versus gating the patient (ABC) versus gating the machine. Consider image-guided radiation (IGRT) strategy (fiducial placement, cone-beam CT, real-time tracking) ■ If abdominal compression, create internal target volume (ITV); if gating is to be used, decide which phase for treatment and contour GTV in that phase ■ Decide on individual patient's motion for PTV expansion and factor in what IGRT modality will be used (cone-beam CT, fiducial markers, real-time tracking) ■ Anticipating individual SBRT strategy is essential for optimizing treatment planning
Margins	■ Decide if target is GTV only or to include elective target (i.e., CTV). CTV can be derived from GTV plus 0.8 cm, if used ■ If three-fraction SBRT is used, consider direct GTV expansion to PTV based on individual motion
Normal tissue	■ Liver is a parallel organ. It has a low radiation dose tolerance per milliliter of tissue and toxicity is volume dependent ■ Evaluate patient's liver volume and Child-Pugh score prior to simulation to think about most appropriate strategy ■ Critical to spare as much liver as possible

Since the liver moves with respiration, the technique of treatment and breathing control listed in Table 14.16 should be anticipated prior to simulation. A patient's status needs to be considered before planning for simulation. It may be difficult for a patient to tolerate 6 weeks of external beam 3D-CRT with abdominal compression but a course of three to five fractions of SBRT may be well tolerated.

Table 14.16 Commonly used breathing control techniques in radiation therapy for upper abdominal malignancies

Technique	Description
Abdominal compression	A mechanical belt or device is placed across the patient's upper abdomen to limit the respiratory excursion so that an internal target volume (ITV) can be created
	The amount of tumor motion is reduced and the target will be treated at all times
Active breathing control (ABC)	A breathing device is placed in the patient's mouth, resulting in a correlation that tells the radiation therapist to turn on the beam at a specified phase
	Often, patients are treated in exhale phase so the ABC device can facilitate this pattern of treatment
Respiratory gating	The treatment machine can be programmed to "beam on" at specified times

Dose and Treatment Delivery

Although published data supports 66 Gy in HCC irradiation using conventional fractionation, residual disease is expected in most patients after 50–70 Gy. Therefore, if a 3D-CRT strategy is favored, radiation should be considered to be combined with TACE (*Aoki K, Okazaki N, Okada S et al (1994) Radiotherapy for hepatocellular carcinoma: clinicopathological study of seven autopsy cases. Hepatogastroenterology 41:427–431*).

There is much interest with regard to SBRT strategies. Two reported schedules for SBRT are listed in Table 14.17. See also Figure 14.5 regarding a patient treated with SBRT.

Table 14.17 Clinical evidences support the use of SBRT in more advanced HCC

Protocols	Criteria	Dose and Fractionation
Indiana University	Child Pugh A	48 Gy in 3 fractions
	Child Pugh B	40 Gy in 5 fractions
PMH	PTV of GTV	24–54 Gy in 6 fractions[a]
	PTV of CTV	24 Gy in 6 fractions

PMH: Princess Margaret Hospital; **RILD**: radiation-induced liver disease

[a]Total dose depending on the estimated risk for RILD, and 6 fractions of SBRT over 2 weeks (on alternating days)

Source: prospective data from Indiana University and PMH, listed in Table 14.13

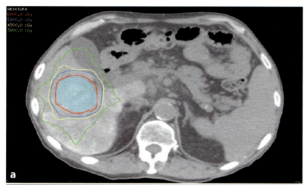

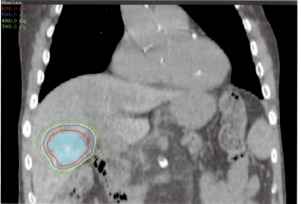

Figure 14.5 a,b a A patient with HCC treated with SBRT for 5 fractions (12 Gy per fraction) with abdominal compression. **b** Dose–volume histogram (DVH) of the same plan

b Dose Volume Histogramm

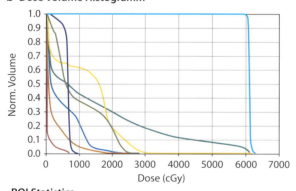

ROI Statistics

Line Type	ROI	Trial	Min.	Max.	Mean	Std. Dev.
■	Cord	appr	98.1	874.2	648.9	116.7
■	L-kidney	appr	10.1	757.3	61.3	120.9
■	PTV	appr	5794.4	6303.1	6123.6	35.9
■	R-kidney	appr	17.1	2995.5	470.9	540.0
■	Stomach	appr	15.0	3027.2	229.0	356.2
■	liver-GTV	appr	15.6	6295.3	1467.9	1795.8

Normal Tissue Tolerance

OARs in radiation therapy of primary liver cancer include small bowel, liver, kidneys, stomach, and spinal cord. Most studies have not specified whether organs are contoured in the free-breathing phase or as planned risk volumes (PRVs) such that the organ is contoured on the phases from the 4D scan. Gated patients typically would have the organs contoured in the appropriate phase corresponding to treatment.

Dose limitation of OARs in the treatment of liver lesions using SBRT over three to six fractions are listed in Table 14.18.

Table 14.18 Dose limitation of OARs in SBRT for liver lesions (over three to six fractions)

OAR	Dose limitation(s)
Spinal cord	■ Maximum dose = 18 Gy[a]
Liver	■ At least 700 ml of normal liver (liver–GTV) should receive total dose of <15 Gy: this is the reported constraint for liver metastases[a] ■ This is based on the surgical data that if a critical volume in the range of 500–600 ml of liver is preserved, there should be adequate reserve to allow regeneration and function; 700 ml is thus more conservative ■ Mean liver dose for HCC <13 Gy in 3 fractions[b]; (<15 Gy in 3 fractions for liver metastases) ■ Mean liver dose for HCC <1 8 Gy in 6 fractions[b], (<20 Gy in 6 fractions for liver metastases). Mean liver dose for HCC, Child-Pugh B is 4–6 Gy per fraction <6 Gy[b]
Small intestine	■ Maximum dose = 30 Gy[a]
Kidney	■ V15 < 35% (bilateral)[a]
Stomach	■ Maximum dose = 30 Gy[a] ■ Volume of stomach >22.5 Gy should be <5 ml[b]

V15: percentage of total kidney volume receiving greater than or equal to 15 Gy

[a]*Source: Rusthoven KE, Kavanagh BD, Cardenes H et al. (2009) Multi-institutional phase I/II trial of SBRT for liver metastases. J Clin Oncol 27:1572–1578*
[b]*Source: Pan C, Kavanagh B, Dowson L et al (2010) Radiation-associated liver injury. Int J Radiat Oncol Biol Phys 76:S94–S100*

Tolerance of normal OARs in conventional fractionated radiation therapy for upper abdominal malignancies including liver cancer is detailed in Table 12.1. Tolerance lowered in the setting of cirrhosis: 5% risk of radiation-induced liver disease (RILD) is mean liver dose 28 Gy at 2 Gy per fraction.

Follow-Up

Close follow-up after completion of treatment for HCC patients is recommended. Schedule and suggested examination during follow-up is presented in Table 14.19.

Table 14.19 Follow-up schedule and examinations

Schedule	Frequency
First follow-up	■ 4–6 Weeks after radiation therapy
Years 0–1	■ Every 3–6 months
Years 2–5	■ Every 6 months
Years 5+	■ Annually
Examinations	
History and physical	■ Complete history and physical examination
Laboratory tests	■ Complete blood counts (*CBC*) and serum chemistry ■ Hepatic and metabolic panels ■ Alpha fetoprotein if initially elevated every 3 months for 2 years, then every 6 months
Imaging studies	■ Three-phase liver CT or MRI with contrast every 3–6 months for 2 years, then annually

Source: NCCN clinical practice guidelines in oncology. Hepatobiliary cancers, v.1.2010. http://www.nccn.org/professionals/physician_gls/PDF/hepatobiliary.pdf. Cited 15 May 2010

Radiation-Induced Adverse Effects

Potential radiation-induced adverse effects include nausea, vomiting, abdominal discomfort/pain, liver dysfunction including RILD, which consists of both a classic and nonclassic subtype (Tables 14.20 and 14.21).

Another potential effect can be hepatitis B reactivation, which can contribute to liver function abnormalities; prophylactic antiretroviral therapy has been associated with reduction of the reactivation.

Table 14.20 Clinical evidences support the use of SBRT in more advanced HCC

Subtypes	Clinical features
Classic	■ Patients develop anicteric hepatomegaly and ascites from 2 weeks to 3 months after treatment ■ Alkaline phosphatase is >2× of the upper limit of normal or >2× of the baseline value ■ Etiology results from occlusion and obliteration of the central veins of the hepatic lobules resulting in secondary hepatocyte necrosis, which can lead to liver failure and death
Non-classic	■ Occurs between 1 week and 3 months ■ Liver transaminases is > 5× of upper limit of normal or a decline in liver function measured by a worsening of Child-Pugh score by 2 or more in the absence of classic RILD ■ Etiology of this is not known

Table 14.21 Radiation-induced liver toxicity (CTEP and CTCAE 3.0)

Grade	Adverse event	Metabolic adverse laboratory value (alkaline phosphatase)
2	Jaundice	>2.5–5.0 × ULN
3	Asterixis	>5.0–20 × ULN
4	Encephalopathy/coma	>20 × ULN
5	Death	

CTEP: Cancer Therapy Evaluation Program; **CTCAE**: Common Terminology Criteria for Adverse Events v 3.0; **ULN**: upper limit of normal

15A Cholangiocarcinoma

Ravi Shridhar[1]

Key Points

- Cholangiocarcinoma (CC) is a malignant neoplasm of bile duct epithelium.
- Intrahepatic CC (ICC) arisees in bile ducts in the liver and extrahepatic CC (ECC) originatees in the bile duct along the hepatoduodenal ligament.
- Worldwide incidence of CC is rising and is the second most common primary malignancy of the liver after hepatocellular carcinoma.
- In the USA, 5,000 new cases are diagnosed annually and this accounts for 3% of gastrointestinal (GI) tract malignancies.
- Approximately 60–70% of CC arise at the bifurcation of the common hepatic duct, 20–30% of CC are ECC, and 5–10% are ICC.
- Risk factors include chronic inflammation such as that occurring in chronic bile duct calculi, choledochal cysts, ulcerative colitis, primary sclerosing cholangitis, liver fluke infections, and hepatitis B or C viral infection.
- Early-stage bile duct cancers are usually asymptomatic.
- Most common presenting symptom is jaundice.
- ICC can present with fever, weight loss and/or abdominal pain, whereas ECC usually present with painless jaundice
- Laboratory tests include liver function tests, CEA and CA 19-9.
- Diagnostic imaging include ultrasound, three-phase computed tomography (CT) scan, magnetic resonance imaging (MRI), and magnetic resonance cholangiography (MRCP) to determine resectability, nodal involvement, and extrahepatic metastases.
- Endoscopic retrograde cholangiopancreatography (ERCP) or percutaneous transhepatic cholangiography (PTC) is recommended for intervention for biliary drainage.
- Better survival is associated with distal tumors rather than mid- or proximal lesions.
- The tumor, node, and metastasis (TNM) system is used for staging.
- Surgery is the only potential cure of CC.   ▶

[1] Ravi Shridhar, MD, PhD (✉)
Email: ravi.shridhar@mofftit.org

J. J. Lu, L. W. Brady (Eds.), *Decision Making in Radiation Oncology*
DOI: 10.1007/978-3-642-13832-4_16, © Springer-Verlag Berlin Heidelberg 2011

Epidemiology and Etiology

The incidence of cholangiocarcinoma is rising in most countries. It is the second most common primary malignancy of the liver, behind hepatocellular carcinoma. Cholangiocarcinoma accounts for 3% of all gastrointestinal (GI) tract malignancies. Incidence of intra-hepatic cholangiocarcinoma (ICC) is rising from 0.32 per 100,000 from 1975 to 1979 to 0.85 per 100,00 from 1995 to 1999. However, the incidence of extra-hepatic cholangiocarcinoma (ECC) is declining. Currently it is 1.2 per 100,000 in men and 0.8 per 100,000 in women.

Risk factors of cholangiocarcinoma are reported in (Table 15A.1).

Table 15A.1 Risk factors of cholangiocarcinoma

Factor	Description
Patient related	**Age and gender:** Male:female ratio is 3:2. Average age at diagnosis is in the seventh decade of life
	Infectious: Hepatitis B and C, liver flukes such as Clonorchis sinensis and Opisthorchis veverrini
	Family medical history: no inherited risk known
	Past medical history: ulcerative colitis, congenital anomalies of the pancreatobiliary tree such as choledochal cysts, hepatolithiasis , primary sclerosing cholangitis, cirrhosis
	Medications: isoniazide and first-generation oral contraceptives
	Genetic predisposition: There is overexpression of epidermal growth factor (EGF) but uncommon expression of Her2neu
Environmental	**Chemical agents:** exposure to Thorotrast, asbestos, vinyl chloride, nitrosamines, dioxin have been associated with cholangiocarcinoma

Anatomy

ICC arises within the liver parenchyma, whereas ECC involves the common bile duct within the hepatoduodenal ligament. Hilar or Klatskin tumors are classified as ECC and are located within 2 cm of the bifurcation of the common hepatic duct (Figure 15A.1).

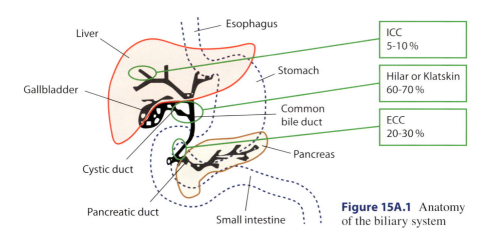

Figure 15A.1 Anatomy of the biliary system

Pathology

Malignant tumors of the bile duct epithelial cells are termed *cholangiocarcinomas* and are most commonly (90%) adenocarcinomas. Most of these tumors are well to moderately differentiated. Other histologies include adenosquamous, leiomyosarcoma, and mucoepidermoid carcinoma (Table 15A.2). Primary neuroendocrine carcinomas and small cell tumors are rare.

Table 15A.2 Subtypes of adenocarcinomas of the bile ducts

Subtype	Description
Sclerosing	■ Account for 90% of adenocarcinomas ■ Extensive desmoplastic reaction ■ Low resectability
Nodular	■ Highly invasive with advanced disease ■ Low resectability and cure rates
Papillary	■ Rare tumors that form obstructive masses ■ High resectability and cure rates

Routes of Spread

Local extension, regional (lymphatic), and distant (hematogenous) metastases are the three major routes of spread in cholangiocarcinoma (Table 15A.3).

Table 15A.3 Routes of spread in cholangiocarcinoma

Route	Description
Local extension	■ Spread along biliary ducts, invade perineural and vascular structures; mucosal extension (10–20 mm) is primarily seen with papillary and nodular tumors. Submucosal or infiltrative extension (6–10 mm) is predominantly seen with sclerosing tumors. Therefore, need 1-cm gross negative margin for submucosal extension and 2 cm for mucosal extension ■ 75% of cases have perineural invasion and this is a negative prognostic factor for survival ■ Hilar or Klatskin tumors directly invade liver parenchyma (80%) and the hepatoduodenal ligament ■ Hilar tumors involving left hepatic duct can involve caudate lobe by direct invasion and hence partial hepatectomy with caudate resection is associated with improved survival ■ ECC can directly invade the pancreas and duodenum and therefore requires a Whipple procedure ■ Portal vein involvement is controversial as a prognostic factor (can result in lobar atrophy as well as contralateral lobar hypertrophy allowing for safer resections)
Regional lymph node metastasis	■ Lymph node involvement is seen in 45–60% of cases at diagnosis and is a negative prognostic factor for survival ■ ECC have a higher incidence of lymph node metastases ■ Hilar or porta hepatis nodes are most frequently involved ■ Para-aortic lymph nodes less frequently involved
Distant metastasis	■ 30% of patients present with distant metastases involving liver, lung, bone, peritoneum, and distant lymph nodes

Diagnosis, Staging, and Prognosis

Clinical Presentation

Commonly observed signs and symptoms are detailed in Table 15A.4.

Table 15A.4 Commonly observed signs/symptoms in cholangiocarcinoma

Type	Details

General	■ ICC often diagnosed by imaging tests are usually present with no symptoms
	■ Advanced ICC may present with right upper quadrant (RUQ) pain, fever, and weight loss
	■ ECC usually present with painless jaundice and with symptoms of itching, clay-colored stools, and dark urine
	■ Portal vein invasion or thrombus may present with signs of portal hypertension like varices and splenomegaly
	■ Most common presenting symptoms
	  1. Jaundice: 84%
	  2. Pruritis: 66%
	  3. Weight loss: 35%
	  4. Hepatomegaly: 25–40%
	  5. Abdominal pain: 30%
	  6. Nausea and vomiting: 20%
	  7. Fever: 10%
	  8. Palpable gallbladder (Courvoisier's sign): rare

Diagnosis and Staging

Table 15A.5 illustrates the diagnostic procedure of cholangiocarcinoma, including suggested examination and tests.

Table 15A.5 Diagnostic workup

Modality	Description
Laboratory values	■ Complete blood count (*CBC*) with differential ■ Comprehensive metabolic panel (*CMP*) to assess renal function and liver status ■ Coagulation studies ■ Tumor markers for CC are controversial. Carcinoembryonic antigen (CEA) and CA19-9 are neither sensitive nor specific. They are elevated in other malignancies including gastric, pancreatic, and colon cancers. CA19-9 is also elevated in patients with biliary obstruction, cholelithiasis, primary sclerosing cholangitis (PSC), and other biliary anomalies

Table 15A.5 *(continued)*

Modality	Description
Ultrasound	■ Initial imaging test for biliary obstruction ■ Sensitivity and specificity for diagnosing ECC is 90% ■ ICC is difficult to distinguish from other solid hepatic masses ■ Helpful for assessing portal venous and hepatic parenchymal involvement ■ Sensitivity improved with elevated CA19-9 levels ■ Strong operator dependence
CT	■ Triple-phase CT scan ■ Used to assess local spread, vascular invasion, lymph node involvement, vascular thrombus, and distant metastases, which will help determine resectability ■ Can also evaluate for lobar atrophy/hypertrophy, biliary dilatation, bile duct wall thickening, capsular invasion ■ ICC appears as hypodense masses with varying degrees of delayed venous enhancement. Enhancing lesions tend to behave more aggressively
MRI/ magnetic resonance cholangiography (MRCP)	■ MRI done in conjunction with MRCP ■ Provides 3D reconstruction of biliary tree ■ Diagnostic accuracy is comparable to ERCP but is non-invasive and strictly a radiologic modality ■ Can assess for vascular invasion, lymph node metastases, and distant metastases ■ ICC appear hypointense on T_1- and hyperintense on T_2-weighted images
Cholangiography	■ Involves use of invasive techniques like ERCP or PTC ■ Provide dynamic images to detect biliary anomalies and determine location and extent of ECC ■ Sensitivity and specificity is 75–80% ■ Can obtain brushings for tissue diagnosis ■ Can also provide relief of biliary obstruction ■ Post-ERCP complications include pancreatitis, bacteriobilia, bleeding, sepsis, vascular injury, and death
EUS	■ Meta-analysis shows sensitivity and specificity of 78% and 84%, respectively ■ Provides ability to perform fine-needle aspiration (FNA) ■ Allows interrogation of organs in direct proximity to the stomach and duodenum
PET	■ Sensitivity and specificity of 90% and 78%, respectively ■ Able to detect lymph node and distant metastases ■ Allows assessment of tumor response to treatment ■ Many false positives in patients with PSC or other inflammatory biliary conditions ■ False-negative results in patients with mucinous tumors

American Joint Committee on Cancer Tumor, Node, and Metastasis Staging

Tables 15A.6 and 15A.7 present the American Joint Committee on Cancer (AJCC) tumor, node, and metastasis staging and grouping.

Table 15A.6 AJCC (7th edn) TNM classification of Cholangiocarcinoma

Stage	Description
Primary tumor (T) ICC	
TX	Primary tumor cannot be assessed
T0	No evidence of primary tumor
T1	Solitary tumor without vascular invasion
T2a	Solitary tumor with vascular invasion
T2b	Multiple tumors with vascular invasion
T3	Tumors perforating the visceral peritoneum or involving the local extrahepatic structures by direct invasion
T4	Tumors with periductal invasion
Primary tumor (T) perihilar CC	
TX	Primary tumor cannot be assessed
T0	No evidence of primary tumor
T1	Tumor confined to the bile duct, with extension up to the muscle layer of fibrous tissue
T2a	Tumor invades beyond the wall of the bile duct to surrounding adipose tissue
T2b	Tumor invades adjacent hepatic parenchyma
T3	Tumor invades the unilateral branches of the portal vein (right or left) or hepatic artery (right or left)
T4	Tumor invades any of the following: main portal vein or its branches bilaterally, common hepatic artery, or the second-order biliary radicals bilaterally; or unilateral second-order biliary radicals with contralateral portal vein or hepatic artery involvement
Primary tumor (T) ECC	
TX	Primary tumor cannot be assessed
T0	No evidence of primary tumor
T1	Tumor confined to the bile duct histologically
T2a	Tumor invades beyond the wall of the bile duct

Table 15A.6 *(continued)*

Stage	Description
Primary tumor (T) ECC	
T3	Tumor invades the gallbladder, pancreas, duodenum, or other adjacent organs without involvement of the celiac axis, or the superior mesenteric artery (*SMA*)
T4	Tumor involves celiac axis or SMA
Regional lymph nodes (N) for ICC	
NX	Regional lymph nodes cannot be assessed
N0	No regional lymph node metastasis
N1[a]	Regional lymph node metastasis
Regional lymph nodes (N) for perihilar CC	
NX	Regional lymph nodes cannot be assessed
N0	No regional lymph node metastasis
N1	Regional lymph node metastasis (nodes along cystic duct, common bile duct, hepatic artery, and portal vein)
N2	Metastases to periaortic, pericaval, SMA, and celiac artery
Regional lymph nodes (N) for ECC	
NX	Regional lymph nodes cannot be assessed
N0	No regional lymph node metastasis
N1[b]	Regional lymph node metastasis
Distant metastasis (M)	
MX	Distant metastasis cannot be assessed
M0	No distant metastasis
M1	Distant metastasis

[a] Tumors is segment 2–3 preferentially drain to lymph nodes along the lesser curvature of the stomach and celiac nodes. Segments 5–8 drain to hilar (hepatic artery, common bile duct, portal vein, and cystic duct) lymph nodes. Segments 2–4 drain to hilar, gastric, and gastrohepatic lymph nodes. Inferior phrenic nodes are regional. Caval and periaortic nodes are M1 disease

[b] For resection, a minimum number of 12 lymph nodes should be removed. Regional lymph nodes are similar to pancreatic head tumors. These include hilar, celiac trunk, pancreaticoduodenal arteries, SMA, and superior mesenteric vein (*SMV*) lymph nodes

Source: TNM staging system for cholangiocarcinoma (2010) In: National Comprehensive Cancer Network (NCCN). Clinical practice guidelines in oncology: cholangiocarcinoma, v. 2.2010, 7th edn

Table 15A.7 Stage grouping of cholangiocarcinoma

Stage Grouping				
ICC				
	T1	T2	T3	T4
N0	I	II	III	IVA
N1	IVA	IVA	IVA	IVA
M1	IVB	IVB	IVB	IVB
ECC				
	T1	T2	T3	T4
N0	IA	IB	IIA	III
N1	IIB	IIB	IIB	III
N2	IV	IV	IV	IV
Perihilar HCC				
	T1	T2a/b	T3	T4
N0	I	II	IIIA	IVA
N1	IIIB	IIIB	IIIB	IVA
N2	IVB	IVB	IVB	IVB
M1	IVB	IVB	IVB	IVB

Source: TNM staging system for cholangiocarcinoma (2010) In: National Comprehensive Cancer Network (NCCN). Clinical practice guidelines in oncology: cholangiocarcinoma, v. 2.2010, 7th edn

Prognosis

Negative prognostic factors include unresectable tumors, margin-positive resection, lymph node positive, and perineural invasion (Table 15A.8). Median survival periods of patients with unresectable disease and metastatic disease are 6–12 months and <6 months, respectively.

For ECC, 5-year survival rates average 15–25%, but are as high as 54% in selected patients who undergo complete resection for node-negative disease.

Table 15A.8 Five-year overall survival, dependent on various prognostic factors

Prognostic factors	Positive (%)	Negative (%)
Margin status	0–12%	19–47%
Nodal status	10–15%	30–40%
Perineural invasion	13%	47%

Treatment

Principles and Practice

Surgery is the only curative treatment modality for CC; however, resectability rates vary by tumor location. The resectability rates for ECC, hilar CC, and ICC are 91, 56, and 60%, respectively. Margin-negative resections are obtained in 20–40% of ICC versus 50% of ECC. Chemoradiation therapy is recommended for margin-positive or node positive resections and unresectable locally advanced tumors. Chemotherapy is reserved for unresectable or metastatic disease. Table 15A.9 details the various treatment modalities and Table 15A.10 references and studies regarding surgery outcomes.

Table 15A.9 Treatment modalities used in Cholangiocarcinoma

Modality	Description
Surgery	
ICC	■ Partial hepatectomy ■ Extended hepatic resection ■ Bile duct resection ■ Regional lymphadenectomy ■ Roux-en-Y hepaticojejunostomy ■ Vascular resection ■ Liver transplantation
Hilar	■ Extended radical resection ■ Partial hepatectomy (caudate lobe resection) ■ Regional lymphadenectomy ■ Liver transplantation
ECC	■ Pancreaticoduodenectomy ■ Regional lymphadenectomy ■ Rarely, partial hepatectomy ■ Liver transplantation
Criteria for unresectability	■ Bilateral hepatic duct involvement up to secondary radicles bilaterally ■ Encasement or occlusion of the main portal vein proximal to its bifurcation ■ Atrophy of 1 liver lobe with encasement of the contralateral portal vein branch ■ Atrophy of 1 liver lobe with contralateral secondary biliary radicle involvement ■ Involvement of bilateral hepatic arteries ■ Multifocal or bilobar liver disease ■ Distant metastases ▶

Table 15A.9 *(continued)*

Modality	Description
Radiation therapy	
External beam	■ 3D conformal or IMRT ■ Used adjuvantly for margin-positive or node-positive resections ■ Used definitively for unresectable, locally advanced tumors ■ Usually done concurrently with fluorouracil (5-FU) or capecitabine ■ Treat tumor plus regional lymphatics including portahepatis, celiac, periduodenal, peripancreatic, and para-aortic regions
Brachytherapy	■ Used to boost tumor after external-beam radiation or for palliation of obstructive symptoms caused by tumor ■ Delivers high doses to the tumor, with rapid falloff of dose to surrounding normal structures ■ Most commonly used source is Ir-192 delivered through externalize biliary catheters
Radio-embolization	■ Beta radiation from yttrium-90 tagged microspheres injected intrahepatically through hepatic artery ■ Used mainly in unresectable disease ■ Treats entire liver with radiation. Most commonly treating 1 lobe at a time, with 4–6 weeks of separation between treatments
Chemotherapy	
Systemic	■ No benefit of adjuvant chemotherapy after surgery ■ Survival benefit for gemcitabine/cisplatin versus gemcitabine alone for unresectable or metastatic disease ■ 5-FU or capecitabine used concurrently with radiation
Chemo-embolization	■ Transarterial injection and embolization via hepatic artery ■ Most commonly used agents include gemcitabine, cisplatin, and doxorubicin

Table 15A.10 Surgery outcomes

Tumor	Series	Number of cases	5-Year OS	R0(%)
ICC	DeOliverira 2007	34	40	–
	Miwa 2006	41	29	–
	Jan 2005	81	15	–
	Ohtsuka 2003	50	23	–
	Uenishi 2001	28	27	–
	Inoue 2000	52	36	–
	Yamamoto 1999	83	23	–
	Madariaga 1998	34	35	–
ECC	DeOliverira 2007	229	23	–
	Cheng 2007	112	25	–
	Murakami 2007	36	50	–
	Yoshida 2002	26	37	–
	Fong 1996	45	27	–
Hilar	Hasegawa 2007	49	40	78%
	DeOliveira 2007	173	10	19%
	Dinant 2006	99	27	31%
	Hemming 2005	53	45	80%
	Rea 2004	46	26	80%
	Kawasaki 2003	79	40	68%
	Kawarada 2002	87	26	64%
	Jarnagin 2001	80	37	78%
	Tabata 2000	75	23	60%
	Kosuge 1999	66	35	52%
	Miyazaki 1998	76	26	71%

References and studies summarized in review by Aljiffry M, Walsh M, Molinari M (2009) Advances in diagnosis, treatment and palliation of cholangiocarcinoma: 1990–2009. World J Gastroenterol 15:4240–4262

Adjuvant Treatment

Table 15A.11 lists various studies with regard to chemotherapy treatment.

Table 15A.11 Chemoradiotherapy outcomes

Trial	Details
Todorki et al[a]	■ Retrospective review of 47 patients with microscopic positive margins (Klatskin tumor) ■ 28 treated with radiation therapy, 19 not treated ■ 5-year overall survival of 33.9 versus 13.5% for RT versus no RT
Gerhards et al[b]	■ 91 Patients with hilar CC ■ 30 Patients with external beam RT (46 Gy) ■ 41 Patients with external beam RT/brachytherapy ■ 20 Patients no adjuvant treatment ■ Median survival of 24 versus 8 months for RT versus no RT
Alden et al[c]	■ 48 Patients with ECC ■ 24 treated with chemoradiotherapy ■ External-beam RT to 46 Gy ■ Brachytherapy to 25 Gy ■ Chemotherapy was 5-FU with or without adriamycin or mitomycin C ■ 2-year survival 30 versus 17% for RT ■ Median survival of 12 versus 5 months for RT ■ 2-year survival >55 versus <55 Gy; 48 versus 0%
Ben-Josef et al[d]	■ 128 Patients with colon metastases or primary hepatobiliary tumors ■ External-beam RT concurrent with hepatic arterial floxuridine ■ RT delivered 1.5–1.65 Gy twice daily to median dose 60.75 (40–90 Gy) ■ Median survival of 16 months ■ 60% progression-free survival at 3 years
Borghero et al[e]	■ 42 Patients treated with chemoradiotherapy who had positive margins or positive nodes ■ 23 Patients with margin-negative and node-negative resections ■ No difference in local control or 5-year overall survival ■ Conclusion is that adjuvant chemoradiation provides equivalent survival for high-risk patients compared with those with R0 resections

Neoadjuvant Treatment

Table 15A.12 details trials on neoadjuvant chemotherapy.

Table 15A.12 Neoadjuvant chemoradiotherapy outcomes

Trial	Details
McMasters et al[a]	■ 91 Patients (51 unresectable/40 resected) ■ Median survival of 22 versus 10 months in favor of resection ■ 9 Patients treated with neo-CRT ■ 3 pathologic complete response ■ All 9 with margin-negative resection versus 50% margin-negative for patients not treated with neo-CRT ■ No increase in surgical complications with neo-CRT
Nelson et al[b]	■ 45 Patients (12 treated neo-CRT versus 33 adjuvant CRT) ■ 5-Year survival of 54 versus 23% for patients treated with neo-CRT versus adjuvant CRT respectively

[a] *Source: McMasters KM, Tuttle TM, Leach SD et al (1997) Neoadjuvant chemotherapy for extrahepatic carcinoma. Am J Surg 74:605–608*
[b] *Source: Nelson JW, Ghafoori AP, Willett CG et al (2009) Concurrent chemoradiotherapy in resected extrahepatic cholangiocarcinoma. Int J Radiat Oncol Biol Phys 73:148–153*

---

[a] *Source: Todoroki T, Ohara K, Kawamoto T et al. (2000) Benefits of adjuvant radiotherapy after radical resection of locally advanced main hepatic duct carcinoma. Int J Radiat Oncol Biol Phys 46:581–587*
[b] *Source: Gerhards MF, van Gulik TM, Gonzale Gonzalez D et al (2003) Results of postoperative radiotherapy for resectable hilar cholangiocarcinoma. World J Surg 27:173–179*
[c] *Source: Alden M, Mohiuddin M (1994) The impact of radiation dose in combined external beam and intraluminal Ir-192 brachytherapy for bile duct cancer. Int J Radiat Oncol Biol Phys 28:945–951*
[d] *Source: Ben-Josef E, Normolle D, Ensminger WD et al (2005) Phase II trial of high-dose conformal radiation therapy with concurrent hepatic artery floxuridine for unresectable intrahepatic malignancies. J Clin Oncol 23:8739–8747*
[e] *Source: Borghero Y, Crane CH, Szklaruk J et al (2008) Extrahepatic bile duct adenocarcinoma: patients at high-risk for local recurrence treated with surgery and adjuvant chemoradiation have an equivalent overall survival to patients with standard-risk treated with surgery alone. Ann Surg Oncol 15:3147–3156*

Liver Transplantation

Table 15A.13 lists studies on liver transplantation.

Table 15A.13 Liver transplantation survival rates

First author and year[a]	Institution	Cases (n)	\multicolumn{4}{c}{Survival (years)}
			I (%)	II (%)	III (%)	V (%)
Without neoadjuvant therapy						
O'Grady 1988	King's College	26	34%	15%	8%	5%
Ringe 1989	Hannover	30	38%	32%		14%
Penn 1991	Cincinnati registry	109		30%		14%
Nashan 1996	Hannover	10	30%			10%
Goss 1997	UCLA	10	90%	83%		83%
Iwatsuki 1998	Pittsburgh	27	60%	36%	36%	36%
Bismuth 2000	Paul Brousse	9			33%	
Meyer 2000	Cincinnati registry	207	72%	48%		23%
Shimoda 2001	UCLA	25	71%	35%		
Robles 2004	Spanish centers	36	82%		53%	30%
Robles 2004	Spanish centers	23	77%		65%	42%
Ghali 2005	Canadian centers	10	90%		30%	
With neoadjuvant chemoradiotherapy						
DeVreede 2000	Mayo Clinic	11	100%	100%	100%	80%
Sudan	Nebraska	11	55%	45%	45%	
Rea et al[b]	Mayo Clinic	38	92%		82%	82%
Rea et al	■ 71 patients with stages I and II hilar CC ■ Chemoradiation was 1.5 Gy BID to 45 Gy with 5FU, followed by 20- to 30-Gy HDR boost, followed by capecitabine until surgery ■ 38 Patients with favorable findings at staging operation who went on to transplant ■ 5-Year actuarial survival rate for all patients who begin neoadjuvant therapy is 58%, and the 5-year survival rate after transplantation is 82% ■ 13% Recurrence rate in transplanted group					

[a] *Studies cited in Castaldo ET, Pinson CW (2007) Liver transplantation for non-hepatocellular carcinoma malignancy. HPB (Oxford) 9:98–103*
[b] *Source: Rea DJ, Heimbach JK, Rosen CB et al (2005) Liver transplantation with neoadjuvant chemoradiation is more effective than resection for hilar cholangiocarcinoma. Ann Surg 242:451–458; discussion 458–461*

Chemotherapy

Results from randomized studies demonstrated no benefit to adjuvant chemotherapy. However, chemotherapy is efficacious in palliative setting for unresectable and metastatic disease (Table 15A.14). Two-drug combination (with antimetabolite and platinum) is superior to single-agent chemotherapy.

Table 15A.14 Chemotherapy for unresectable or metastatic cholangiocarcinoma

Trial	Details
Volle et al	■ Randomized 324 patients to gemcitabine (Gem) alone versus gemcitabine/cisplatin (GemCis) ■ Analysis included patients from randomized phase II study yielding 410 patients (204 Gem versus 206 GemCis) ■ Metastatic disease (75%), locally advanced (25%); gallbladder (36%), bile duct (59%), ampulla (5%) ■ Median overall survival (OS) was greater with GemCis than with Gem, 11.7 versus 8.2 months ($p = 0.002$) ■ Median progression-free survival (PFS) was greater with GemCis than with Gem, 8.5 versus 6.5 months ($p = 0.003$)

Source: Valle JW, Wasan HS, Palmer DD et al (2009) Gemcitabine with or without cisplatin in patients (pts) with advanced or metastatic biliary tract cancer (ABC): results of a multicenter, randomized phase III trial (the UK ABC-02 trial). J Clin Oncol 27:Abstract 4503

Embolization

Techniques include intrahepatic arterial injection of embolization particles alone, combined with chemotherapy, or linked with yttrium-90. Radioembolization outcomes are reported in Table 15A.15.

Table 15A.15 Radioembolization outcomes

Trial	Details
Saxena et al[a]	■ 25 Patients with unresectable ICC treated with resin-based Y90 spheres (SIRS spheres) ■ Median survival was 9.3 months ■ Peripheral tumor type and ECOG performance status 0 predicted for better survival ■ By RECIST, 6 (24%) patients with partial response; 11 (48%) patients with stable disease; 5 (20%) patients with progressive disease ■ Most common toxicities were fatigue (64%), abdominal pain (40%), grade 3 bilirubin, and albumin (8%)
Ibrahim et al[b]	■ 24 Patients with unresectable ICC treated with Y90 glass microspheres (Theraspheres) ■ Median survival was 14.9 months ■ On imaging follow-up of 22 patients, 6 patients (27%) with partial response, 15 patients (68%) with stable disease, and 1 (5%) patients with progressive disease by RECIST criteria ■ By EASL guidelines, 17 patients (77%) showed >50% tumor necrosis on imaging follow-up; 2 patients (9%) demonstrated 100% tumor necrosis ■ Median survival for patients with an ECOG performance status of 0, 1, and 2 was 31.8, 6.1, and 1 month, respectively ($p < 0.0001$) ■ Median survival for patients without and with portal vein thrombosis (PVT) was 31.8 and 5.7 months, respectively ($p < 0.0003$) ■ Median survival for patients with peripheral versus periductal-infiltrative tumors was 31.8 and 5.7 months, respectively ($p < 0.0005$)

ECOG: Eastern Cooperative Oncology Group; **RECIST**: response evaluation criteria in solid tumors; **EASL**: European Association for the Study of the Liver

[a] *Source: Saxena A, Bester L, Chau T et al (2010) Yttrium-90 radiotherapy for unresectable intrahepatic cholangiocarcinoma: a preliminary assessment of this novel treatment option. Ann Surg Oncol 17:484–491*

[b] *Source: Ibrahim SM, Mulcahy MF, Lewandowski RJ et al (2008) Treatment of unresectable cholangiocarcinoma using yttrium-90 microspheres: Results from a pilot study. Cancer 113:2119–28*

Radiation Therapy Techniques

Radiation Therapy for Adjuvant Therapy

Simulation and Field Arrangements

Radiation fields should encompass tumor bed plus regional lymph nodal areas for locoregional control (see section on staging, above, for regional lymphatics at risk). A CT scan (3- to 5-mm cut) with intravenous and oral contrast should be performed from the carina to the bottom of L5. Organs at risk (OARs; see Chap. 13, "Pancreatic Cancer," Table 13.13) should be delineated. Four-dimensional (4D) CT scans should be performed to assess tumor motion by respiration.

Dose and Treatment Delivery
Conventional fractionation to a total dose of 45–50.4 Gy is recommended after R0 resection, using high-energy (≥10 MVx) photon. For R1 or R2 resection, a boost to residual tumor with a 2cm margin (surgical clips) to 54–60 Gy is recommended

Intensity-Modulated Radiation Therapy
The benefit of intensity-modulated radiation therapy (IMRT) and the delineation of clinical target volume (CTV) for treatment have not been fully addressed. If used, tumor or tumor bed and subclinical target volumes including lymphatic draining regions (porta hepatic, periduodenal, peripancreatic, periaortic, pericaval, celiac, and superior mesenteric) should be delineated as CTV.

Radiation Therapy for Unresectable Disease

Simulation and Target Volume Delineation

Simulation in unresectable cases is similar to that for adjuvant treatment. Fusion of positron-emission (PET)-CT scan in the treatment planning position can allow for more accurate delineation of GTV and gross nodal disease if they are fluorodeoxyglucose (FDG) avid. Comparing to conventional technique, 3D-CRT or IMRT directed to the gross tumor volume (GTV) with a margin can reduce the dose to the OARs, thereby improving the therapeutic ratio and facilitating dose escalation. Definitions of GTV (or GITV if using 4D-CT), CTV, and planning target volume (PTV) in 3D-CRT and IMRT are as follow:

- GTV: gross tumor on imaging studies and accounting for respiratory motion (GITV)
- CTV: GTV plus regional lymphatics plus 1 cm or GITV plus regional lymphatics plus 0.5 cm (with daily image guidance)
- PTV: CTV plus 0.5–1 cm.

Dose and Treatment Delivery

A total dose of 50.4–59.4 Gy in 30–33 fractions with seven to nine co-planar fields can be used according to the shape of the PTV (Figure 15A.2). If external biliary catheters traverse the tumor, treat the PTV to 45–50.4 Gy in 1.8-Gy fractions, followed by high-dose rate (HDR) brachytherapy boost of 10–20 Gy total. Alternatively, dose-painting IMRT can be utilized where the GTV plus small margin is treated to 60 Gy in 2-Gy fractions concurrently with regional lymphatics being treated to 51–54 Gy in 1.7- to 1.8-Gy fractions. All treatment is done concurrently with fluoropyrimidine-based chemotherapy.

Normal Tissue Tolerance

OARs in both adjuvant and definitive settings, include small bowel, liver, kidneys, stomach, and spinal cord, as detailed in Chapter 12, "Gastric Cancer," Table 12.18.

Follow-Up

The poor prognosis of cholangiocarcinoma dictates that close follow-up after completion of treatment is needed. Schedule and suggested examinations during follow-up are presented in Table 15A.16.

Common radiation-induced adverse effects include nausea, vomiting, abdominal discomfort/pain, radiation-induced liver disease, etc. Due to the poor prognosis, reports on long-term complication are rare.

Table 15A.16 Follow-up schedule and examinations

Schedule	Frequency
First follow-up	■ 4–6 Weeks after radiation therapy
Years 0–1	■ Every 3–4 months
Years 2–5	■ Every 6 months
Years 5+	■ Annually
Examinations	
History and physical	■ Complete history and physical examination
Laboratory tests	■ Complete blood counts (CBC) and serum chemistry ■ Liver and renal function tests ■ CA 19-9 (if clinically indicated)
Imaging studies	■ Chest X-ray (if clinically indicated) ■ CT of the abdomen and pelvis (if clinically indicated)

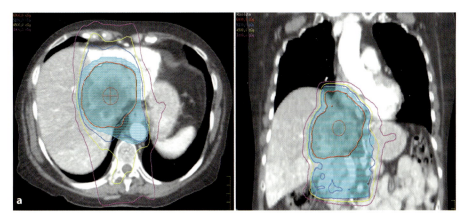

b Dose Volume Histogram

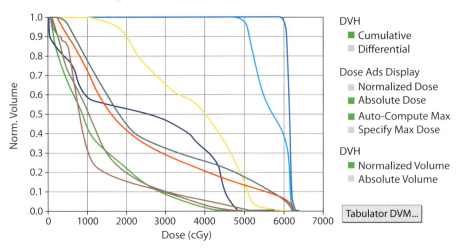

DVH
- ■ Cumulative
- ▫ Differential

Dose Ads Display
- ▫ Normalized Dose
- ■ Absolute Dose
- ■ Auto-Compute Max
- ▫ Specify Max Dose

DVH
- ■ Normalized Volume
- ▫ Absolute Volume

Tabulator DVM...

ROI Statistics

Line Type	ROI	Trial	Min	Max	Mean	Std. Cev	% Out- side crid	% > Max	Generalized CUD
▬	Cord	appr60Gy	35.9	4941.4	2286.2	1824.9	0.00 %	0.00 %	2344.06
▬	Heart	appr60Gy	171.7	6260.6	2307.2	1764.6	0.00 %	0.00 %	2307.22
▬	Lt Kidney	appr60Gy	76.1	4871.5	1147.4	1000.9	0.00 %	0.00 %	1146.9
▬	PTV51	appr60Gy	3641.4	6389.2	5681.8	422.3	0.00 %	0.00 %	5683.59
▬	PTV60	appr60Gy	5624.7	6389.2	6134.0	54.4	0.00 %	0.00 %	6135.14
▬	RT Kidney	appr60Gy	76.2	4708.6	1193.2	1031.2	0.00 %	0.00 %	1192.15
▬	Stomach	appr60Gy	863.3	6111.1	3684.4	1212.7	0.00 %	0.00 %	3684.6
▬	bowel	appr60Gy	64.6	5548.9	1333.0	1137.7	0.00 %	0.00 %	1332.82
▬	liver-gtv	appr60Gy	201.1	6389.2	2542.3	1827.5	0.00 %	0.00 %	2542.39

Figure 15A.2 **a** Dose-painted IMRT for a patient with unresectable ICC with hilar lymphadenopathy. Seven coplanar fields used to avoid excessive dose to liver, bilateral kidneys, and small intestine. Radiation treatments were concurrent with capecitabine. Prescribed dose was 60 Gy (2 Gy per fraction) to tumor (PTV60) and 51 Gy (1.7 Gy per fraction) to the lymphatics (PTV51) (hilar, periaortic, pericaval, celiac, SMA) in 30 fractions. **b** DVH of the same plan

15B Gallbladder Carcinoma

Steven E. Finkelstein[1] and Sarah E. Hoffe[2]

Key Points

- Cancer of the gallbladder is rare worldwide, with a higher incidence in Asia, Eastern Europe, and South America. It is twice as common in women as in men, and the mean age at diagnosis is ~70 years.

- Gallstones and chronic inflammation are predisposing factors. In addition, ~50% of gallbladder cancers are diagnosed incidentally in gallbladders removed because of cholelithiasis.

- Early-stage diseases usually have no specific symptoms; thus, early diagnosis is uncommon. Common signs and symptoms in advanced cases incorporate those signs and symptoms seen in benign gallbladder disease.

- Accurate diagnosis is based on history and physical examination, laboratory, and imaging studies. Endoscopic retrograde cholangiopancreatography (ERCP) and percutaneous transhepatic cholangiography (PTHC) can be used to determine the location of biliary obstruction and perform drainage, as well as to obtain pathological diagnosis.

- Stage at diagnosis is the most important prognosticator and predicts the resectability of the tumor. Gallbladder cancer spreads via lymphatics and hematogenous routes in the early course of the disease.

- Overall survival of patients with T1N0 disease is ~50%, but prognoses of more advanced cases are dismal. The overall median survival is ~10 months.

- Commonly observed metastatic sites include liver, peritoneum, and lung. Metastasis to other organs/tissues is uncommon.

- Treatment of gallbladder cancer depends on the stage at diagnosis. Surgery is the only curative treatment for localized diseases. T1, T2, and some T3 gallbladder cancer are resectable. Completeness of resection (R0 versus R1 or R2 resection) is prognostically important.

- Adjuvant chemoradiation therapy may improve survival in patients with T2–3 and N+ diseases. For marginally resectable or unresectable diseases (i.e., T4 tumors), neoadjuvant treatment using gemcitabine followed by chemoradiation (fluorouracil [5-FU]-based) may improve resectability. Chemotherapy and palliative radiation therapy are the mainstay treatment for metastatic gallbladder cancer.

[1] Steven E. Finkelstein, MD (✉)
Email: steven.finkelstein@moffitt.org

[2] Sarah E. Hoffe, MD
Email: sarah.hoffe@moffitt.org

J. J. Lu, L. W. Brady (Eds.), *Decision Making in Radiation Oncology*
DOI: 10.1007/978-3-642-13832-4_17, © Springer-Verlag Berlin Heidelberg 2011

Epidemiology and Etiology

A number of risk factors have been identified for gallbladder cancer (Table 15B.1). Chronic inflammation of the gallbladder, which can be associated with gallstones, is a leading cause.

Table 15B.1 Risk factors of gallbladder cancer

Factor	Description
Patient related	**Age and gender:** Women are more commonly diagnosed than men are, with a female to male ratio of >2:1. The average age at diagnosis is 73 years
	Lifestyle: Obesity is a risk factor. This risk factor also increases the potential for a patient to develop gallstones, which is associated with gallbladder cancer
	Family medical history: Family history of gallbladder cancer is thought to increase risk
	Past medical history: gallstones, gallbladder polyps, calcified gallbladder also known as porcelain gallbladder. Patients who are chronically infected with salmonella (bacterium that causes typhoid) or typhoid carriers are at increased risk. Choledochal cysts and other bile duct anatomic abnormalities associated with bile reflux
	Genetic predisposition: The highest incidence in the USA is seen in Mexican and Native Americans, while African-Americans have the lowest incidence. Since the incidence is greater in women, studies are now evaluating the expression of estrogen receptor (ER) beta to explore association with prognosis
Environmental	**Industrial chemicals:** Animal studies suggest nitrosamine exposure. Studies also suggest that workers in the rubber and textile industries have a higher risk. More data are needed to confirm these factors

Anatomy

The human gallbladder measures 8 cm in length and 4 cm in diameter when it is fully distended. It functions to store bile, which is produced in the liver. Bile contains substances that allow fats to be emulsified. The gallbladder releases bile when food-containing fat enters the digestive tract.

The gallbladder has three parts: a fundus, body, and neck, which tapers and connects to the biliary tree via the cystic duct (Figure 15B.1). It lies under the liver in line with Cantlie's line, which forms the physiologic division of the liver into right and left lobes. The gallbladder straddles the Couinaud segments IVb and V, such that partial hepatic resection of these areas is often required.

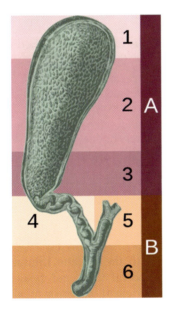

Figure 15B.1 Structures of gallbladder and bile ducts. *A* Gallbladder: *1* fundus, *2* body, *3* neck; *B* bile ducts (extrahepatic): *4* cystic duct, *5* common hepatic duct, *6* common bile duct

Pathology

Carcinomas account for 98% of gallbladder cancers, and ~80% are adenocarcinoma of ductal origin. Microscopic appearance of these adenocarcinomas can range from papillary to poorly differentiated and undifferentiated. Other histologies include squamous cell or mixed tumors. Squamous cell carcinomas have a low metastatic potential, unlike their poorly differentiated adenocarcinoma counterparts. Rare histologies have been reported, such as primary neuroendocrine cancers including carcinoid and small cell.

Routes of Spread

The predominant pattern of spread in gallbladder cancer is locoregional (Table 15B.2). The majority of cancers are found to have direct extension into the liver.

Table 15B.2 Routes of spread in gallbladder cancer

Route	Description
Local extension	■ Direct involvement of adjacent liver can occur and is not considered distant metastasis ■ Direct involvement can also occur to other adjacent organs such as colon, duodenum, stomach, common bile duct, abdominal wall, and diaphragm, and is reflected in the T stage ■ There is no serosa on the gallbladder on the side attached to the liver
Regional lymph node metastasis	■ Regional nodes for gallbladder cancer are restricted to the hepatic hilus. This includes nodes along the common bile duct, hepatic artery, portal vein, and cystic duct ■ Distant nodes include the celiac, periduodenal, peripancreatic, and superior mesenteric artery nodes
Distant metastasis	■ The most common sites of hematogenous metastasis are peritoneum, liver, lungs, and pleura

Lymph Node Metastasis

Regional nodal involvement can occur with spread to the hepatic hilum. Nodes along the common bile duct, hepatic artery, portal vein, and cystic duct are considered regional N1 nodes. Periaortic, pericaval, superior mesenteric artery, and/or celiac artery lymph nodes are considered regional N2 nodes. Any involvement of regional N2 nodes places the patient into the stage IVB category.

Diagnosis, Staging, and Prognosis

Clinical Presentation

As many as 50% of gallbladder cancer cases are found at pathologic analysis after simple cholecystectomy for presumed benign disease. Early gallbladder cancers are usually asymptomatic. In cases more advanced, symptoms are similar to those of benign gallbladder diseases (Table 15B.3).

Table 15B.3 Commonly observed signs and symptoms in gallbladder cancer

Type	Description
Symptoms	■ Abdominal pain ■ Jaundice ■ Anorexia ■ Weight loss ■ Nausea and vomiting
Signs	■ Abdominal tenderness ■ Palpable abdominal mass ■ Hepatomegaly ■ Jaundice ■ Fever

Diagnosis and Staging

Figure 15B.2 illustrates the diagnostic procedure of gallbladder cancer, including suggested examination and tests. The difficulty in diagnosing gallbladder cancer arises because the signs and symptoms can mimic those of benign disease.

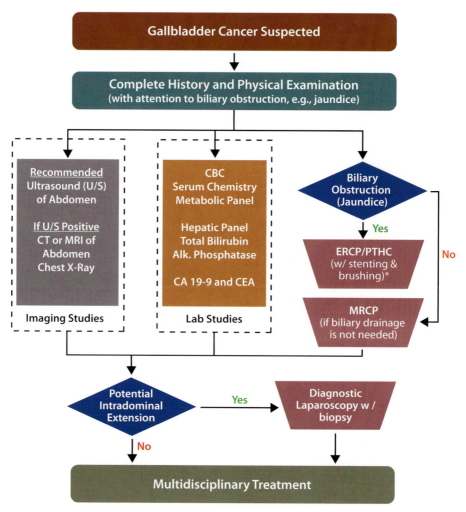

Figure 15B.2 A proposed algorithm for diagnosis and staging for gallbladder cancer. During ERCP or PTHC, brushings can be done to sample the bile to examine tumor cells within the fluid. A fine-needle aspiration (FNA) biopsy can be done at the time of endoscopic ultrasound or at a diagnostic laparoscopy. If biliary drainage is not needed, an MRCP can be performed to evaluate the gallbladder and adjacent ductal system. *ERCP* endoscopic retrograde cholangiopancreatography, *PTHC* percutaneous transhepatic cholangiography, *MRCP* MRI cholangiopancreatography

Tumor, Node, and Metastasis Staging

Diagnosis and clinical staging depends on findings from history and physical examination, imaging, and lab tests. Pathological staging depends on findings during surgical resection and pathological examination, in addition to those required in clinical staging.

The 7th edition of the tumor, node, and metastasis (TNM) staging and grouping system of the American Joint Committee on cancer (AJCC) is presented in Tables 15B.4 and 15B.5.

Table 15B.4 AJCC TNM classification of gallbladder carcinoma

Stage	Description
Primary tumor (T)	
TX	Primary tumor cannot be assessed
T0	No evidence of primary tumor
Tis	Carcinoma in situ
T1	Tumor invades lamina propria or muscular layer
T1a	Tumor invades lamina propria
T1b	Tumor invades muscular layer
T2	Tumor invades perimuscular connective tissue; no extension beyond serosa or into liver
T3	Tumor perforates the serosa (visceral peritoneum) and/or directly invades the liver and/or one other adjacent organ or structure, such as the stomach, duodenum, colon, pancreas, omentum, or extrahepatic bile ducts
T4	Tumor invades main portal vein or hepatic artery or invades two or more extrahepatic organs or structures
Regional lymph nodes (N)	
NX	Regional lymph nodes cannot be assessed
N0	No regional lymph node metastasis
N1	Metastases to nodes along the cystic duct, common bile duct, hepatic artery, and/or portal vein
N2	Metastases to periaortic, pericaval, superior mesenteric artery, and/or celiac artery lymph nodes
Distant metastasis (M)	
MX	Distant metastasis cannot be assessed
M0	No distant metastasis
M1	Distant metastasis

Source: Edge SB, Byrd DR, Compton CC et al (2009) American Joint Committee on Cancer, American Cancer Society. AJCC cancer staging manual, 7th edn. Springer, Berlin Heidelberg New York

Table 15B.5 Stage grouping of gallbladder carcinoma

Stage Grouping				
	T1a/b	T2	T3	T4
N0	I	II	IIIA	IVA
N1	IIIB	IIIB	IIIB	IVA
N2	IVB	IVB	IVB	IVB
M1	IVB	IVB	IVB	IVB

Source: Edge SB, Byrd DR, Compton CC et al (2009) American Joint Committee on Cancer, American Cancer Society. AJCC cancer staging manual, 7th edn. Springer, Berlin Heidelberg New York

Prognosis

Stage at diagnosis and completeness of surgical resection are strong prognosticators for gallbladder cancer. The 5-year survival is ~50% for T1 tumors; however, prognosis is usually dismal in advanced disease.

The results of a review of 435 patients are presented in Tables 15B.6 and 15B.7.

Table 15B.6 Results of the Memorial Sloan–Kettering Cancer Center series of 435 gallbladder cancer cases

Trial	Findings
Duffy et al	■ Surgery: ~50% of diseases were diagnosed incidentally at laparoscopic cholecystectomy ■ Re-exploration showed residual disease in ~75% of patients; 123 patients underwent curative resections ■ Adjuvant therapy: Of the 123 patients after curative resection, 6.5% of patients were treated with adjuvant chemotherapy, 6.5% adjuvant chemoradiation alone, and 6.5% both chemoradiation and systemic chemotherapy Efficacy of adjuvant therapy remained unknown due to limited number of patients ■ Survival: Median survival was significantly better for patients who had no disease on re-exploration (72 months) compared with those with residual disease (14.6 months). ■ MS were 12.9 and 5.8 months for stages I–III, and IV diseases, respectively.

MSKCC: Memorial Sloan–Kettering Cancer Center; **MS**: medial survival

Source: Duffy A, Capanu M, Abou-Alfa GK et al (2008) Gallbladder cancer (GBC): 10-year experience at Memorial Sloan–Kettering Cancer Centre (MSKCC). J Surg Oncol 98:485–489

Table 15B.7 Treatment modalities used in gallbladder cancer

Modality	Description
Cholecystectomy/en bloc hepatic resection/regional node dissection	
Indications	■ The only curative treatment modality ■ For T1 disease, simple cholecystectomy ■ For T2 or T3 disease, radical cholecystectomy with en bloc hepatic resection and regional node dissection ■ Incidentally diagnosed disease (T2 or above) requires re-resection ■ Patients who undergo re-resection experience the same survival as those who undergo primary resection
Facts	■ Mortality is low in experienced hands ■ Completeness of resection (R0 versus R1/R2) is a strong prognostic indicator
Radiation therapy	
Indications	■ Adjuvant treatment after resection (with 5-FU-based chemotherapy) ■ Neoadjuvant radiation (with 5-FU) either upfront or after systemic gemcitabine-based therapy ■ Definitive treatment with a 5-FU-based regimen either up front for unresectable disease or after systemic gemcitabine-based chemotherapy ■ Palliative treatment to primary or metastatic foci
Techniques	■ EBRT using 3D-CRT or IMRT ■ Motion management strategies accounting for respiration ■ Consideration of daily image guidance strategies
Chemo-/targeted therapy	
Indications	■ Adjuvant treatment after surgery (with EBRT) ■ After adjuvant chemoradiation ■ Treatment with concurrent EBRT for unresectable disease, either up front or after gemcitabine initial therapy ■ Mainstay treatment for palliative therapy
Medication	■ Gemcitabine is the mainstay medication for chemotherapy in advanced gallbladder/hepatobiliary cancer ■ It significantly improves treatment outcome in patients with advanced hepatobiliary cancer

Sources: Valle JW, Wasan H, Johnson P et al (2009) Gemcitabine alone or in combination with cisplatin in patients with advanced or metastatic cholangiocarcinomas or other biliary tract tumors: a multicentre randomized phase II study – the UK ABC-01 Study. Br J Cancer 101:621–627; Jang JS, Lim HY, Hwang IG et al (2010) Gemcitabine and oxaliplatin in patients with unresectable biliary cancer including gallbladder cancer: a Korean Cancer Study Group phase II trial. Cancer Chemother Pharmacol 65:641–647

Treatment

Principles and Practice

Surgery remains the cornerstone of therapy in this disease. The oncologic goal would be to achieve an R0 resection with a radical cholecystectomy with negative margins, and to avoid an R1 (microscopically positive margins) and R2 (grossly positive margins) resection.

A proposed treatment algorithm based on the best available clinical evidence is presented in Figure 15B.3. Treatment modalities and strategies are listed in Table 15B.8.

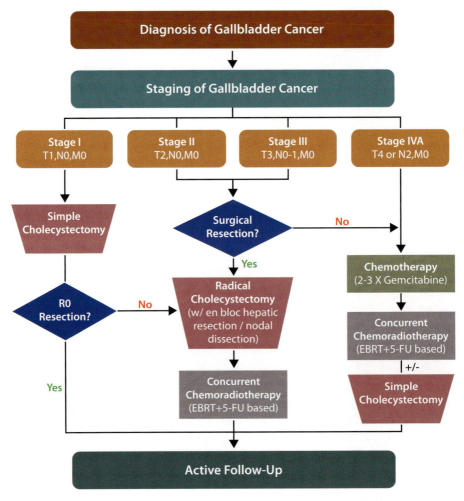

Figure 15B.3 A proposed treatment algorithm for treatment of gallbladder adenocarcinoma

Table 15B.8 Treatment strategies for *resectable* gallbladder cancer and supporting clinical evidence

Non-randomized Trial	Description
Mayo Clinic (Kresl et al)a	▪ 21 consecutive patients (majority had pathologic stages III–IV disease who were treated with adjuvant chemo-RT ▪ Median dose was 54 Gy using EBRT ▪ 5-Year OS was 65% for stages I–III versus 0% for stage IV ($p < 0.02$) ▪ 5-Year local control rate was 100% for EBRT doses >54 Gy versus 65% for lower doses
Mayo Clinic (Gold et al)b	▪ Retrospective review of 73 R0 resections of gallbladder carcinoma cases included T1–3, N0–1 diseases ▪ 25 Patients received adjuvant chemoradiation: EBRT median dose 50.4 Gy with concurrent 5-FU ▪ Median OS was 4.8 years for adjuvant therapy versus 4.2 years after surgery alone ($p = 0.56$) ▪ After adjusting for stage parameters and histology, there is the suggestion that adjuvant chemoradiation might improve OS for these patients
Dukec	▪ Retrospective review of patients who underwent surgery and adjuvant therapy over 23-year period ▪ 22 Patients with primary and non-metastatic gallbladder cancer were identified, who were treated ▪ 18 Patients received EBRT plus 5-FU chemotherapy: Median radiation dose 45Gy ▪ 5-Year actuarial local control rate was 59% ▪ 5-Year actuarial OS, DFS, MFS rates were 37, 33, and 36%, respectively. MS for all patients 1.9 years
SEERd	▪ SEER database queried from 1992 to 2002 for retrospective analysis of patients with gallbladder carcinoma ▪ The end point of the study was OS ▪ There were 3,187 cases in the registry: of the surgical group, 35, 36, 6, and 21% had stages I, II, III, and IV, respectively ▪ Adjuvant RT was used in 17% of cases ▪ MS improved with adjuvant RT (14 versus 8 months) ($p < 0.001$) ▪ The survival benefit was only seen in those patients presenting with regional spread and with tumors infiltrating the liver ▶

Table 15B.8 *(continued)*

Non-randomized Trial	Description
Prediction model[e]	■ Regression model constructed to enable individualized predictions of the net survival benefit of adjuvant RT ■ Multivariate Cox proportional hazards model was constructed using data from 4,180 patients from 1988 to 2003 in the SEER database ■ On multivariate analysis, the model showed that age, sex, papillary histology, stage, and adjuvant RT were significant predictors of overall survival ■ The model predicts that adjuvant RT provides a survival benefit in node positive or ^{3}T2 disease

RT: radiation therapy; **EBRT:** external-beam RT; **MS:** median survival; **OS:** overall survival; **DFS:** disease-free survival; **MFS:** metastatic-free survival

[a] *Source: Kresl JJ, Schild SE, Henning GT et al (2002) Adjuvant EBRT with concurrent chemotherapy in the management of gallbladder carcinoma. Int J Radiat Oncol Biol Phys 52:167–175*

[b] *Source: Gold DG, Miller RC, Haddock MG et al (2009) Adjuvant therapy for gallbladder carcinoma: the Mayo Clinic Experience. Int J Radiat Oncol Biol Phys 75:150–155*

[c] *Source: Czito BG, Hurwitz HI, Clough RW et al (2005) Adjuvant EBRT with concurrent chemotherapy after resection of primary gallbladder carcinoma: a 23-year experience. Int J Radiat Oncol Biol Phys 62:1030–1034*

[d] *Source: Mojica P, Smith D, Ellenhorn J et al (2007) Adjuvant RT is associated with improved survival for gallbladder carcinoma with regional metastatic disease. J Surg Oncol 96:8–13*

[e] *Source: Wang SJ, Fuller CD, Kim JS et al (2008) Prediction model for estimating the survival benefit of adjuvant RT for gallbladder cancer. J Clin Oncol 26:2112–2117*

Treatment of Resectable Gallbladder Cancer (T1–3, N0–1, M0)

Most patients with this disease present at an advanced stage, thus only about a third of patients are surgical candidates. Multidisciplinary review of imaging studies can facilitate understanding of the extent of disease and whether the disease is operable. Staging laparoscopy may be useful in this setting because there is a high rate of occult metastasis.

Adjuvant Treatment

Clinical evidence for adjuvant therapy in resectable gallbladder cancer is presented below. There are no randomized trials, and data are from single-institutional series.

Neoadjuvant Treatment

Although neoadjuvant chemotherapy or chemoradiation may benefit marginally resectable gallbladder cancer, there is no clear consensus on the optimal strategy.

Possible strategies would initiate with conformal external beam radiation targeting gross disease and regional lymph nodes, with concurrent fluorouracil (5-FU)-based chemotherapy.

Alternatively, chemoradiation could be delivered after an initial gemcitabine-based chemotherapy of two to three cycles. This may facilitate improved treatment geometry and determine whether the patient will be found to have occult metastatic progression during this time. If neoadjuvant chemotherapy proceeds well, consolidation chemoradiation would be recommended.

Treatment of Non-metastatic but Unresectable Gallbladder Cancer (T4, N0–1, M0)

Most patients with locoregionally advanced gallbladder cancer are unresectable. The efficacy of combined chemoradiation therapy has been suggested with single institutional reports (Table 15B.9). Efficacy of gemcitabine-based combinations has been reported as well.

Table 15B.9 Clinical evidence for the treatment of *unresectable* locoregionally advanced gallbladder cancer

Trial	Description
University of Texas at San Antonio[a]	■ Single institutional review of 24 patients with primary disease were treated with image guided IMRT between 2001 and 2005 ■ Evaluated biliary adenocarcinomas, including gallbladder and extrahepatic cholangiocarcinomas ■ Data from a series of 24 patients treated conventionally from 1995 to 2005 were compared ■ A higher mean dose was given to patients treated with IMRT versus patients treated conventionally, 59 versus 48 Gy ■ IMRT patients had a median survival of 17.6 versus 9.0 months in the conventional group
UK ABC-01[b]	■ Evaluated the activity of gemcitabine (G) and cisplatin/gemcitabine (C/G) in patients with locally advanced or metastatic advanced biliary cancers ■ Randomized 86 patients to either G (1,000 mg/m2 on days 1, 8, and15 every 28 days) or C (25 mg/m2), followed by G (1,000 mg/m2 on days 1 and 8, every 21 days) ■ Treatment was for 6 months or disease progression ■ Median time to progression (TTP) (8 versus 4 months) and 6 month PFS (57.1 versus 45.5%) favored combined chemotherapy

IMRT: intensity-modulated radiation therapy

[a] *Source: Fuller CD, Dang ND, Wang SJ et al (2009) Image guided IMRT for biliary adenocarcinomas: Initial clinical results. Radiother Oncol 92:249–254*

[b] *Source: Valle JW, Wasan H, Johnson P et al (2009) Gemcitabine alone or in combination with cisplatin in patients with advanced or metastatic cholangiocarcinomas or other biliary tract tumors: a multicentre randomized phase II study – the UK ABC-01 Study. Br J Cancer 101:621–627*

Radiation Therapy Techniques

Radiation Therapy for Adjuvant Therapy

Simulation and Field Arrangements

Techniques of computed tomography (CT) simulation are similar to those used in radiation therapy for cholangiocarcinoma.

Given abdominal motion with respiration, motion management strategy should be used prior to simulation, as detailed in the "Simulation and Field Arrangements" section of Chap. 14, "Hepatocellular Carcinoma."

Dose and Treatment Delivery

Conventional fractionation to a total dose of 45–50.4Gy is recommended after R0 resection, using high-energy (≥10 MVx) photons. Boost to 54 Gy to residual tumor (surgical clips) is recommended after R1 or R2 resection, as long as constraints can be met.

Intensity-Modulated Radiation Therapy
With intensity-modulated radiation therapy (IMRT), the option of dose painting can be utilized so that the site of highest risk (the preoperative site of disease) can receive 2.0 Gy per fraction, while the elective sites receive 1.8 Gy per fraction.

Target volumes and delineation techniques are detailed in Table 15B.10. Figure 15B.4 presents a case of T2N1M0 gallbladder treated with surgery and adjuvant IMRT.

Table 15B.10 Target volumes used in adjuvant treatment

Target volume	Description
Preoperative GTV	■ Review preoperative CT/MRI and determine the initial extent of disease ■ Compare the preoperative films with the postoperative location of clips ■ Delineate the preoperative gross tumor volume ■ Consider 4D CT simulation or respiratory gating techniques upfront to account for respiratory motion
CTV	■ Delineate the tumor bed encompassing the preoperative GTV as above ■ Delineate the nodes which have traditionally been included in adjuvant field design: porta hepatis, periocholedochal, celiac, and pancreaticoduodenal ■ Consider whether an internal CTV will be used or whether CTV in phase used for gated treatment will be delineated
PTV	■ Determine amount of respiratory movement with 4D CT if available. If not, take patient to fluoroscopy and image motion of clips ■ If movement >5 mm, decide if treatment will be delivered with 3D-CRT or IMRT with respiratory motion strategies: abdominal compression, gating the patient or gating the machine ■ Individualize PTV margin based on treatment strategy ■ All fields should be irradiated on daily basis if 3D conformal plan ■ If IMRT plan, take motion into account for planning and delivery ■ Most series treated in the adjuvant setting have used 45 Gy, with multiple field techniques followed by a boost to a reduced field of 5.4–9.0 Gy

3D-CRT: three-dimensional conformal radiation therapy

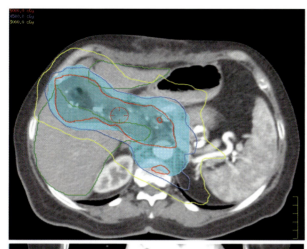

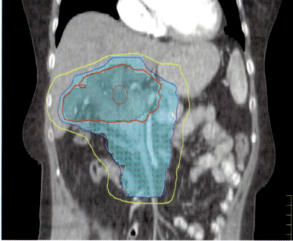

Figure 15B.4 Transverse and coronal view of a 64-year-old female patient with poorly differentiated T2N1M0 resected adenocarcinoma of the gallbladder. Postoperative multileaf collimator (MLC)-based IMRT radiation was delivered with dose painting: Preoperative GTV received 50 Gy and CTV received 45Gy in 25 fractions, using daily image guidance with cone beam CT and abdominal compression. Abdominal compression used because maximal motions of targets on 4D CT scan was 1.0 cm. Patient treated concurrently with continuous infusion 5-FU, and only complained of fatigue during radiation

Radiation Therapy for Unresectable Disease

Simulation and Target Volume Delineation

Either three-dimensional (3D) conformal techniques or IMRT techniques are preferable to minimize the dose to the normal tissue in the upper abdomen. Simulation and target volume delineation techniques are similar to those used in adjuvant radiation therapy.

Dose and Treatment Delivery

Microscopic disease should be treated to 45–50.4 Gy in standard fractionation. Gross disease should be treated to higher doses, preferably at least 50–54 Gy. Higher doses of up to 59.4 Gy can be considered if normal tissue constraints are not exceeded.

Normal Tissue Tolerance

Organs at risk (OARs) in radiation therapy of upper abdominal cancers are detailed in Chapter 12, "Gastric Cancer."

Follow-Up

The dismal prognosis of gallbladder cancer dictates close follow-up after completion of treatment. Schedules and suggested examinations during follow-up are similar to those after treatment for cholangiocarcinoma, and are presented in Table 15B.11.

Table 15B.11 Follow-up schedule and examinations

Schedule	Frequency
First follow-up	■ 4–6 Weeks after radiation therapy
Years 0–1	■ Every 3–4 months
Years 2–5	■ Every 6 months
Years 5+	■ Annually
Examinations	
History and physical	■ Complete history and physical examination
Laboratory tests	■ Complete blood counts (*CBC*) and serum chemistry ■ Liver and renal function tests ■ CA 19-9 (if clinically indicated)
Imaging studies	■ Chest X-ray (if clinically indicated) ■ CT of the abdomen and pelvis (if clinically indicated)

16

Rectal Cancer

Edward Kim[1] and Luther W. Brady[2]

Key Points

- Colorectal cancer is the third most commonly diagnosed malignancy in the USA, and ~41,000 new cases of rectal cancer were diagnosed in the USA in 2009.

- Typical presenting symptoms include frank bleeding from the rectum, constipation, diarrhea, narrowing of stool caliber, and pain.

- The majority of colorectal cancers are sporadic, with only ~5% of patients possessing known hereditary syndromes such as hereditary non-polyposis colorectal cancer (HNPCC) or familial adenomatous polyposis (FAP).

- Accurate clinical staging by physical examination, endoscopic ultrasound, and computed tomography (CT) imaging is critical in selecting patients who may benefit from neoadjuvant chemoradiation.

- Stage at presentation is highly prognostic.

- Preoperative radiation therapy (with and without chemotherapy) has been shown to improve local control and survival over surgery alone for locally advanced tumors.

- Postoperative chemoradiation therapy has been shown to improve local control and survival over surgery alone.

- Neoadjuvant chemoradiation for locally advanced rectal cancers has been demonstrated to improve local control over postoperative chemoradiation and is the current standard of care for patients with locally advanced rectal cancers.

- Patients with limited metastatic disease to the liver that are able to undergo resection may have a 15–20% chance of long-term survival.

[1] Edward Kim, MD
Email: edykim@uw.edu

[2] Luther W. Brady, MD (✉)
Email: lbrady@drexelmed.edu

J. J. Lu, L. W. Brady (Eds.), *Decision Making in Radiation Oncology*
DOI: 10.1007/978-3-642-13832-4_18, © Springer-Verlag Berlin Heidelberg 2011

Epidemiology and Etiology

There were an estimated 40,870 cases of rectal cancer diagnosed in the USA in 2009. The majority of newly diagnosed colorectal cancers are sporadic (~75%). Earlier diagnoses can occur in men and women with genetic disorders that carry a predisposition for colorectal cancers such as hereditary non-polyposis colorectal cancer (HNPCC) or familial adenomatous polyposis (FAP).

Table 16.1 Risk factors of rectal cancer

Factor	Description
Patient related	**Age and gender:** typically diagnosed in patients older than 50 years of age. Slightly more common in male patients
	Lifestyle: possibly associated with high-fat and low-residue diets
	Past personal or family medical history: ~15–20% of patients with a family history of malignancy or personal history of polyps, ~ 5% with FAP or HNPCC, and ~1% associated with inflammatory bowel disease, particularly ulcerative colitis
Genetic predispositions	**FAP:** mutation in the APC gene on chromosome 5 or MUTYH on chromosome 1. Patients develop hundreds of polyps throughout the small and large intestine. Risk of colorectal cancer is 100% without intervention. Consider prophylactic colectomy
	Gardner's syndrome: phenotypic variant of FAP
	HNPCC: Also known as Lynch syndrome, caused by mutations in DNA mismatch repair genes, with an 80% lifetime risk of colorectal cancer and increased risk of ovarian and endometrial cancer
	Peutz-Jeghers syndrome: Patients form polyps throughout the intestines, with ~50% lifetime risk of cancer

HNPCC: hereditary non-polyposis colon cancer

A number of risk factors have been identified for rectal cancer (Table 16.1). Certain factors may indicate a higher probability of HNPCC, and their pathologic specimens should be tested for microsatellite instability or immunohistochemistry to identify protein expression for the mismatch genes known to be mutated in HNPCC (*MLH1, MSH2, MSH6,* and *PMS2*). These factors are summarized in the Table 16.2.

Table 16.2 Factors indicate a higher probability of HNPCC

Type	Description
Bethesda Criteria for testing tumors for MSI	■ Colorectal cancer in a patient younger than 50 years of age
	■ Presence of synchronous or metachronous HNPCC-associated tumors, regardless of age (colorectal, endometrial, gastric, ovarian, pancreas, ureter, renal pelvis, biliary tract, brain, and small intestine malignancies)
	■ Colorectal cancer with features suggestive of MSI in a patient younger than 60 years of age: tumor-infiltrating lymphocytes, Crohn's-like lymphocytic reaction, mucinous/signet ring differentiation, or medullary growth pattern)
	■ Colorectal cancer in a patient with 1 or more 1st-degree relatives with an HNPCC related cancer with 1 of the cancers diagnosed before age 50
	■ Colorectal cancer in a patient with 2 or more 1st- or 2nd-degree relatives with HNPCC-related cancers, regardless of age
Revised Amsterdam Criteria for HNPCC	■ At least 3 relatives must have a cancer associated with HNPCC (colorectal, endometrial, small bowel, ureter, renal pelvis) and all of the following factors: ■ One must be a 1st-degree relative of the other 2 ■ At least 2 successive generations are affected ■ At least 1 of the relatives with cancer associated with HNPCC should be diagnosed before the age of 50 ■ FAP should be excluded

HNPCC: hereditary non-polyposis colorectal cancer; **MSI**: microsatellite instability; **FAP**: familial adenomatous polyposis 0

Anatomy

The rectum extends from the top of the anorectal ring distally to the puborec-talis muscle palpable on digital rectal examination (Figure 16.1). Historically, tumors below the peritoneal reflection have been treated as *rectal cancers,* while tumors above the reflection have been treated as *colon cancers.* Euro-pean and North American trials, respectively, have used a cutoff of 16 or 12 cm above the anal verge to define rectal tumors.

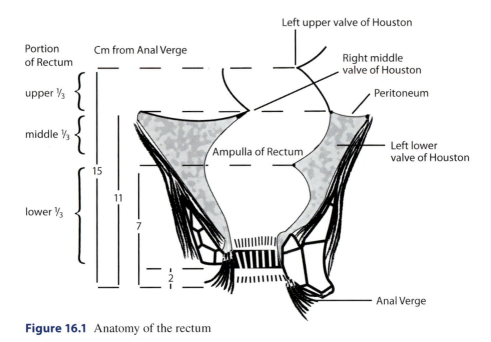

Figure 16.1 Anatomy of the rectum

Pathology

More than 90% of rectal cancers are adenocarcinoma, and thus form the focus of this chapter. Colloid histology is seen in 15–20% of cases, but this does not affect prognosis, and signet ring cell histology has been associated with a poorer prognosis.

Other histologies include carcinoid, leiomyosarcomas, lymphomas, and squamous cell cancers.

Routes of Spread

Local extension, regional (lymphatic), and distant (hematogenous) metastases are the three major routes of spread in rectal cancer. Common sites of distant metastasis include liver and lung (Table 16.3; Figure 16.2).

Table 16.3 Routes of distant spread in rectal cancer

Tumor	Routes
Proximal tumors	More likely to drain via the superior rectal vessels to the inferior mesenteric vessels and ultimately, the portal vein and liver
Distal tumors	More likely to travel along the internal iliac vessels to the upper pelvic nodes and then the para-aortic nodes
Large primary	Involvement of the external iliac and inguinal nodes is unlikely, except for T4 lesions or lesions that involve the anal canal

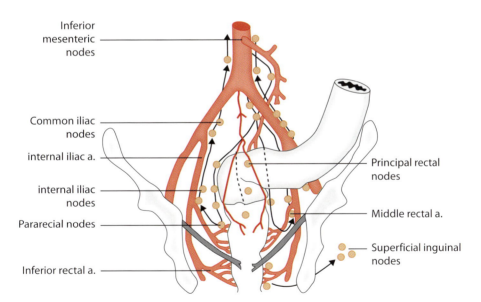

Figure 16.2 Possible routes of spread of rectal cancer via lymph nodes

Lymph Node Metastasis

Perirectal lymphatics typically travel along the obturator nodes, internal iliac vessels, and common iliac vessels. Therefore, the internal iliac and obturator nodes are commonly included in radiation portals. Similarly, the presacral nodes are at risk and must be adequately covered by radiation portals. The external iliacs are not typically at risk and therefore are not included, except for patients with locally advanced/T4 disease.

Diagnosis, Staging, and Prognosis

Clinical Presentation

Common presenting symptoms of rectal cancer include frank rectal bleeding, constipation, diarrhea (particularly for obstructive lesions), narrowing of stool caliber, tenesmus, rectal urgency, urinary symptoms, buttock pain, or sciatic pain, suggestive of locally advanced disease.

Diagnosis and Staging

Figure 16.3 illustrates the diagnostic algorithm of rectal cancer, including suggested examination and tests.

Patients who satisfy the Bethesda or Amsterdam criteria, have more than ten adenomas, multiple hamartomatous polyps, or have a family history of a known hereditary cancer syndrome should undergo genetic evaluation (Table 16.4).

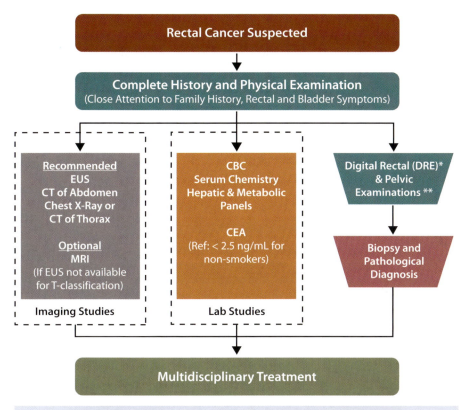

Figure 16.3 Proposed algorithm for diagnosis and staging of rectal cancer

Table 16.4 AJCC TNM classification of rectal cancer (clinical or pathological)

Stage	Description
Primary tumor (T)[a]	
TX	Primary tumor cannot be assessed
T0	No evidence of primary tumor
Tis	Carcinoma in situ, intraepithelial or invasion of the lamina propria
T1	Tumor invades submucosa
T2	Tumor invades muscularis propria
T3	Tumor invades through the muscularis propria into perirectal tissue
T4a	Tumor penetrates to the surface of the visceral peritoneum
T4b	Tumor directly invades or is adherent to other organs or structures
Regional lymph nodes (N)[b]	
NX	Regional lymph nodes cannot be assessed
N0	No regional lymph node metastasis
N1a	Metastasis in 1 node
N1b	Metastasis in 2–3 regional nodes
N1c	Tumor deposits in the subserosa, mesentery, or nonperitonealized perirectal tissues without regional nodal metastasis
N2a	Metastasis in 4–6 regional nodes
N2b	Metastasis in 7 or more regional nodes
Distant metastasis (M)	
MX	Distant metastasis cannot be assessed
M0	No distant metastasis
M1a	Metastasis confined to one organ site (liver, lung, ovary, nonregional lymph node)
M1b	Metastases in more than one organ/site or the peritoneum

[a]The use of "m" denotes multiple primaries; "r" denotes recurrent disease; "y" if tumor is staged after neoadjuvant chemoradiation (and not at initial presentation); "L0" or "L1" denotes with or without lymphatic vessel invasion, respectively; "V0," "V1," or "V2" denotes no, microscopic, or macroscopic venous invasion, respectively

[b]Regional nodes include perirectal, presacral, lateral sacral, inferior mesenteric, internal iliac, sacral promontory, superior rectal, middle rectal, and inferior rectal; at least 10–14 nodes should be studied for accurate pN staging in patients who have not undergone neoadjuvant therapy

Tumor, Node, and Metastasis Staging

Diagnosis and clinical staging depends on findings from history and physical examination, imaging, and laboratory tests. Pathological staging depends on findings during surgical resection and pathological examination, in addition to those required in clinical staging.

The 7th edition of the tumor, node, and metastasis (TNM) staging and grouping system of the American Joint Committee on Cancer (AJCC) is presented in Tables 16.4 and 16.5. If patients receive neoadjuvant treatment, the tumor regression grade should be noted as in Table 16.6.

Table 16.5 AJCC stage grouping of rectal cancer (clinical or pathological)

Stage Grouping					
	T1	T2	T3	T4a	T4b
N0	I	I	IIA	IIB	IIC
N1	IIIA	IIIA	IIIB	IIIB	IIIC
N2a	IIIA	IIIB	IIIB	IIIC	IIIC
N2b	IIIB	IIIB	IIIC	IIIC	IIIC
M1a	IVA	IVA	IVA	IVA	IVA
M1b	IVB	IVB	IVB	IVB	IVB

Source: Edge SB, Byrd DR, Compton CC et al (2009) American Joint Committee on Cancer, American Cancer Society. AJCC cancer staging manual, 7th edn. Springer, Berlin Heidelberg New York

Table 16.6 Tumor regression after neoadjuvant chemoradiation therapy for rectal cancer

Grade	Result
0	Complete response No viable cancer cells
1	Moderate response Single cell or small groups of cancer cells
2	Minimal response Residual cancer outgrown by fibrosis
3	Poor response Minimal or no tumor kill, extensive residual cancer

Prognosis

Stage at presentation is the most important prognostic factor for rectal cancer. Other adverse prognostic factors include serum carcinoembryonic antigen (CEA) level, and presence of obstructive or perforated lesions. The 5-year overall survival rates for nonmetastatic rectal cancer are presented in Table 16.7.

Table 16.7 Overall survival for patients with rectal cancer

Stage	Dukes	Modified Astler–Coller (*MAC*)	5-Year survival (%)
I	A	A	81%
		B1	76%
IIA		B2	64%
IIB	B	B2	56%
IIC		B3	45%
IIIA		C1	72%
		C1	74%
IIIB		C2	44–55%
	C	C1/C2	43–44%
		C1	42–53%
IIIC		C2	44%
		C2	25–32%
		C3	12–24%

Source: Edge SB, Byrd DR, Compton CC et al (2009) American Joint Committee on Cancer, American Cancer Society. AJCC cancer staging manual, 7th edn. Springer, Berlin Heidelberg New York

Treatment

Principles and Practice

Surgery is the only curative treatment modality for rectal cancer. Radiation therapy and chemotherapy play important roles as neoadjuvant or adjuvant treatment for patients with locally advanced disease or patients who undergo limited surgical intervention (Table 16.8).

Table 16.8 Treatment modalities used in rectal cancer

Type	Description
Surgery	
Indications for transanal excision	■ For small tumors (<3 cm) within 8 cm of the anal verge, mobile (nonfixed), well-differentiated histology (grades 1–2) that involve <30% of the circumference of the lumen ■ No lymphovascular invasion (LVI) or perineural invasion ■ Negative margins ≥3 mm are required
Indications for LAR	■ Trans-abdominal approach that resects the tumor and mesorectum but leaves the anal sphincter intact ■ Appropriate for patients that can be resected with at least a 2-cm distal margin ■ Modern techniques include total mesorectal excision (TME), en bloc resection of the rectal mesentery to the sacrum including blood supply and lymphatics
Indications for APR	■ Reserved for low rectal lesions involving the sphincter or levator muscles ■ Removal of the tumor, mesorectum, levator muscles, and anus, with permanent colostomy
Radiation therapy	
Indications	■ Neoadjuvant chemoradiation therapy (preferred and considered standard) for locally advanced disease improves resectability, reduces the risk of locoregional recurrence after surgery, and potentially increases the chance of a sphincter-sparing procedure for patients with low-lying lesions ■ Adjuvant treatment with concurrent chemotherapy for resected rectal cancer to decrease the risk of local recurrence in $T3^+$ or N^+ diseases ■ Palliative treatment to primary or metastatic foci
Techniques	■ EBRT using 3D-CRT ■ Intensity-modulated radiation therapy (IMRT) may be considered in certain cases but is not currently recommended for routine use by NCCN ▶

Table 16.8 *(continued)*

Type	Description
Chemo-/targeted therapy	
Indications	■ Neoadjuvant treatment prior to surgery (with concurrent EBRT) ■ Adjuvant treatment with concurrent EBRT for resected rectal cancer ■ Mainstay treatment for palliative therapy
Medications (cytotoxic)	■ Continuous infusion 5-FU (225–250 mg/m²/day) is given concurrently with radiation as a radiosensitizer ■ Capecitabine (825 mg/m² twice daily) has been used to substitute for 5-FU, due to ease of administration and the results of phase II studies that have shown comparable pathological response rates ■ No large randomized study has compared 5-FU with capecitabine-based chemoradiation regimens ■ Improved pathologic control rates when capecitabine is given 1 h prior to radiation has been suggested ■ FOLFOX (5-FU plus oxaliplatin–based chemotherapy) or FOLFIRI (5-FU plus irinotecan-based chemotherapy) have been used in the adjuvant and metastatic setting
Medications (molecular targeted)	■ Anti-VEGF agents such as bevacizumab have shown efficacy in combination with conventional chemotherapy in the adjuvant and metastatic setting ■ Anti-EGFR agents such as cetuximab and panitumumab have shown efficacy in k-ras wild-type patients both as a single agent and in combination with traditional chemotherapy. These agents are not efficacious in k-ras mutant patients ■ The use of targeted therapy agents with radiation has been investigated, but this is not standard practice

LAR: low, anterior resection; **APR**: abdominoperineal resection; **EBRT**: external-beam radiation therapy; **VEGF**: vascular endothelial growth factor; **EGFR**: epidermal growth factor receptor

A proposed treatment algorithm based on the best available clinical evidence is presented in Figure 16.4.

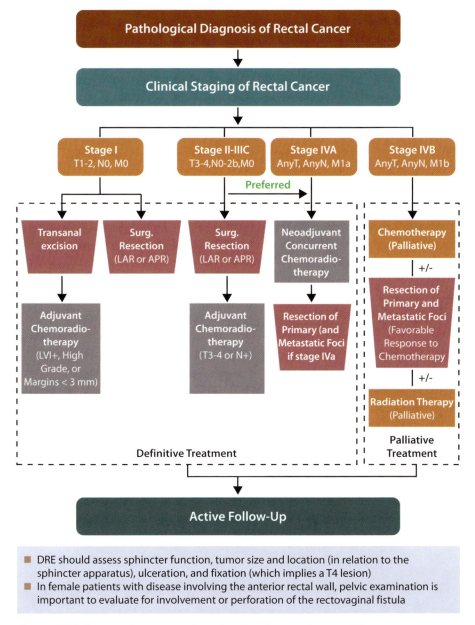

Figure 16.4 Proposed treatment algorithm for adenocarcinoma of the rectum

Treatment of Stage I (T1–2N0M0) Rectal Cancer

Surgical intervention can consist of transanal excision for patients with stage I rectal cancers that meet the following criteria:

- Size <3 cm and within 8 cm from the anal verge, low grade, without lymphovascular invasion (LVI)
- Occupy <30% of the circumference
- Mobile (nonfixed)

Patients who have any of the following risk factors should either undergo low, anterior resection (LAR) or abdominoperineal resection (APR), or receive postoperative chemoradiotherapy due to a higher risk of local recurrence with transanal excision alone:

- Margins <3 mm
- High-grade histology
- Presence of lymphovascular/perineural invasion

(*Paty PB, Nash GM, Baron P et al (2002) Long-term results of local excision for rectal cancer. Ann Surg 236:522–529; Steele GD Jr, Herndon JE, Bleday R et al (1999) Sphincter-sparing treatment for distal rectal adenocarcinoma. Ann Surg Oncol 6:433–441*).

Treatment of Stage II–IIIc (T3N0–T4N2b) Rectal Cancer

Patients with T3 or greater or node-positive disease are typically offered preoperative chemoradiation therapy to downstage disease, reduce the risk of local recurrence after surgical resection, and potentially increase the odds of performing a sphincter-sparing procedure for patients with low-lying tumors (Table 16.9; Figure 16.5).

Table 16.9 Selected clinical evidence (randomized clinical trial) for neoadjuvant and/ or adjuvant chemoradiation therapy for locally advanced rectal cancer treatment

Randomized trial	Description
Swedish Rectal Cancer Trial[a]	■ Randomized trial evaluating the efficacy of hypofraction-ated pre-op. RT versus surgery alone ■ 1,168 Patients randomized, and 908 received definitive surgery ■ 454 Patients received 25 Gy of RT in 5 fractions (5Gy × 5) within 1 week preoperatively, and 454 received surgery alone ■ Median follow-up time was 13 years ■ The OS rates (38 versus 30%, $p = 0.008$) and cancer-specific survival rate (72 versus 62%, $p = 0.03$), and local recurrence rate (9 versus 26%, $p < 0.001$), respectively, all favored the pre-op. RT group
NCCTG[b]	■ Randomized trial compared protracted venous infusion versus bolus 5-FU used with concurrent RT in stage II and III rectal cancer treatment ■ 606 Patients were randomized to protracted venous infusion versus bolus 5-FU; patients also received systemic chemotherapy with semustine plus 5-FU or with 5-FU alone in a higher dose, administered before and after the pelvic RT ■ The median follow-up was 46 months among surviving patients ■ Protracted venous infusion improved time to relapse ($p = 0.01$) and OS ($p = 0.005$) ■ There was no evidence of a beneficial effect in the patients who received semustine plus 5-FU
German Rectal Cancer Trial[c]	■ Randomized trial compared pre- versus post-op. CRT in patients with T3/4 or N⁺ rectal cancer ■ No difference in OS but an improvement in local control with pre-op. therapy was shown ■ Treatment regimen and outcome detailed in Figure 16.5 ▶

Table 16.9 *(continued)*

Randomized trial	Description
EORTC 22921[d]	▪ Randomized trial compared pre-op. RT, pre-op. CRT, pre-operative RT and post-op. chemotherapy, or pre-op. CRT and post-op. chemotherapy in 1,011 cT3 or cT4 resectable rectal cancer patients ▪ Primary endpoint was OS ▪ RT consisted of 45 Gy over a period of 5 weeks; Chemotherapy used 5-FU (350 mg/m^2/day) and leucovorin (20 mg/m^2/day), for 5 days per cycle ▪ 2 Courses of chemotherapy were combined with pre-op. RT in the group receiving pre-op. CRT and the group receiving pre-op. CRT and post-op. chemotherapy; 4 courses were planned post-op. in the group receiving pre-op. RT and post-op. chemotherapy and the group receiving pre-op. CRT and post-op. chemotherapy ▪ The 5-year cumulative local recurrence rates were 8.7, 9.6, and 7.6% in the groups that received chemotherapy preoperatively, postoperatively, or both, respectively, and 17.1% in patients did not receive chemotherapy ($p = 0.002$) ▪ No significant difference in OS between the groups received pre-op. ($p = 0.84$) and those received post-op. ($p = 0.12$) chemotherapy ▪ 5-FU-based chemotherapy given pre-op. or post-op. does not significantly improve OS if added to preoperative radiotherapy ▪ However, chemotherapy confers a significant benefit in local control, regardless of whether it is administered before or after surgery

pre-op: preoperative; **post-op**: postoperative; **APR**: abdominal perineal resection; **LAR**: low-anterior resection; **CRT**: concurrent chemoradiation therapy; **RT**: radiation therapy; **DFS**: disease-free survival; **OS**: overall survival; **NCCTG**: North Central Cancer Treatment Group; **EORTC**: European Organization for Research and Treatment of Cancer

[a] *Sources: Folkesson J, Birgisson H, Pahlman L et al (2005) Swedish Rectal Cancer Trial: long lasting benefits from RT on survival and local recurrence rate. J Clin Oncol 23:5644–5650*

[b] *Source: O'Connell MJ, Martenson JA, Wieand HS et al (1994) Improving adjuvant therapy for rectal cancer by combining protracted-infusion 5-FU with RT after curative surgery. N Engl J Med 331:502–507*

[c] *Source: Sauer R, Becker H, Hohenberger W et al (2004) Preoperative versus postoperative chemoradiotherapy for rectal cancer. N Engl J Med 351:1731–1740*

[d] *Source: Bosset JF, Collette L, Calais G et al (2006) Chemotherapy with preoperative radiotherapy in rectal cancer. N Engl J Med 355:1114–1123*

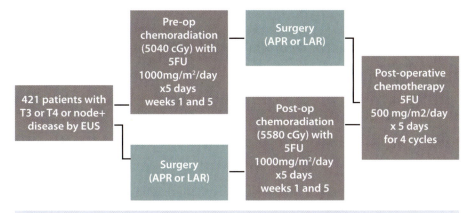

Overall, no difference in overall survival between pre- and post-operative chemoRT (76% vs 74%, $p = 0.80$) but local relapse rates were 6% in the pre-op chemoRT arm vs 13% in the post-op arm, $p = 0.01$

Figure 16.5 Schema of the German rectal cancer trial

Treatment of Stage IV (M1) Diseases

The management of stage IV patients depends on the extent of metastatic disease.

Patients with limited metastatic disease involving one site (stage IVa) may be curable if their metastases are surgically resectable. Patients with large, symptomatic primary lesions amenable to surgical resection may benefit from aggressive local therapy with preoperative chemoradiation therapy, followed by surgical resection of both the primary and metastatic lesions.

Approximately 15–20% of patients with surgically resectable liver metastases may achieve long-term survival (*Tomlinson JS, Jarnagin WR, DeMatteo RP et al (2007) Actual 10-year survival after resection of colorectal liver metastases defines cure. J Clin Oncol 25:4575–4780*).

Radiation Therapy Techniques

Radiation Therapy for Neoadjuvant or Adjuvant Therapy

Simulation and Field Arrangements

Patients may be treated supine or prone, though placing the patient prone with a belly board may help move small bowel out of the pelvis. Computed tomography (CT)-based treatment planning is preferred to ensure adequate coverage of the tumor and regional nodes and improve dose homogeneity. A rectal marker or rectal contrast can help delineate the location of the tumor. Fusion of the treatment planning CT with other imaging modalities (magnetic resonance imaging [MRI] or positron-emission tomography [PET]) may also help identify the tumor location. Simulating and treating a patient with a full bladder may also reduce the dose to small bowel and bladder.

Patients who are being treated after an APR should have the perineal incision marked with a wire and included in the treatment fields. A three-field arrangement (two laterals and a posterior–anterior [PA]) allows some sparing of the anterior pelvic structures such as small bowel, bladder, and the external genitalia. Wedges or other beam modifiers are used on the lateral beams to improve dose homogeneity.

Field setup is illustrated in Figures 16.6 and 16.7, and Table 16.10, and should consider surgical clips to define gross tumor or tumor bed.

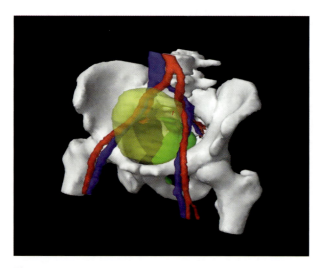

Figure 16.6 Example of a 3D rendering of pelvic anatomy, showing the iliac vessels in *red* (artery) and *blue* (vein) as well as the rectum (*green*) and bladder (*yellow*). When a patient is treated with a full bladder, a significant amount of small bowel can be displaced out of the pelvis, thus reducing bowel toxicity

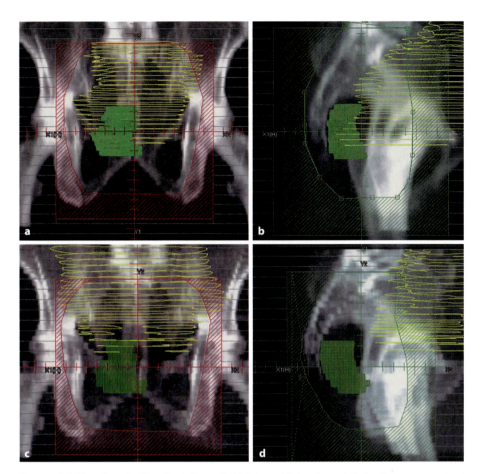

Figure 16.7 a–d **a, b** Standard three-field PA and lateral portals in the same patient simulated supine and prone on a belly board. **c, d** The GTV is contoured green and small bowel is yellow Treating a patient prone with a belly board may also move small bowel away from the pelvis.

Source: Huth BJ, Brady LW. Rectal Cancer. In: Lu JJ, Brady LW (eds.) (2008) Radiation oncology: An Evidence-Based Approach. Springer, Berlin Heidelberg New York

Table 16.10 Treatment fields used for radiation therapy for locally advanced rectal cancer

Fields	Borders
AP/PA or PA	▪ Superior: between L5 and S1 ▪ Inferior (in pre-op. setting): 3–5 cm below the palpable disease ▪ Inferior (in post-op. setting): include perineum after APR or 2–3 cm beyond the anastomosis after LAR ▪ Lateral: 1.5–2 cm lateral to the pelvic brim
Lateral	▪ Superior/Inferior: as AP/PA fields ▪ Anterior (T3 disease): 2- to 3-cm margin to the anterior of rectum or posterior margin of the pubic symphysis to cover internal iliac nodes (which ever is more anterior) ▪ Anterior (T4 disease): 2- to 3-cm margin to the anterior of rectum or anterior margin of the pubic symphysis to cover external iliac nodes (which ever in more anterior) ▪ Posterior: 1 cm behind the anterior edge of the sacrum, or many will include the entire sacrum
Boost	Gross tumor or tumor bed plus 3 cm in all directions

Rectal cancer with anal canal involvement should consider inguinal lymph node irradiation

pre-op: preoperative; **post-op**: postoperative; **APR**: abdominal perineal resection; **LAR**: low-anterior resection

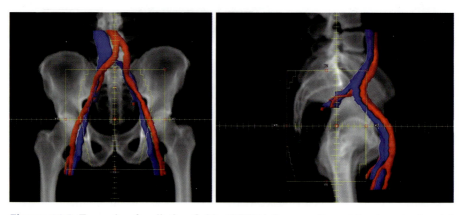

Figure 16.8 Example of radiation fields (AP/PA) for neoadjuvant treatment of rectal cancer. Note the sacrum is completely included on the lateral field to ensure coverage of the presacral space

Three-dimensional conformal radiation treatment (3D-CRT) portals are outlined in the figure above (Figure 16.8). The external iliac nodal chains are typically only included for T4 lesions.

Dose and Treatment Delivery

For neoadjuvant therapy, conventional fractionation to a total dose of 45 Gy to the entire pelvis, followed by a boost of 5.4 Gy to the tumor bed is recommended, using high-energy (≥6 MV) photons. Patients with T4 disease or low-lying tumors may be boosted to a total dose of 54 Gy.

For postoperative radiation, conventional fractionation to a total dose of 45 Gy to the entire pelvis, followed by a boost of 5.4 Gy to the tumor bed is recommended, using high-energy (≥6 MV) photons. Boost to a total of 54 Gy if positive margin present.

Intensity-Modulated Radiation Therapy

Intensity-modulated radiation therapy (IMRT) may offer the potential to reduce toxicity, but there are no set standards regarding its use. Different IMRT volume–based dose constraints have been proposed for bowel and bladder, but there is no set consensus. IMRT-based sparing of the iliac crests may also reduce bone marrow toxicity, but there are no consensus guidelines. Currently, IMRT is not recommended by the National Comprehensive Cancer Network (NCCN) for routine use. The Radiation Therapy Oncology Group (RTOG) has published a consensus contouring atlas to help standardize treatment volumes (*Myerson RJ, Garofalo MC, El Naqa I et al (2009) Elective clinical target volumes for conformal therapy in anorectal cancer: a radiation therapy oncology group consensus panel contouring atlas. Int J Radiat Oncol Biol Phys 74:824–830*).

Normal Tissue Tolerance

Organs at risk (OARs) in radiation therapy of rectal cancer, in both neoadjuvant and adjuvant settings, usually include small bowel, bladder, and bone (femoral head) (Table 16.11).

Table 16.11 Dose limitation of OARs in radiation therapy for upper abdominal malignancies

OAR	Dose limitations
Bladder	■ <50 Gy
Small intestine	■ <50 Gy ■ Restrict the volume of small bowel exceeding 15 Gy to 120 ml or less if small bowel is outlined ■ If the entire peritoneal cavity in which small bowel can move is outlined, restrict the amount exceeding 45 Gy to <195 ml
Femoral heads	■ <50 Gy

Sources: Kavanaugh BD, Pan CC, Dawson L et al (2010) Radiation dose–volume effects in the stomach and small bowel. Int J Radiat Oncol Biol Phys 76:S101–S107; Emami B, Lyman J, Brown A et al (1991) Tolerance of normal tissue to therapeutic irradiation. Int J Radiat Oncol Biol Phys 21:109–122

Follow-Up

Active follow-up after definitive treatment for rectal cancer is recommended. Schedule and suggested examinations during follow-up is presented in Table 16.12.

Common radiation-induced adverse acute effects include diarrhea, abdominal discomfort/pain, increased frequency of urination, dysuria, and skin irritation. Possible chronic or late toxicities include loose stools, rectal urgency, infertility, ovarian dysfunction for premenopausal women, vaginal stenosis, pelvic hair loss, dry ejaculation for men, femoral head fracture, and a small risk of late, secondary radiation-related malignancy.

Table 16.12 Follow-up schedule and examinations

Schedule	Frequency
First follow-up	■ 4–6 Weeks after radiation therapy
Years 1–2	■ Every 3–4 months
Years 3–5	■ Every 6 months
Years 5+	■ Annually
Examinations	
History and physical	■ Complete history and physical examination
Laboratory tests	■ Complete blood counts (CBC) and serum chemistry ■ Liver and renal function tests ■ CEA (if elevated before treatment)
Imaging studies	■ CT of the chest/abdomen/pelvis annually for 3 years ■ More frequent studies as indicated for patients at high risk for recurrence
Other procedures	■ Proctoscopy every 6 months × 5 years after LAR ■ Colonoscopy should be performed at 1 year, or within 3–6 months if omitted prior to treatment

Source: NCCN guidelines for treatment of rectal cancer, V2.2010. http://www.nccn. org/professionals/physician_gls/PDF/rectal.pdf. Cited 20 May

17

Anal Cancer

Qing Zhang[1,] Shen Fu[2]
and Luther W. Brady[3]

Key Points

- Squamous cell carcinoma (SCC) of the anal canal is a relatively rare malignancy, with an increasing incidence.

- Symptoms of anal cancer depend on the location of the primary disease and its extent. Common signs and symptoms include rectal bleeding, rectorrhagia, anal mass, and pain. Inguinal lymph adenopathy is common in diseases more advanced.

- Histological confirmation of diagnosis is essential. Tissue for pathology can be obtained from primary tumor under proctoscopy or fine-needle aspiration (FNA) or simple excision of inguinal lymph adenopathy.

- Accurate diagnosis and staging are based on history and physical examination, laboratory tests, and imaging studies. For high-risk patients including homosexual males or potentially with HIV infection, HIV test, and CD4 counts are of value for determining on the optimal treatment strategy.

- Stage at diagnosis is the most important prognostic factor. Other adverse prognostic factors in addition to advanced stage include male gender, age ≥65, hemoglobin levels ≤10 g/l at presentation, and poor performance status. Subtypes of SCC have no prognostic significance. The 5-year overall survival rates of patients with well or poorly differentiated disease are roughly 75 and 25%, respectively.

- Concurrent chemoradiation therapy is the mainstay treatment, and surgery has limited role in definitive therapy of anal cancer.

- Radiation therapy (with concurrent chemotherapy) plays a major role in anal canal carcinoma. Intensity-modulated radiation therapy (IMRT) is an option to protect normal tissues and allows the delivery of the entire radiation course in a single phase. Break during radiation should be minimized, and split-course radiation technique should be avoided as it may increase local failure and colostomy rates.

- 5-Fluorouracil (5-FU) and mitomycin are the standard chemotherapy regimen used concurrently with radiation therapy. Cisplatin and 5-FU are commonly used in salvage treatment. Neoadjuvant chemotherapy provides no additional benefit for disease-free survival (DFS) or function preservation.

- Complete response may take up to 12 months to achieve. Biopsy of a persistent but nonprogressive anal lesion within 3 months after treatment is not recommended, as slow regression of gross primary disease is common.

[1] Qing Zhang, MD (✉)
Email:
zhangqingcyw@ hotmail.com

[2] Shen Fu, MD
Email:
shen_fu@hotmail.com

[3] Luther W. Brady, MD
Email:
luther.brady@ drexelmed.edu

J. J. Lu, L. W. Brady (Eds.), *Decision Making in Radiation Oncology*
DOI: 10.1007/978-3-642-13832-4_19, © Springer-Verlag Berlin Heidelberg 2011

Epidemiology and Etiology

Carcinoma of the anal canal is a rare disease, accounts for 1–2% of all gastrointestinal malignancies and ~4% of anal–rectal cancers. There is a clear increasing trend of the disease in the Western countries. In 2010, approximately 5,260 new cases of anal cancer will be diagnosed in USA.

The etiology of disease has not been clearly identified; however, a number of risk factors have been identified for anal carcinoma (Table 17.1). The most significant risk factors include human papilloma virus (HPV) infection, immunosuppression, and smoking.

Table 17.1 Risk factors of anal cancer

Stage	Description
Patient-related factors	**Age and gender:** median age of diagnosis is ~62 years; approximately two thirds of the newly diagnosed epidermoid carcinoma and 40% of adenocarcinoma occur in female patients. Male:female ratio is 1:1.5–2
	Lifestyle: cigarette smoking is associated with a fourfold increase of risk. A history of anal intercourse before 30 years old and multiple sexual partners (>10) are also identified as increased risks for anal carcinoma
	Infection: ~85% of cases demostrate human papilloma virus (*HPV*) infection. High risk subtypes include type-16, -18, -31, -33, and -35. Human immunodeficiency virus (*HIV*) or HPV infections may lead to immunodeficiency and further increase the risk of anal carcinoma
	Immunosuppression: a tenfold risk is seen in immunosuppressed patients, particularly in patients whose CD4 count is less than 200, and those on immunosuppression after organ transplants
	Past medical history: sexually transmitted disease and cancer of the cervix, vagina, or vulva, as well as benign lesions of the anus (such as chronic anal–rectal inflammation)

Anatomy

The anal canal extends from anorectal ring superiorly to anal verge distally, with an average length of 4 cm (4.2 cm in male, 3.8 cm in female). It is surrounded by the internal and external anal sphincter muscle.

The superior border is the palpable upper border of the anal sphincter and puborectalis muscle of the anorectal ring, which is located ~2 cm superior to the dentate line. The transitional zone of the anus between the dentate line and anorectal ring is where the vertical mucosal folds where columnar epithelium of the rectum meets the squamous epithelium of the anus. It includes the columns of Morgagni. The distal end, i.e., anal verge is the junction of the nonkeratinized squamous epithelium of the anal canal and the keratinized and hair-bearing skin (Figure 17.1).

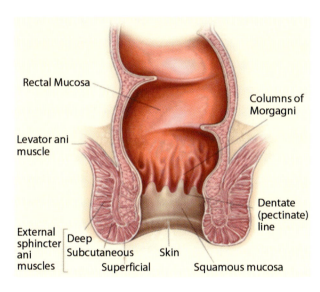

Figure 17.1 Diagram of the anal canal

Source: Ryan DP, Compton CC, Mayer RJ (2000) Carcinoma of the anal canal. N Engl J Med 342:792–800. Used with permission from the Massachusetts Medical Society

Pathology

Commonly diagnosed carcinoma of the anal canal include:
- Keratinizing squamous cell carcinoma (SCC): more common subtype of SCC of anal canal, usually originated inferior to the dentate line
- Nonkeratinizing SCC: usually arise from the transitional zone above the dentate line
- Adenocarcinoma: may arise from rectal type mucosa or anal glands, usually originated above the dentate line

Approximately 80% of anal cancers are of squamous origin, and 10% are adenocarcinoma. Other uncommonly diagnosed anal malignancies include neuroendocrine carcinoma, carcinoid tumors, basal cell carcinomas, extra-mammary Paget's disease, mucinous carcinoma, undifferentiated carcinoma, lymphoma, melanoma, and sarcoma. Malignancies of the perianal skin are managed according to skin cancers.

Routes of Spread

Local extension, regional (lymphatic) and distant (hematogenous) metastases are the three major routes of spread in anal cancer (Table 17.2).

Table 17.2 Routes of spread in anal cancer

Stage	Description
Local extension	■ Early invasion into the sphincter muscles and peri-anal connective tissues is common, ~30% of cases present with sphincter involvement ■ Tumor may further extend beyond the canal into rectal, perineum, prostate, perineal fossa, perianal skin, or pelvic wall ■ Tumor invasion into the vaginal septum (~10%) or vaginal mucosa is more common than extent to the prostate ■ Anal-vaginal fistula is seen in <5% of cases
Regional lymph node metastasis	■ Lymphatic spread may occur early in disease ■ Overall lymph node spread is seen in 25% of cases at diagnosis ■ Perirectal, pelvic, and inguinal lymph node involvement are seen in 50, 30, and 20% of cases, respectively ■ Pattern of lymphatic spread depends on the location of the primary tumors (Table 17.3; Figure 17.2) ■ Delayed inguinal lymph node metastasis is seen in approximately 10–25% of patients
Distant metastasis	■ Distant metastasis is relatively rare, and extrapelvic metastasis is seen in <10% of patients before treatment ■ The most common route of hematogenous metastasis is through the portal venous system as well as lymphatic drainage ■ Common sites of metastasis include liver, lungs, and extrapelvic lymph nodes

Lymph Node Metastasis

The lymphatic drainage of anal canal is rich, and numerous lymphatic con-
nections exist between various levels of anal canal. The regional nodes for
the anal canal include perirectal (anal- and perirectal, and lateral sacral), internal iliac (hypogastric), and superficial inguinal nodes (Table 17.3; Figure
17.2). There is an intramural system linking the lymphatics of the anal canal
and rectum.

Table 17.3 Lymphatic drainage of various levels of anal canal

Anatomic level	First echelon lymph node group(s)
Distal rectum and proximal anal canal	■ Anorectal, perirectal, and lateral sacral nodes ■ Superior hemorrhoidal nodes
Anal canal proximal to dentate line	■ Pudendal, internal iliac, and obturator nodes ■ Inferior and middle hemorrhoidal nodes
Anal canal distal to dentate line	■ Inguinal and femoral nodes

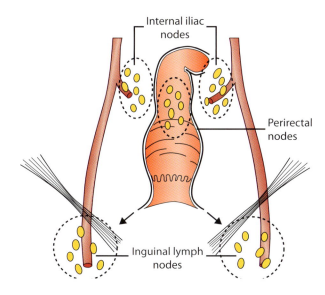

Figure 17.2 Regional lymph nodes of anal canal.

Source: Edge SB, Byrd DR, Compton CC et al (2009) American Joint Committee on Cancer, American Cancer Society. AJCC cancer staging manual, 7th edn. Springer, Berlin Heidelberg New York, used with permission from Springer

Diagnosis, Staging, and Prognosis

Clinical Presentation

Signs and symptoms of anal cancer depend on the location and extent of the primary disease. Commonly observed signs and symptoms of anal cancer include bleeding (~45% cases at presentation), rectorrhagia, and anal pain/mass. Anal incontinence is associated with tumor invasion into anal sphincter (~5% cases). Other symptoms include alternative in bowel habit, tenesmus, and pruritus.

Diagnosis and Staging

Figure 17.3 illustrates a diagnostic algorithm of anal cancer, including suggested examination and tests.

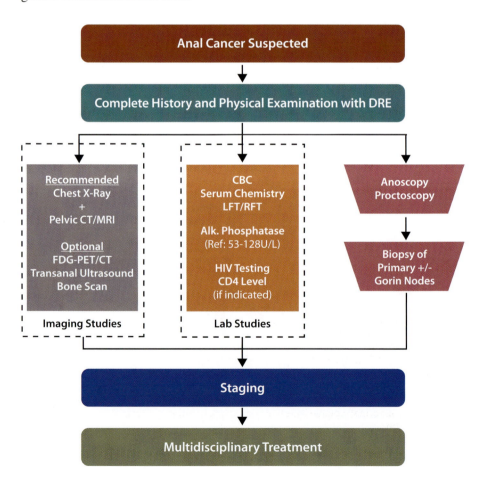

Tumor, Node, and Metastasis Staging

Diagnosis and clinical staging depends on findings from history and physical examination, imaging, and lab tests. As the primary management of anal canal carcinoma includes chemoradiation therapy without surgery, the staging is typically based on clinical findings with biopsies of the primary tumor and regional lymph node.

The 7th edition of the tumor, node, and metastasis (TNM) staging system of American Joint Committee on Cancer (AJCC) is presented in Tables 17.4 and 17.5.

Table 17.4 AJCC TNM classification of anal cancer

Stage	Description
Primary tumor (T)	
TX	Primary tumor cannot be assessed
T0	No evidence of primary tumor
Tis	Carcinoma in situ
T1	Tumor ≤2 cm in greatest dimension
T2	Tumor >2 cm but ≤5 cm in greatest dimension
T3	Tumor >5 cm in greatest dimension
T4	Tumor of any size invades adjacent organ(s), e.g., vagina, urethra, bladder ▶

Figure 17.3 Proposed algorithm for diagnosis and staging of anal cancer

- Histological confirmation is essential, and tissue for pathology diagnosis can be obtained via biopsy of the primary tumor under proctoscopy or fine-needle aspiration (FNA) or simple excision of enlarged groin lymph nodes is also recommended
- Magnetic resonance imaging (MRI) is more sensitive than enhanced computer tomography (CT) to evaluate the extent of tumor. Neither CT nor MRI is reliable for detecting metastasis to internal iliac and superior hemorrhoidal lymph nodes (~50% of the involved nodes are <0.5 cm)
- Fluorodeoxyglucose–positron-emission tomography (FDG-PET) is more sensitive for detecting abnormal inguinal lymph nodes than conventional CT and physical examination
- For high-risk patients of HIV infection including homosexual males, HIV, and CD4 counts are of value to determining the optimal and tolerable treatment strategy

Table 17.4 *(continued)*

Stage	Description
Regional lymph nodes (N)	
NX	Regional lymph nodes cannot be assessed
N0	No regional lymph node metastasis
N1	Metastasis in perirectal lymph node(s)
N2	Metastasis in unilateral internal iliac and/or inguinal lymph node(s)
N3	Metastasis in perirectal and inguinal lymph nodes and/or bilateral internal iliac and/or bilateral internal iliac and/or inguinal lymph nodes
Distant metastasis (M)	
MX	Distant metastasis cannot be assessed
M0	No distant metastasis
M1	Distant metastasis (including seeding of the peritoneum and positive peritoneal cytology)

Source: Edge SB, Byrd DR, Compton CC et al (2009) American Joint Committee on Cancer, American Cancer Society. AJCC cancer staging manual, 7th edn. Springer, Berlin Heidelberg New York

Table 17.5 Stage grouping of anal cancer

Stage Grouping				
	T1	T2	T3	T4
N0	I	II	II	IIIA
N1	IIIA	IIIA	IIIA	IIIB
N2	IIIB	IIIB	IIIB	IIIB
N3	IIIB	IIIB	IIIB	IIIB
M1	IV	IV	IV	IV

Source: Edge SB, Byrd DR, Compton CC et al (2009) American Joint Committee on Cancer, American Cancer Society. AJCC cancer staging manual, 7th edn. Springer, Berlin Heidelberg New York

Prognoses

Staging at diagnosis is the most important prognostic factor of anal cancer. Patients with T1N0 cancer have a significantly better prognosis than those with larger tumors. Adverse prognostic factors include male gender, age ≥65 years, hemoglobin levels ≤10 g/l at presentation, nodal metastasis at presentation, and poor performance status, and the presence of HIV infection or AIDS, especially if CD4 counts are less than 200 µl.

Subtypes of SCC have no prognostic significance. However, the 5-year overall survival rates of patients with well or poorly differentiated disease are roughly 75 and 25%, respectively (Table 17.6).

Table 17.6 Five-year overall survival (OS) rates of anal cancer patients, based on histology type

Stage	Squamous (%)	Nonsquamous (%)
I	71.4%	59.1%
II	63.5%	52.9%
IIIA	48.1%	37.7%
IIIB	43.2%	24.4%
IV	20.9%	7.4%

Source: National Cancer Database: cases diagnosed between 1998 and 1999

Principles and Practice

Nonmetastatic SCC and adenocarcinoma of the anal canal are usually treated with radiation therapy in tandem with chemotherapy, and surgery has limited role in its treatment (Table 17.7).

A proposed treatment algorithm based on the best available clinical evidence is presented in Figure 17.4.

Table 17.7 Treatment modalities used in anal cancer

Type	Description
Radiation therapy	
Indications	■ EBRT with concurrent chemotherapy is the mainstay treatment for localized anal cancer ■ RT alone can be reserved for stage T1N0M0 disease ■ Palliation to primary or metastatic foci
Techniques	■ EBRT using three-dimensional conformational RT (*3D-CRT*) or IMRT ■ Brachytherapy has no role in the treatment and is associated with high incidence of anal necrosis
Chemotherapy	
Indications	■ Standard treatment (with EBRT) for nonmetastatic disease except for T1N0M0 ■ Mainstay treatment for palliative therapy ■ Neoadjuvant chemotherapy has no local control and survival benefit (results of RTOG 98-11 Trial) ■ No evidence to support adjuvant chemotherapy after definitive chemoradiation therapy
Medications	■ 2 Cycles of 5-FU (1,000 mg/m^2 days 1–4, continuous infusion) plus mitomycin C (10 mg/m^2 bolus on day 1) in weeks 1 and 5 as standard regimen ■ Cisplatin-based chemotherapy (with RT) may produce similar DFS to standard regimen ■ Cisplatin plus 5-FU is used in salvage treatment
Surgery	
Indications	■ Has limited role in the primary treatment of anal cancer ■ Local excision can be considered only for selected patients with well differentiated early-stage (T1N0M0) SCC that is <40% circumferential involvement and no sphincter involvement ■ Abdominal peritoneal resection (*APR*) is reserved for salvage after primary chemoradiotherapy failure
Facts/issues	■ 5-Year OS after curative or local resection is ~50% ■ Reserved for salvage (APR) after chemoradiation failure, with a salvage rate approached ~50%

EBRT: external-beam radiation therapy; **RT**: radiation therapy

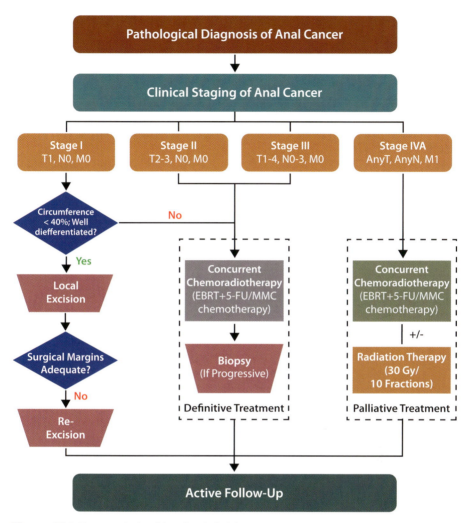

Figure 17.4 Proposed algorithm for definitive treatment of anal cancer

Treatment of T1N0M0 Anal Cancer

Selected patients with limited T1N0M0 anal cancer (well-differentiated disease of less than 40% circumference) can be treated with wide local excision. If incomplete resection (including positive margin) is expected, radiation therapy should be considered instead. Radiation therapy with or without chemotherapy (depends on the extent of disease) is a valid treatment option for T1N0M0 anal cancer.

Treatment of T2–4 or N⁺ Anal Cancer Without Metastasis

Concurrent chemoradiation therapy is the mainstay treatment of this group of patients. It provides similar outcome in terms of overall survival as compared with surgery (abdominal perineal resection [APR]), but allows sphincter preservation after treatment. Results of randomized clinical trials have confirmed the benefit of concurrent chemoradiation therapy over radiation alone (Table 17.8).

Results of an Intergroup trial demonstrated that mitomycin C (MMC) is needed (Table 17.9).

Table 17.8 Randomized trials comparing concurrent chemoradiation therapy versus radiation therapy alone

Randomized trial	Description
UKCCCR Trial[a]	■ Randomized 585 patients to either radiation therapy (RT) alone or concurrent chemoradiation therapy (CRT) ■ RT alone used 45 Gy in 20 or 25 fractions over 4–5 weeks ■ CRT used 5-FU (1,000 mg/m2 days 1–4 or 750 mg/m2 days 1–5 continuous infusion) plus mitomycin C (12 mg/m^2 bolus on day 1) during the first and last week of RT (same RT regimen) ■ 3-Year local control rates (61 versus 36%, $p < 0.001$) ■ Addition of chemotherapy produced a reduction of 46% in local failure ($p < 0.0001$) ■ No benefit of OS observed with CRT
Bartelink et al (EORTC)[b]	■ Randomized 101 patients with T3–4N0–3 or T1–2N1–3 anal cancer to either RT alone or CRT ■ RT alone used 45 Gy at 1.8 Gy/day over 5 weeks ■ CRT used 5-FU (750 mg/m^2 days 1–5 and days 29–33) plus mitomycin C (15 mg/m^2 bolus on day 1) (same RT regimen) ■ Both the 5-year locoregional control rates (68 versus 50%, $p = 0.02$), colostomy-free survival rates (72 versus 40%, $p = 0.002$) favored the CRT group ■ CRT significantly increase the complete remission rate to 80% as compared with 54% from RT alone ■ No benefit of OS observed with CRT

CRT: concurrent chemoradiation therapy; **DFS**: disease-free survival; **OS**: overall survival; **EORTC**: European Organization for Research and Treatment of Cancer

[a]*Source: UKCCCR Anal Cancer Trial Working Party (1996) Epidermoid anal cancer: results from the UKCCCR randomized trial of RT alone versus RT, 5-FU, and mitomycin. Lancet 348:1049–1054*

[b]*Source: Bartelink H, Roelofsen F, Eschwege F et al (1997) CRT is superior to RT alone in the treatment of locally advanced anal cancer: results of a phase III randomized trial of the EORTC Radiotherapy and Gastrointestinal Cooperative Groups. J Clin Oncol 15:2040–2049*

Table 17.9 Randomized trials comparing different chemotherapy regimens used with concurrent radiation therapy

Randomized trials	Description
Flam et al (Intergroup Trial) (Figure 17.5)[a]	■ Aimed to determine the MMC in the standard treatment regimen for anal cancer, and to assess the role of salvage therapy in patients who have residual tumor following definitive chemoradiation ■ Randomized 310 patients to RT to 45–50.4 Gy to pelvic field plus either 5-FU or 5-FU plus MMC ■ Chemotherapy included 5-FU (1,000 mg/m^2/day for 4 days) or same 5-FU regimen plus MMC (10 mg/m^2 per dose for 2 doses). ■ Posttreatment biopsies (at ~6 weeks) were positive in 15 and 7.7% of patients in the 5-FU or MMC arm, respectively (p = NS). These patients were treated with a salvage RT (9 Gy) with 5-FU plus cisplatin (100 mg/m^2) ■ No significant difference in OS at 4 years, but colostomy rates were lower (9 versus 22%, p = 0.002), colostomy-free survival higher (71 versus 59%, p = 0.014), and DFS higher (73 versus 51%, p = 0.0003) in the MMC arm ■ Toxicity was greater in the MMC arm (23 versus 7%, grades 4–5 toxicity, p < 0.001) ■ Of 24 assessable patients who underwent salvage therapy, 12 (50%) were rendered disease free
RTOG 9811[b]	■ Randomized 682 patients with anal cancer to 5-FU plus MMC used concurrently with RT or induction 5-FU plus cisplatin, followed by concurrent 5-FU plus cisplatin and RT ■ Chemotherapy regimens were A: 5-FU (1,000 mg/m^2 days 1–4 and 29–32) plus MMC (10 mg/m^2 days 1 and 29) or ■ B: 5-FU (1,000 mg/m^2 days 1–4, 29–32, 57–60, and 85–88) plus cisplatin (75 mg/m^2 on days 1, 29, 57, and 85) ■ RT dose was 45–59 Gy in both arms, but RT started on day 57) in arm B ■ 5-Year DFS, OS were 56 versus 48%, 69 versus 69%, respectively, in both arms (p = NS) ■ 5-Year colostomy rate was 10 versus 20% for arms A and B, respectively (p = 0.12) ■ Grades 3–4 hematologic toxicity was lower in arm B (67 versus 47%, p = 0.0004) ■ Induction 5-FU and cisplatin, followed by 5-FU and cisplatin and RT failed to improve DFS or OS

MMC: mitomycin C; **DFS**: disease-free survival; **OS**: overall survival; **RTOG**: Radiation Therapy Oncology Group; **ECOG**: Eastern Cooperative Oncology Group

[a] *Source: Flam M, John M, Pajak TF et al (1996) Role of MMC in combination with 5-FU and RT, and of salvage chemoradiation in the definitive nonsurgical treatment of epidermoid carcinoma of the anal canal: results of a phase III randomized intergroup study. J Clin Oncol 14:2527–2539*
[b] *Source: Ajani JA, Winter KA, Gunderson LL et al (2006) Intergroup RTOG 98-11: a phase III randomized study of 5-FU, MMC, and RT vs. 5-FU, cisplatin and RT in carcinoma of the anal canal. J Clin Oncol 24:4009*

Neoadjuvant and Adjuvant Treatment

Results of Radiation Therapy Oncology Group (RTOG) Trial 9811 have demonstrated that neoadjuvant chemotherapy provides no additional benefit for disease-free survival (DFS) or function preservation as compared with standard concurrent chemoradiation therapy (Table 17.9).

The current standard treatment algorithm incorporating concurrent chemoradiation therapy based on the Intergroup trial is detailed in Figure 17.5. However, whether to biopsy the primary disease at 6 weeks after chemoradiation therapy is debatable (*Cummings BJ, Keane TJ, O'Sullivan B et al (1991) Epidermoid anal cancer: treatment by RT alone or by RT and 5-FU with and without MMC. Int J Radiat Oncol Biol Phys 21:1115–1125*).

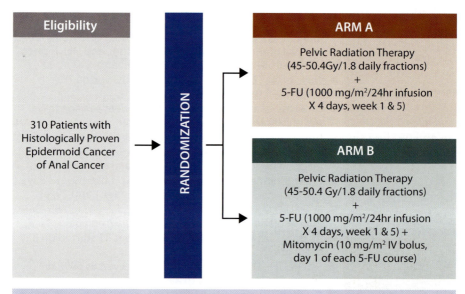

Eligibility

310 Patients with Histologically Proven Epidermoid Cancer of Anal Cancer

RANDOMIZATION

ARM A

Pelvic Radiation Therapy (45-50.4Gy/1.8 daily fractions)
+
5-FU (1000 mg/m²/24hr infusion X 4 days, week 1 & 5)

ARM B

Pelvic Radiation Therapy (45-50.4 Gy/1.8 daily fractions)
+
5-FU (1000 mg/m²/24hr infusion X 4 days, week 1 & 5) + Mitomycin (10 mg/m² IV bolus, day 1 of each 5-FU course)

RESULTS
Colostomy rates were 9 vs. 23% (p=0.002), colostomy-free survival rates were 71 vs. 59% (p=0.014) and DFS rates were 73 vs. 51% (p=0.0003). All favored 5-FU+Mitomycin group

Figure 17.5 Treatment schema (excluding salvage treatment) and results of the Intergroup trial

Salvage Treatment

Recurrent or persistent disease after definitive chemoradiation therapy can be salvaged by APR. For patients with positive inguinal lymph adenopathy, groin dissection after APR is indicated. Salvage APR is associated with a 5-year survival of ~50%.

Radiation Therapy Techniques

Radiation Therapy for Definitive Therapy

Simulation and Field Arrangements

Radiation fields should encompass tumor bed plus regional lymph node areas (including inguinal nodes) for locoregional control.

The patient should be placed in the supine position, with a full bladder and a radio-opaque marker at the anal verge of the edge of the tumor. Three-dimensional conformal planning using CT simulation with small bowel contrast is highly recommended.

Various technique of exist for conventional radiation, and the anterior/posterior (AP/PA) technique is detailed here (Table 17.10). Radiation therapy can be divided into three phases directed to the entire pelvic field (Figure 17.6): cone-down pelvic field (Figure 17.7), and tumor bed only.

Table 17.10 Fields of radiation therapy in conventional treatment of anal cancer

Fields	Borders
AP/PA fields (whole pelvis)	■ Superior: top of S1 ■ Inferior: the lower of anal verge or tumor with 3 cm margin ■ Anterior lateral: to include lateral inguinal nodes with 1.5-cm margin, determined by bony landmark or lymphangiogram ■ Posterior lateral: 1.5 cm lateral to the widest bony margin of the true pelvis
AP/PA fields (cone-down pelvis)	■ Superior: inferior border of sacroiliac joint ■ Inferior: same as in the whole-pelvis field ■ Anterior lateral: same as in the whole-pelvis field ■ Posterior lateral: same as in the whole-pelvis field
Tumor bed boost field(s)	■ Primary tumor: gross tumor with 2- to 2.5-cm margin ■ Lymph adenopathy: gross disease with 2-cm margin

The radiation dose to the initial whole-pelvic field is 30.6 Gy, followed by 14.4 Gy to the cone-down pelvic field, and a boost of 9–14.4 Gy to the tumor bed(s)

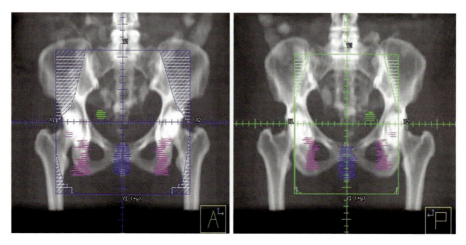

Figure 17.6 Initial radiation fields (AP/PA) to cover the entire pelvis

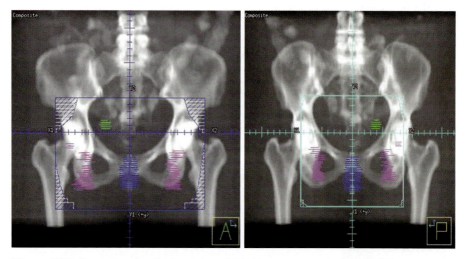

Figure 17.7 Cone-down radiation fields (AP/PA) to cover the inferior pelvis

The inguinal lymph node distribution is illustrated in Figure 17.8. The lateral inguinal lymph node regions are included in the AP but not PA fields, thus requiring supplemental inguinal electron fields (medial boarder to match the exit of PA field) to ensure the full radiation dose. The depth of the femoral vessel ranges from 2 to 18.5 cm.

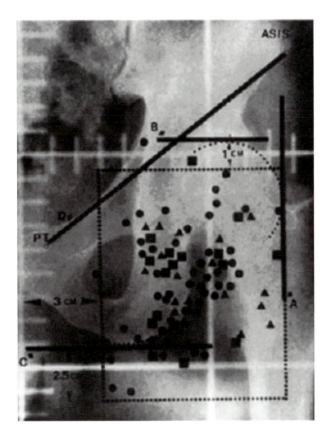

Figure 17.8 Topographic distribution of inguinal lymph node metastases in patients with carcinoma of the anus and lower rectum (*circles, n = 50*), vulva vagina–cervix (*triangles, n = 17*), and urethra (*squares, n = 17*). The field arrangement described provided adequate coverage of 86% of all inguinal lymph nodes

Source: Wang CJ, Chin YY, Leung SW et al (1996) Topographic distribution of inguinal lymph nodes metastasis: significance in determination of treatment margin for elective inguinal lymph nodes irradiation of low pelvic tumors. Int J Radiat Oncol Biol Phys 35:133–136, used with permission from Elsevier

Dose and Treatment Delivery

High-energy (15 MV) linear accelerator is recommended. Conventional fractionation to a total dose of 30.6 Gy to the entire pelvis, followed by 14.4 Gy to the inferior pelvis is usually recommended to cover pelvic and inguinal lymph nodes. Total dose to the supplemental inguinal lymph node region is 36 Gy in clinically N0, and 45 Gy in N+ disease.

Boost to 54–59.4 Gy to gross tumor, with a 2–2.5 cm margin is recommended for patients with T3 or T4, N+ patients, or T2 disease with gross residual after 45 Gy.

Break during radiation therapy for skin toxicity should not exceed 10 days. A split course of radiation therapy is not recommended; although it is associated with lower incidence of severe toxicity, it may increase local failure and colostomy rates (*John M, Pajak T, Flam M et al (1996) Dose escalation in chemoradiation for anal cancer: preliminary results of RTOG 92-08. Cancer J Sci Am 2:205–211*).

Intensity-Modulated Radiation Therapy for Anal Cancer Treatment

Intensity-modulated radiation therapy (IMRT) is an option to protect normal tissues and allows the delivery of the entire radiation course in a single phase. IMRT with chemotherapy is effective in anal cancer treatment and can reduce toxicity. Treatment plan should include the anorectum and primary disease with a margin, posterior pelvic, internal iliac, and inguinal lymph nodes (Figures 17.9 and 17.10).

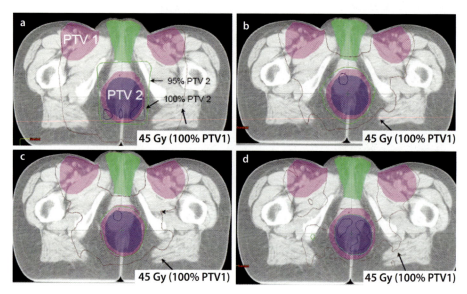

Figure 17.9 a–d Dose distributions by treatment arm on the same axial CT slice through both target volumes (*PTV1* and *PTV2*) and the external genitalia in a female patient. This CT slice shows the sparing of the genitalia by the 45-Gy isodose curve in arms **a**, **b**, and **d** (IMRT) as compared with arm **a** (3D-CRT). *Adapted from Menkarios C, Azria D, Laliberté D et al (2007) Optimal organ-sparing intensity-modulated radiation therapy (IMRT) regimen for the treatment of locally advanced anal canal carcinoma: a comparison of conventional and IMRT plans. Radiat Oncol 2: 41*

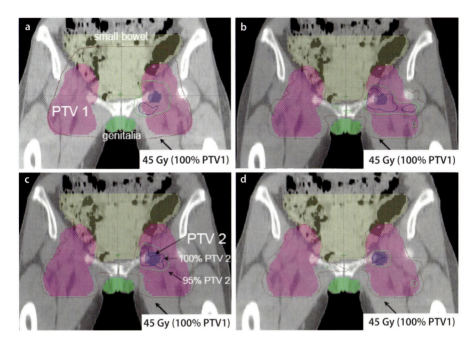

Figure 17.10 a–d Dose distributions by treatment arm on the same coronal CT slice through both target volumes and avoidance structures. This CT slice also shows the sparing of the external genitalia, small bowel, and iliac crests in arms **b**, **c**, and **d** (IMRT) as compared with arm **a** (3D-CRT)

Normal Tissue Tolerance

Organs at risk (OARs) in radiation therapy of anal cancer include small bowel, bladder, rectum, skin, vagina, bone including femoral head, and other normal tissues/organs in the treatment fields. Dose limitations of OARs are detailed in Chapters 16, 22, and 23 for rectal, cervical, and vulva cancers, respectively.

Follow-Up

Most recurrences occur within the 3 years after chemoradiation therapy, and lifelong follow-up is usually recommended. Schedule and suggested examination during follow-up is presented in Table 17.11.

Table 17.11 Follow-up schedule and examinations

Schedule	Frequency
First follow-up	■ 8 Weeks after completion of treatment
Years 0–1	■ Every 3–4 months
Years 2–5	■ Every 6 months
Years 5+	■ Annually
Examinations	
History and physical	■ Complete history and physical examination ■ Digital rectal examination (*DRE*) and proctoscopy ■ Examination of bilateral inguinal lymph nodes
Laboratory tests	■ Lab tests are recommended if clinically indicated
Imaging studies	■ CT of the abdomen and pelvis (every 6 months for 5 years) ■ Chest X-ray (if clinically indicated)

Source: Zhang Q, Abitbol A (2008) Cancer of the anal canal. In: Lu JJ, LW Brady (eds) Radiation oncology: an evidence-based approach. Springer, Berlin Heidelberg New York

As slow regression of gross primary disease is common, and complete response may take up to 12 months to achieve in anal cancer, biopsy of a persistent anal lesion within 3 months after treatment is not recommended unless disease progression occurs. Common chemoradiation-induced acute adverse effects include neutropenia, thrombocytopenia, confluent moist desquamation, pubic hair loss, fatigue, diarrhea, nausea, vomiting, dysuria, and urinary urgency/frequency.

Severe long-term side effects are uncommon, but may include rectal bleeding, chronic diarrhea, anal ulceration/fistula/stricture, anal incontinence, skin fibrosis and telangiectasia, vaginal stenosis/atrophy (females), impotence and sterility, and a very small chance of pelvic bone or femoral fracture, femoral head necrosis, soft tissue edema, and second primary tumor.

Side effects and complications of radiation and chemotherapy are more prominent in patients with HIV infection and AIDS, especially in patients whose CD4 counts are less than 200 μl.

Index of Volumes 1 and 2